SURGICAL
APPROACHES
TO THE
SPINE

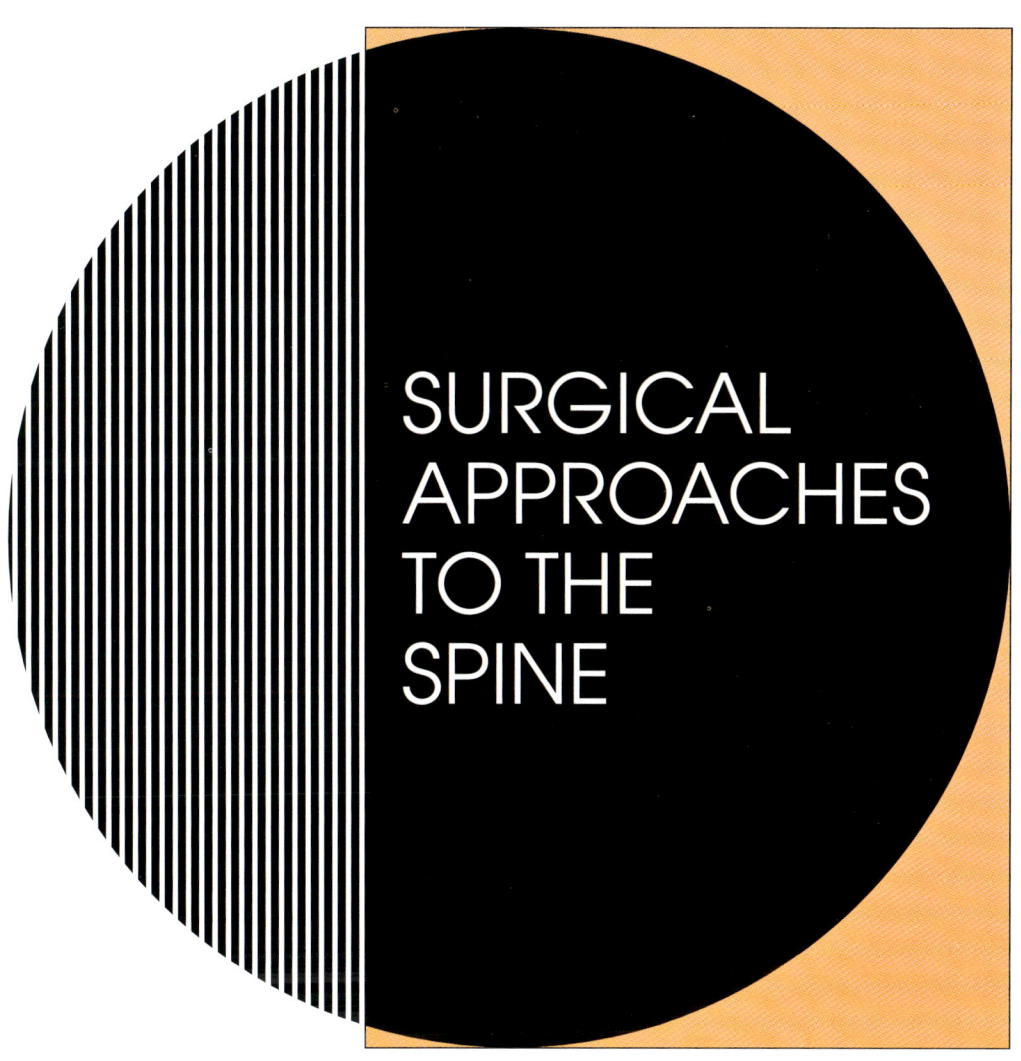

SURGICAL APPROACHES TO THE SPINE

Todd J. Albert, MD
Assistant Professor,
Department of Orthopaedic Surgery,
Thomas Jefferson University;
Attending Surgeon,
Rothman Institute,
Pennsylvania Hospital,
Philadelphia, Pennsylvania

Richard A. Balderston, MD
Professor and Vice Chairman
Department of Orthopaedic Surgery,
Thomas Jefferson University;
Chief, Scoliosis Service,
Rothman Institute,
Pennsylvania Hospital,
Philadelphia, Pennsylvania

Bruce E. Northrup, MD
Clinical Associate Professor,
Department of Neurosurgery,
Thomas Jefferson University,
Philadelphia, Pennsylvania

Illustrations by
Philip M. Ashley, C.M.I.

W.B. SAUNDERS COMPANY
A Division of Harcourt Brace & Company
Philadelphia London Toronto Montreal Sydney Tokyo

W.B. SAUNDERS COMPANY
A Division of Harcourt Brace & Company

The Curtis Center
Independence Square West
Philadelphia, Pennsylvania 19106

Library of Congress Cataloging-in-Publication Data

Albert, Todd J.
  Surgical approaches to the spine / Todd J. Albert, Richard A. Balderston, Bruce E. Northrup; artist, Philip M. Ashley.

    p.   cm.

  ISBN 0-7216-4554-2

  1. Spine—Surgery.   2. Anatomy, Surgical and topographical.
     I. Balderston, Richard A.   II. Northrup, Bruce.   [DNLM:
  1. Spine—surgery.   2. Spine—anatomy & histology.   WE 725 A333s
  1997]

  RD768.A43 1997   617.3'75059—dc20

  DNLM/DLC   96-29395

SURGICAL APPROACHES TO THE SPINE   ISBN 0-7216-4554-2

Copyright © 1997 by W.B. Saunders Company

All rights reserved. No part of this publication may be reproduced or transmitted in any form or by any means, electronic or mechanical, including photocopy, recording, or any information storage and retrieval system, without permission in writing from the publisher.

Printed in the United States of America

Last digit is the print number: 9   8   7   6   5   4   3   2   1

To Lauren, Stuart, Elliot, and Emily—Your undying devotion motivates me constantly.

To Dick Rothman for being a mentor, a friend, and an inspiration.
TODD J. ALBERT

To my wife Claudia and my children Jessica and Phillip—with their understanding and compassion this work was possible.
RICHARD A. BALDERSTON

With love to my wife Fran Northrup and my children Michael Northrup and Nicole Northrup for their encouragement and support.
BRUCE E. NORTHRUP

Contributors

Phillip R. Adams, M.D.
Clinical Associate Professor of Surgery,
Division of Cardiovascular Surgery,
University of Texas Medical
  School–Houston,
Houston, Texas
Alternative Anterior Lumbar Exposures

Todd J. Albert, M.D.
Assistant Professor,
Department of Orthopaedic Surgery,
Jefferson Medical College of Thomas
  Jefferson University.
Attending Physician,
Rothman Institute,
Pennsylvania Hospital,
Philadelphia, Pennsylvania
*Relevant Cervical Anatomy; Anterior
  Middle and Lower Cervical Exposures;
  Lateral Retropharyngeal Approach to the
  Upper Cervical Spine (The Whitesides
  Approach); Thoracotomy; Posterior
  Lumbar Approach; Autologous Bone
  Graft*

Howard S. An, M.D.
Associate Professor of Orthopaedic
  Surgery,
Department of Orthopaedic Surgery,
Medical College of Wisconsin.
Director of Spine Surgery,
MCW Clinics at Froedtert,
East Medical College of Wisconsin
  Physicians and Clinics,
Milwaukee, Wisconsin
Posterior Cervical Exposures

Thomas G. Andreshak, M.D.
Clinical Instructor,
Medical College of Ohio.
Attending Surgeon,
St. Vincent Medical Center,
Toledo, Ohio
Posterior Cervical Exposures

Richard A. Balderston, M.D.
Professor and Vice Chairman,
Department of Orthopaedic Surgery,
Jefferson Medical College of Thomas
  Jefferson University.
Chief of Orthopaedic and Scoliosis Service,
Rothman Institute, Pennsylvania Hospital,
Philadelphia, Pennsylvania
Thoracotomy; Posterior Lumbar Approach

Robert E. Booth, M.D.
Clinical Professor of Orthopaedic Surgery,
Jefferson Medical College of Thomas
  Jefferson University,
Philadelphia, Pennsylvania
Posterior Lumbar Approach

Howard B. Cotler, M.D.
Clinical Associate Professor of Orthopaedic
  Surgery,
University of Texas Medical
  School–Houston,
Houston, Texas
Alternative Anterior Lumbar Exposures

Jerome M. Cotler, M.D.
Everett J. & Marian Gordon Professor of
  Orthopaedic Surgery,
Jefferson Medical College of Thomas
  Jefferson University,
Philadelphia, Pennsylvania
Autologous Bone Graft

Sanford E. Emery, M.D.
Assistant Professor,
Department of Orthopaedics,
University Hospitals of Cleveland/
  Case Western Reserve University,

Cleveland, Ohio
Anterior Retroperitoneal Lumbar Exposures

Steven R. Garfin, M.D.
Professor and Chair,
Department of Orthopaedics,
University of California,
San Diego,
Medical Center,
San Diego, California
Wiltse Paravertebral Muscle Posterolateral Exposures

Harry N. Herkowitz, M.D.
Chairman,
Department of Orthopaedic Surgery,
and Director,
Spine Surgery Fellowship Program,
William Beaumont Hospital,
Royal Oak, Michigan
Anterior Exposures of the Cervicothoracic Junction and Upper Thoracic Spine

William M. Keane, M.D.
Professor and Chairman,
Otolaryngology, Head and Neck Surgery, Thomas Jefferson
University Hospital, Philadelphia, Pennsylvania
Anterior Upper Cervical Exposures; Relevant Cervical Anatomy

David L. Kramer, M.D.
Spine Fellow,
Rothman Institute and Thomas Jefferson University Hospital,
Philadelphia, Pennsylvania
Posterior Lumbar Approach

Lawrence T. Kurz, M.D.
Department of Orthopaedic Surgery,
William Beaumont Hospital,
Royal Oak, Michigan
Anterior Exposures of the Cervicothoracic Junction and Upper Thoracic Spine

Srdjan Mirkovic, M.D.
Assistant Professor,
Department of Orthopaedic Surgery,
Northwestern University School of Medicine.
Attending Staff, Orthopaedic Associates of Chicago, Northwestern Memorial Hospital, Chicago, Illinois
Wiltse Paravertebral Muscle Posterolateral Exposures

Bruce E. Northrup, M.D.
Clinical Associate Professor,
Department of Neurosurgery,
Thomas Jefferson University,
Philadelphia, Pennsylvania

Bernard A. Rawlins, M.D.
Assistant Professor of Surgery (Orthopaedics),
Cornell University Medical College.
Assistant Attending Physician,
Hospital for Special Surgery,
New York Hospital–Cornell Medical Center,
New York, New York
Thoracotomy

David Rosen
Resident in Otolaryngology
Thomas Jefferson University Hospital
Philadelphia, Pennsylvania
Anterior Upper Cervical Exposures

Marc R. Rosen, M.D.
Department of Otorhinolaryngology,
Pennsylvania Hospital,
Philadelphia, Pennsylvania
Anterior Upper Cervical Exposures; Relevant Cervical Anatomy

Alexander R. Vaccaro, M.D.
Associate Professor,
Department of Orthopaedic Surgery,
Jefferson Medical College of Thomas Jefferson University.
Attending Physician,
Rothman Institute,
Philadelphia, Pennsylvania
Costotransversectomy

Cathleen S. Van Buskirk, M.D.
Spine Fellow,
Rothman Institute,
Philadelphia, Pennsylvania
Autologous Bone Graft

Thomas E. Whitesides, Jr., M.D.
Professor,
Department of Orthopaedics,
Emory University School of Medicine,
Atlanta, Georgia
Lateral Retropharyngeal Approach to the Upper Cervical Spine (The Whitesides Approach)

Foreword

A cornerstone of each and every surgeon's ability to operate is knowledge of and familiarity with anatomic structures and landmarks. To lack these is to invite complications and disaster.

This textbook is not just another addition to the already existing texts covering this subject. Rather, the editors have assembled a group of spine surgeons—highly expert, with considerable experience—to discuss complex surgical anatomy, provide technical descriptions of the surgical approaches, and identify the potential complications of these approaches.

In addition, the 238 full-color illustrations provide the reader with a comprehensive three-dimensional guide to the anterior and posterior exposures of the cervical, thoracic, and lumbar spine. These illustrations were drawn by the artist Philip M. Ashley in close association with one of the editors, Dr. Todd J. Albert.

Given the fact that spine surgeons know what they want to do when they arrive, this text provides an exquisite "road map" to the spine with the requisite "danger signs" along the way.

Reflecting for a moment as a charter member of the Scoliosis Research Society, early in my career I would have greatly benefited from a text such as this and, more importantly, my patients would have benefited.

The text is organized with a consistent format throughout and includes approaches not only to the spine but also to the iliac crest and fibula. It is not constructed to discuss specific diseases, conditioning, or problems of the spine, but rather to present the reader with time-tested and true surgical approaches to the spine—accomplished in a comprehensive, extremely well-illustrated, consistent manner.

Surgical Approaches to the Spine is, indeed, a contribution to the literature. The ultimate outcome for the reader will be an improvement in the care of his or her patient.

C. McCollister Evarts, M.D.

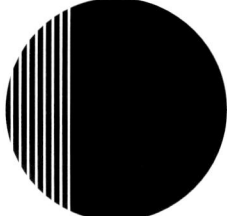

Preface

Orthopaedic surgeons spend a lifetime developing decision matrices for choice of surgical approach. An equal amount of time may be consumed contemplating complications when approaches lead to an anomalous spinal nerve or to rare arterial courses. Within the field of orthopaedic surgery, perhaps only musculoskeletal oncological surgery rivals spine surgery when it comes to the importance of surgical approaches. The pathology that must be addressed in choosing approaches may involve the anterior, middle, or posterior column of osseous structures, as well as intradural or extradural extensions. The surgeon must not only plan for adequate exposure of the specific areas of pathology but also must expose enough additional area so that working space and possibly fixation points for instrumentation may be adequately visualized. In addition, should complications arise, a plan for additional exposure to neutralize these situations must be developed.

Surgeons may learn about live anatomic exposure through a variety of techniques. There is no substitute for a training period during which the surgical student is in close proximity to the surgical teacher and the live patient. Surgeons must think three-dimensionally and may utilize other tools to construct their own three-dimensional mental image as they perform an operation. When appropriate, it is our philosophy in this book to combine intraoperative photos, photos of anatomic specimens, and artist's drawings of important anatomic structures to aid the surgeon in synthesizing a mental image before each surgery.

In this book we will touch on some of the relative merits of each approach. However, it is well beyond the scope of this text to discuss operative indications in general, especially those related to degenerative disease. As most spinal surgeons come to realize, the majority of degenerative spinal entities are not pathologic, and most pathologic entities that may indeed be the cause of patient symptoms do not require surgery.

The repair of symptomatic spinal disease can be most rewarding for patient and surgeon. We hope that this text will aid the surgeon in providing a smoother operation and a much safer experience for the patient.

Todd J. Albert
Richard A. Balderston
Bruce E. Northrup

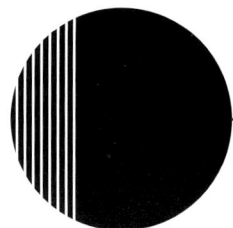

Contents

CHAPTER 1
RELEVANT CERVICAL ANATOMY... 1
Todd J. Albert, Marc R. Rosen, and William M. Keane

CHAPTER 2
ANTERIOR MIDDLE AND LOWER CERVICAL EXPOSURES............... 9
Todd J. Albert

CHAPTER 3
ANTERIOR UPPER CERVICAL EXPOSURES 25
Marc R. Rosen, William M. Keane, and David Rosen

CHAPTER 4
LATERAL RETROPHARYNGEAL APPROACH TO THE UPPER
CERVICAL SPINE (THE WHITESIDES APPROACH) 53
Todd J. Albert and Thomas E. Whitesides, Jr.

CHAPTER 5
ANTERIOR EXPOSURES OF THE CERVICOTHORACIC JUNCTION
AND UPPER THORACIC SPINE 61
Lawrence T. Kurz and Harry N. Herkowitz

CHAPTER 6
POSTERIOR CERVICAL EXPOSURES..................................... 81
Thomas G. Andreshak and Howard S. An

CHAPTER 7
THORACOTOMY 115
Bernard A. Rawlins, Todd J. Albert, and Richard A. Balderston

CHAPTER 8
COSTOTRANSVERSECTOMY 133
Alexander R. Vaccaro

CHAPTER 9
ANTERIOR RETROPERITONEAL LUMBAR EXPOSURES.................. 145
Sanford E. Emery

CHAPTER 10
ALTERNATIVE ANTERIOR LUMBAR EXPOSURES 157
Phillip R. Adams and Howard B. Cotler

CHAPTER 11
POSTERIOR LUMBAR APPROACH 173
David L. Kramer, Robert E. Booth, Todd J. Albert, and Richard A. Balderston

CHAPTER 12
WILTSE PARAVERTEBRAL MUSCLE POSTEROLATERAL EXPOSURES 193
Srdjan Mirkovic and Steven R. Garfin

CHAPTER 13
AUTOLOGOUS BONE GRAFT 201
Cathleen S. Van Buskirk, Jerome M. Cotler, and Todd J. Albert

INDEX 221

CHAPTER 1

RELEVANT CERVICAL ANATOMY

Todd J. Albert, M.D.
Marc R. Rosen, M.D.
William M. Keane, M.D.

The cervical region contains those structures that connect the head with the rest of the body. The cortical blood supply and neural pathways course through the neck; those organs vital to speech and deglutition are contained here. Located deep in the neck is the cervical spine. This structure brings mobility and stability to the cervical region while protecting the spinal cord. Although the anatomy of the region is quite complex, five fascial layers invest all of its structures, creating compartments that facilitate surgical exposure.

Familiarity with the one superficial and four deep layers of the cervical fascia is paramount to understanding surgical exposure. The fascial layers consist of (1) the superficial fascia, which contains the platysma; (2) the superficial layer of the deep fascia surrounding the sternocleidomastoid and overlying the anterior and external jugular veins; (3) the middle layer of deep fascia, investing the strap muscles and forming the visceral fascia that encloses the trachea, esophagus, and recurrent nerve; (4) the alar fascia, which fuses in the midline to the visceral fascia and forms the two carotid sheaths; and (5) the deepest prevertebral fascia, which covers the spine, longus coli, and scalenus muscles (Figure 1–1).

The sternocleidomastoid muscle is the most prominent muscle of the cervical region. It courses in a transverse manner from the mastoid tip to the clavicular and sternal areas, where it divides into two heads: the clavicular head and sternal head. This important landmark separates the neck into an anterior and posterior triangle. The anterior triangle is

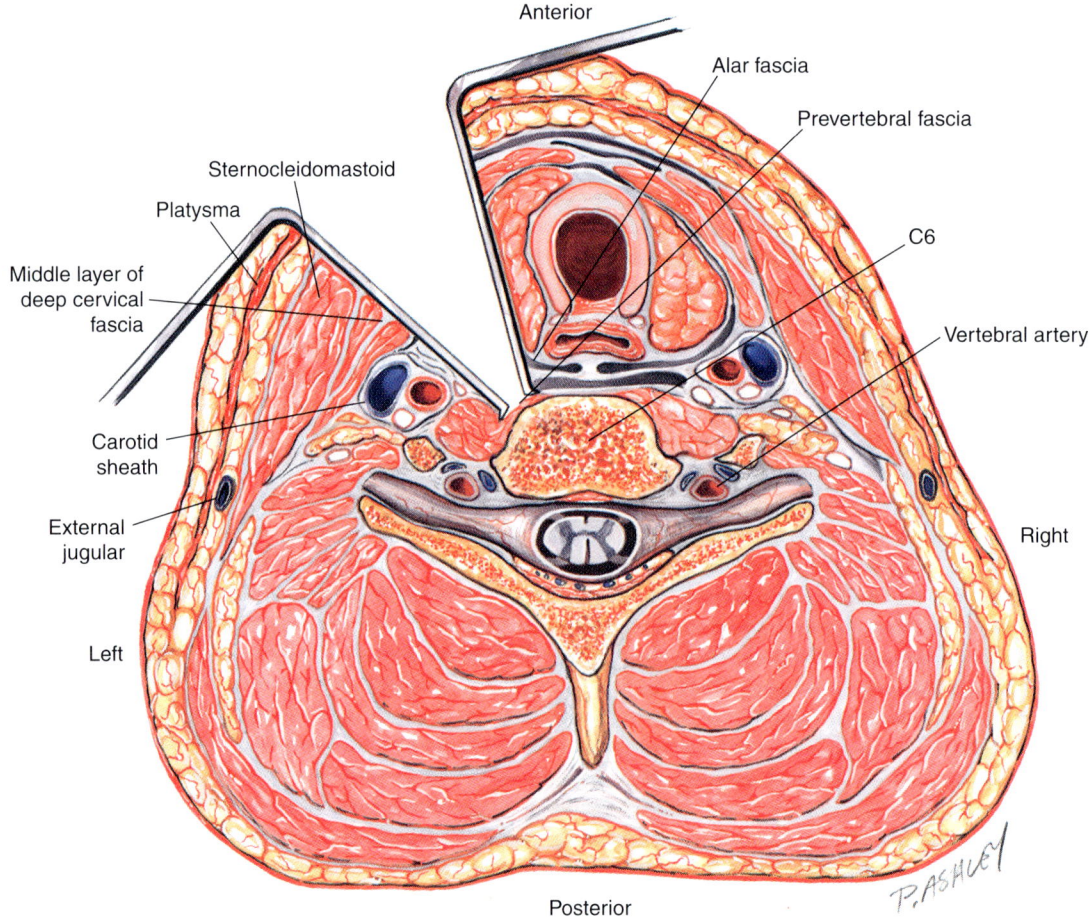

● **Figure 1-1.** Cross-sectional view at C6 vertebral body level.

the one most frequently entered during cervical spine surgery. As the sternocleidomastoid muscle is retracted posteriorly, the carotid sheath is seen just deep and running in a nearly parallel plane. The omohyoid muscle courses in a posterolateral direction from the hyoid bone in the inferior portion of the anterior cervical triangle. The anterior and posterior bellies of the digastric muscle attach to the hyoid bone in a sling-like manner and define the inferior limits of the submandibular triangle (Figure 1–2).

As the dissection is carried more medially toward the visceral compartment of the neck, the strap of muscles of the larynx is encountered. Anatomically the muscles are divided into superficial and deep layers. The superficial layer includes the sternohyoid and omohyoid muscles. The deep layer consists of the thyrohyoid and sternohyoid muscles. The omohyoid muscle, which is frequently encountered during anterior dissection of the spine, is invested by the middle layer of the deep cervical fascia (see Figure 1–1).

The carotid and vertebral arteries carry the crucial blood supply to the brain. The carotid artery also supplies the visceral compartments of the neck. A number of other vessels course transversely through the cervical region (Figure 1–3). These are frequently encountered during cervical spine surgery and may need to be ligated to improve exposure. As the surgical dissection is carried from an inferior to superior direction, the middle thyroid vein is seen at the level of C5 (Figure 1–4). With more superior dissection, the first division of the carotid artery, the superior thyroid artery, comes into view. The superior thyroid vein and superior laryngeal nerve are in close proximity to this artery as they course from a lateral to medial direction in the transverse plane. The lingual artery is typically one interspace above the superior laryngeal nerve and is deep but proximate to the hypoglossal nerve. The facial artery is superior and more superficial than the lingual artery, and is intimately associated with the posterior limit of the submandibular gland. This vessel is often ligated when high cervical exposure is required.

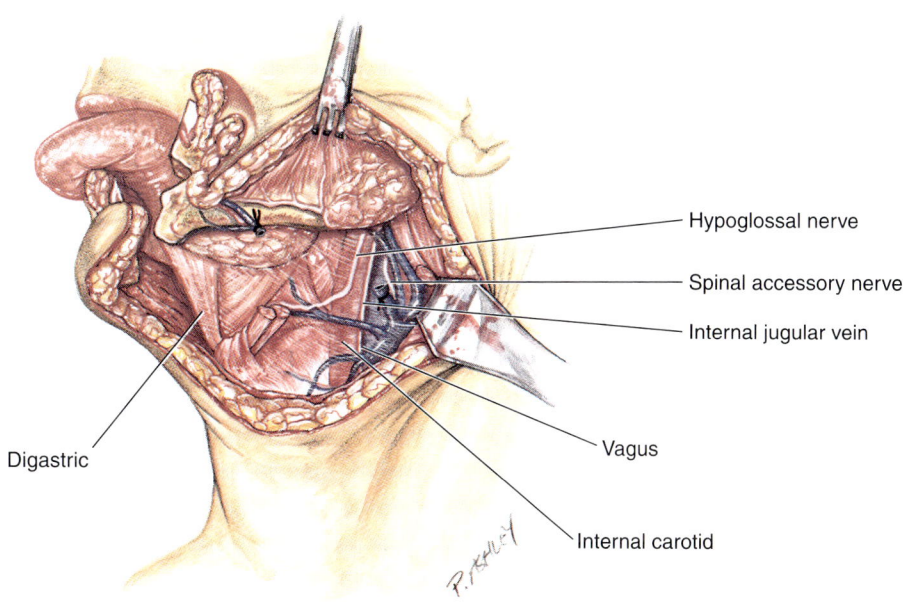

● **Figure 1–2.** Inferior view of the submandibular triangle.

A number of nerves cross the anterior cervical triangle transversely and therefore are subject to the risk of injury during dissection in this region. The superficial ansa hypoglossus divides into superficial and deep branches. These nerves, which supply function to the strap muscles of the larynx, are often sacrificed during exposure of the cervical spine. This produces minimal morbidity.

The left recurrent laryngeal nerve descends from the skull base with the vagus nerve within the carotid sheath. It leaves the vagus nerve within the thorax as it loops under the aortic arch beneath the ligamentum arteriosum and ascends back into the neck within the tracheoesophageal groove. The right recurrent laryngeal nerve also descends from the skull base with the vagus nerve in the carotid sheath and loops around the subclavian artery as it ascends into the neck within the tracheoesophageal groove.

In a few patients a nonrecurrent laryngeal nerve may be encountered on the right side. The aberrant nerve may be noted to cross in a transverse direction at the level of the thyroid gland. Both recurrent laryngeal nerves are covered by the visceral fascia.

The superior laryngeal nerve passes in a transverse direction from the vagus nerve in close proximity to the superior laryngeal artery and vein at the level of the third cervical vertebra. The nerve then divides into an internal and external branch. This nerve innervates the cricothyroid muscle. If it is injured, hoarseness and voice fatigue may result. The hypoglossal nerve descends from the skull base near to the carotid sheath. It then courses transversely as it crosses the carotid artery near the superior thyroid artery and vein and passes deep to the digastric sling at the level of the hyoid bone (Figure 1–5).

Injury to this nerve may result in paralysis of the ipsolateral tongue musculature, creating difficulties with speech and swallowing.

The marginal mandibular nerves are the most superficial and superiorly positioned nerves of the cervical region and are at risk for injury during cervical spine surgery. This

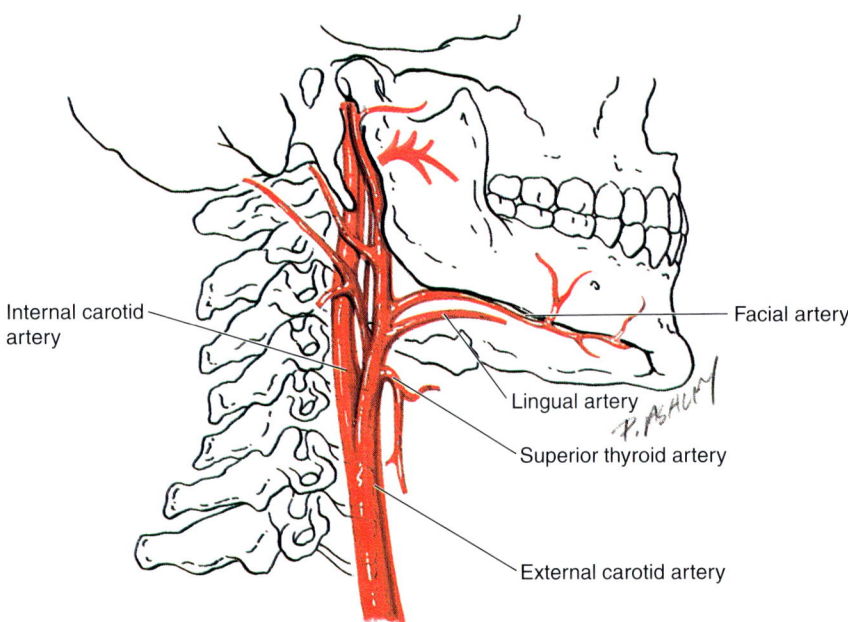

● **Figure 1–3.** Schematic of branches of carotid system.

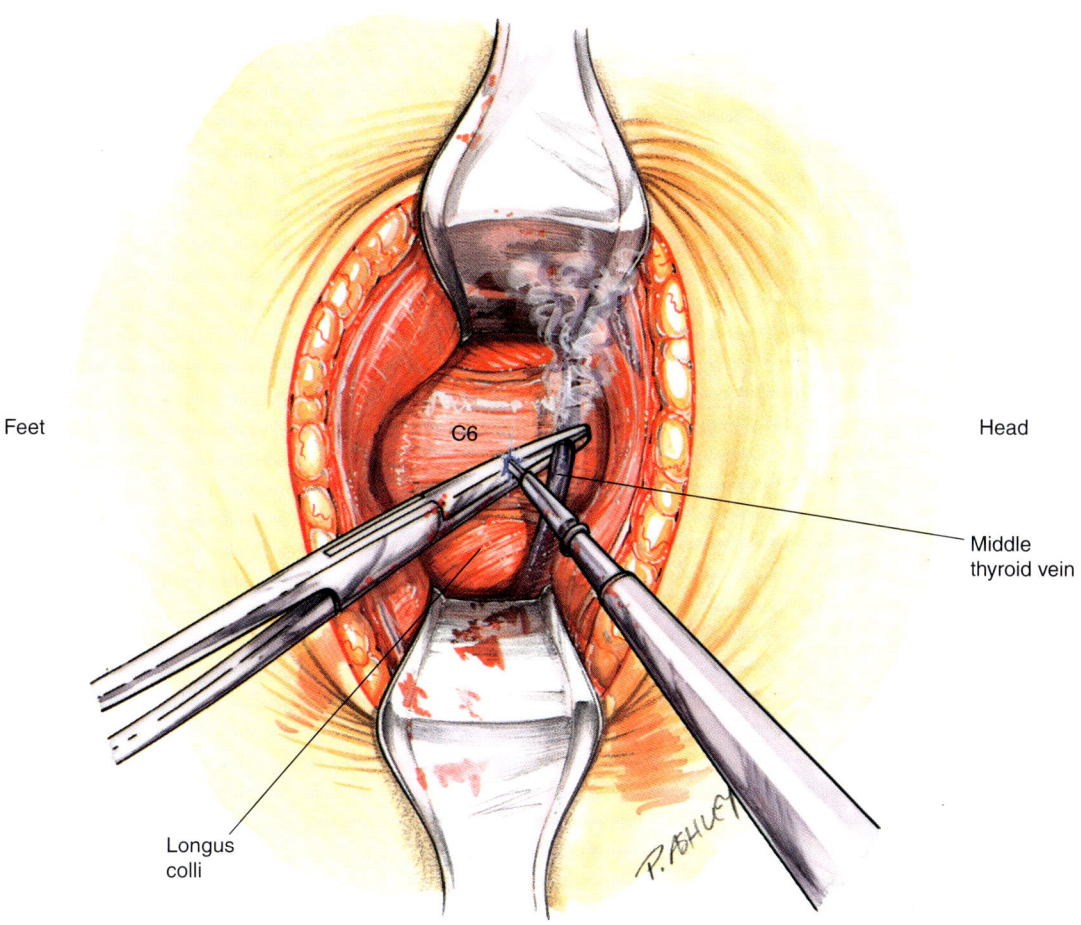

● **Figure 1-4.** Division of the middle thyroid vein at the inferior aspect of C5 vertebral body.

division of the facial nerve extends into the cervical region just below the angle of the mandible and courses in a plane beneath the platysma muscle toward the submandibular triangle (Figure 1–6).

The careful identification and preservation of these nerves is important during cervical spine surgery. Inadvertent clamping or sectioning of the nerves results in permanent injury, while overly aggressive traction produces neuropraxia, which may last for months or years. The maintenance of a soft tissue buttress between the nerve and retractor is helpful in avoiding compression injury. Excessive traction is to be avoided.

The cervical sympathetic ganglion passes in a vertical direction near the lateral aspect of the vertebral bodies in close proximity to the prevertebral musculature and extends from the thoracic inlet to the second cervical vertebra. There are usually three prominent ganglionic enlargements: the superior, middle, and inferior ganglions. The superior ganglion is identified at the level of the second or third cervical vertebral bodies. The middle ganglion is variable in its presence and can be identified at the level of C6. The inferior ganglion is located near the first thoracic vertebra and forms the stellate ganglion. Injuries to these structures may result in ipsilateral myosis and lid ptosis, also known as Horner's syndrome.

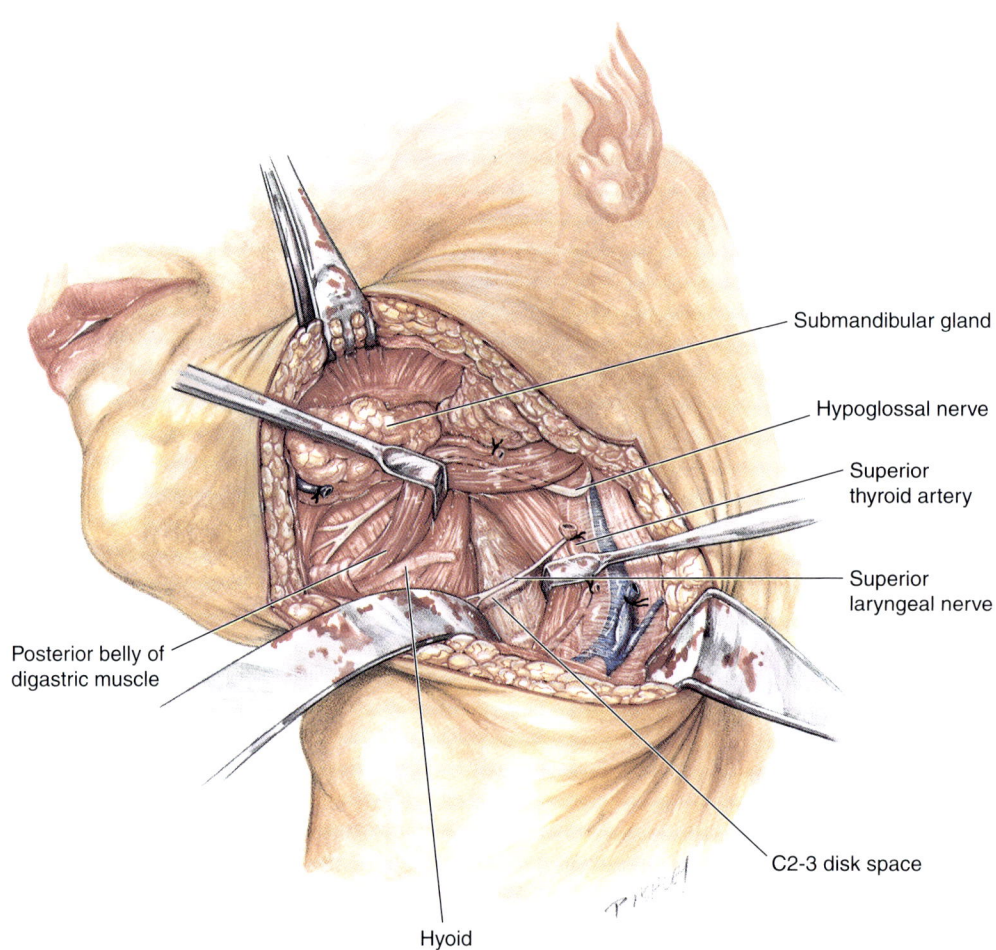

● **Figure 1-5.** High retropharyngeal approach after dissection.

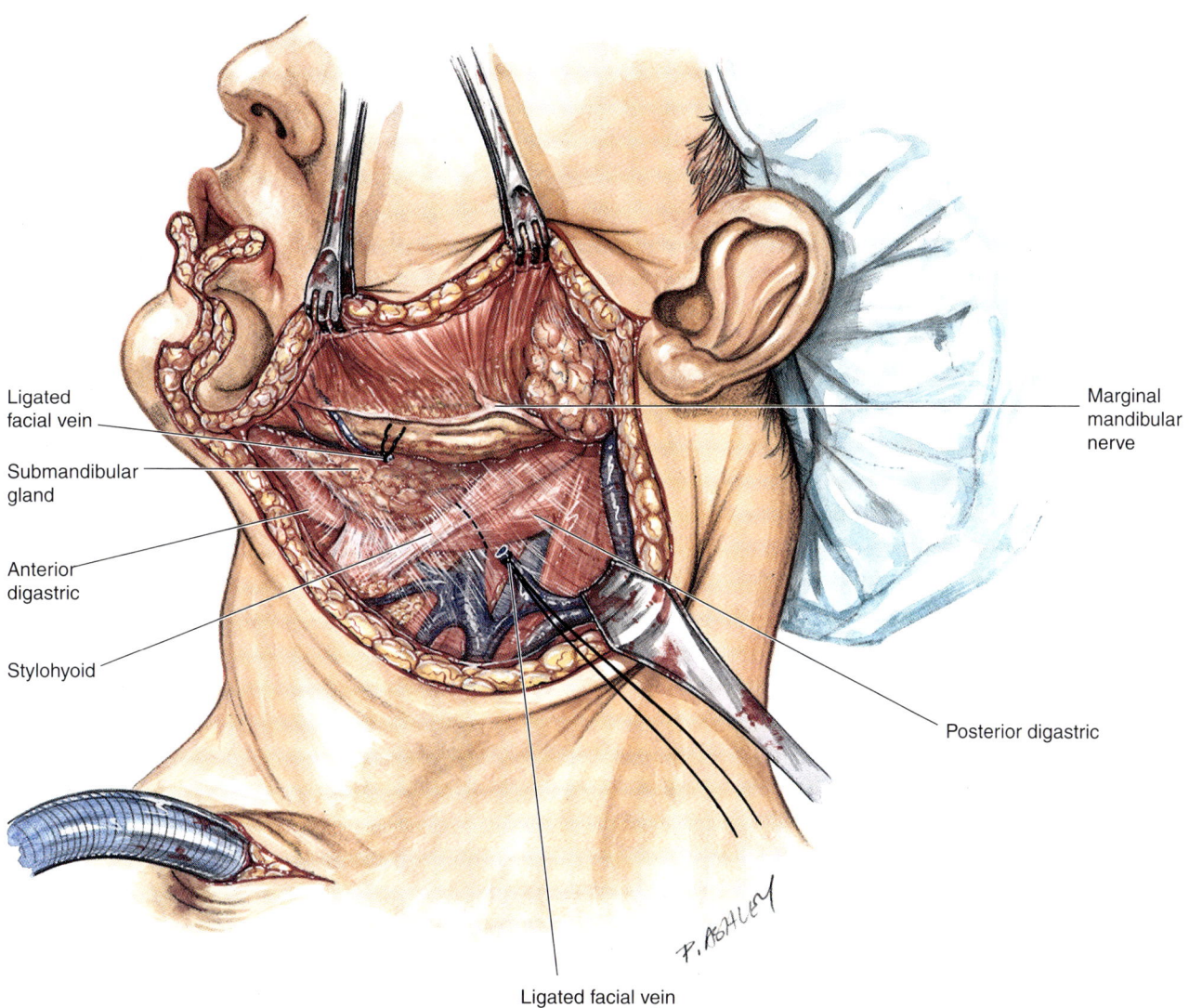

● **Figure 1-6.** Facial vein divided and retracted superiorly to protect marginal mandibular nerve.

The vertebral artery, although not typically identified or injured during anterior cervical spine surgery, is an important structure. This first branch of the subclavian artery enters the transverse foramen of the 6th cervical vertebra and ascends the neck through successive vertebral transverse foramina to the first cervical vertebra. After leaving the transverse foramen of the atlas, it curves posterioromedially over the posterior ring of the atlas and penetrates the posterior atlanto-occipital ligament prior to ascending through the foramen magnum. Intracranially, it joins the contralateral vertebral artery, forming the basilar artery, and communicates with the circle of Willis. The vertebral vein accompanies the artery in close proximity. A portion of the sympathetic chain may also be identified in the most superior limits of this posterior dissection.

CHAPTER 2

ANTERIOR MIDDLE AND LOWER CERVICAL EXPOSURES

Todd J. Albert, M.D.

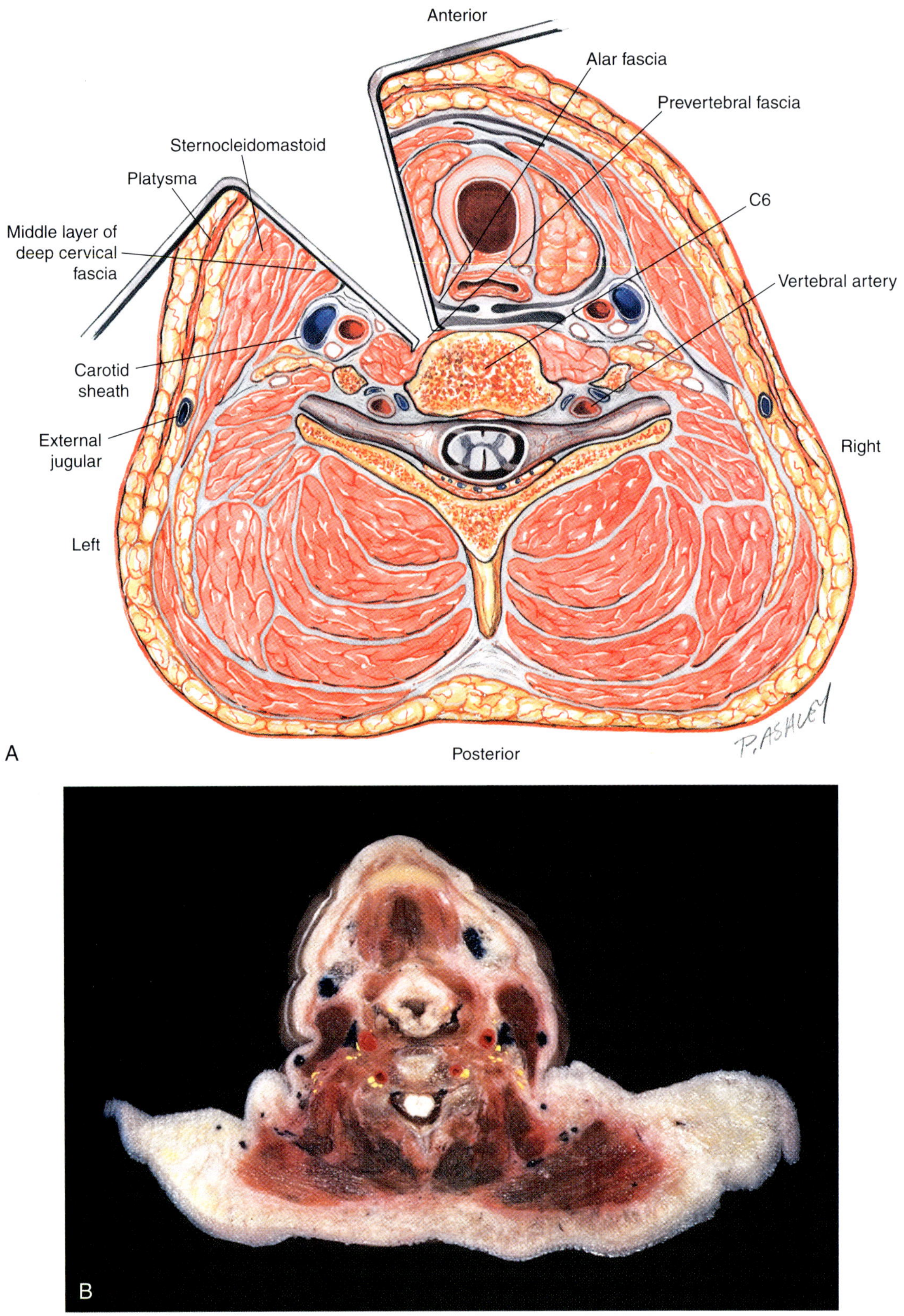

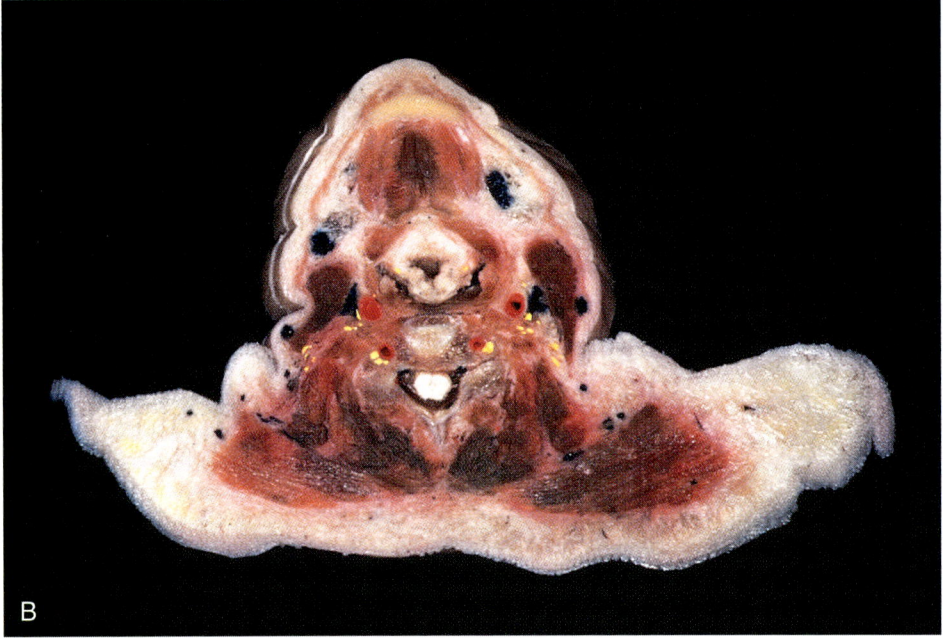

● **Figure 2-1.** *A*, Cross-sectional view at C6 vertebral body level. *B*, Cross-sectional cadaveric prosection at approximate level of C4-5.

The anterior approach between C2 and T1 exploits the interval between the sternocleidomastoid and carotid sheath laterally and the trachea and esophagus medially in a bloodless plane traversing the four levels of cervical fascia (Figure 2–1). The technique is potentially extensile and atraumatic and allows removal of diseased intervertebral disks, vertebral bodies, and other spinal pathologic processes, such as tumors or infected tissue. This approach was first described in the orthopaedic literature by Southwick and Robinson as well as by Bailey and Badgley. This safe approach, when extended, can expose up to seven vertebral bodies and allow for removal of multiple disks and vertebral bodies along with strut grafting and potential internal fixation anteriorly in the cervical spine. Its main function is anterior decompression of the spinal cord and nerve roots, although access to the anterior spine for any reason can be accomplished through this approach.

Surgical Technique

External traction is not used when performing this surgery, other than in the case of multiple vertebral body removal. Internal intervertebral distraction or distraction across two disk spaces with a distractor for a one-level corpectomy is adequate. For procedures involving more than one vertebral body being resected, the patient is placed in Gardner-Wells tong traction with the neck extended. Before the operation is begun, the patient is checked to ensure that he or she can extend the neck for intubation purposes. If there is any degree of myelopathy or neurologic changes with awake extension of the neck, an awake intubation is performed. Appropriate spinal cord monitoring is in place before the start of the procedure.

If the patient can extend the neck without myelopathic symptoms, asleep intubation is performed. After intubation and with appropriate spinal cord monitoring, a towel rolled

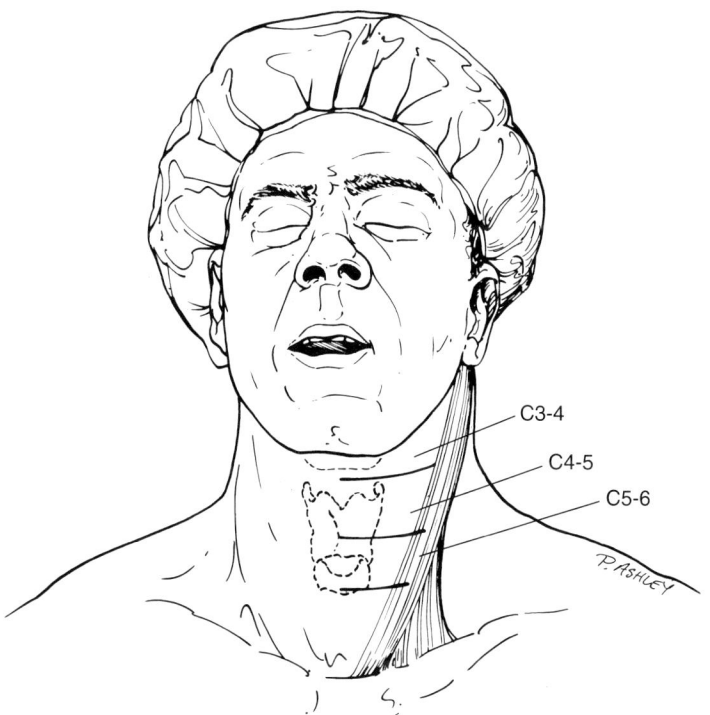

● **Figure 2-2.** Landmarks for transverse incision for the anterolateral exposure to the cervical spine. Frontal view.

longitudinally is placed in the inner scapular area to allow further neck extension. A bump is placed under the hip if the iliac crest is to be taken and the patient is large or if the anterior-superior iliac spine is difficult to palpate. The entire anterior neck from lateral to the sternocleidomastoid on both sides down to below the clavicle is prepped, as is the iliac crest if an iliac crest bone graft is to be used. If a fibular graft is to be used, the leg is prepped as described elsewhere. For up to three disk levels to be operated on without instrumentation, a transverse incision is employed. For three disk levels with instrumentation or for more than two body level corpectomies, a longitudinal incision centered along the anterior aspect of the sternocleidomastoid is used. The level for a transverse incision is determined by superficial landmarks (Figure 2–2). When the neck is in a significantly extended position, these landmarks are often displaced. To accommodate for this, the incision is moved slightly higher in the neck. As a general rule, one is usually *lower* than is expected. Sometimes in the asleep patient, the carotid tubercle (Chassaignac's tubercle) can be palpated on the transverse process of C6 as a landmark. The incision for one- to two-level diskectomy is approximately 2 to 3 inches long and begins at the midline of the neck and goes to, but not past, the sternocleidomastoid. Extension of the incision past the sternocleidomastoid can

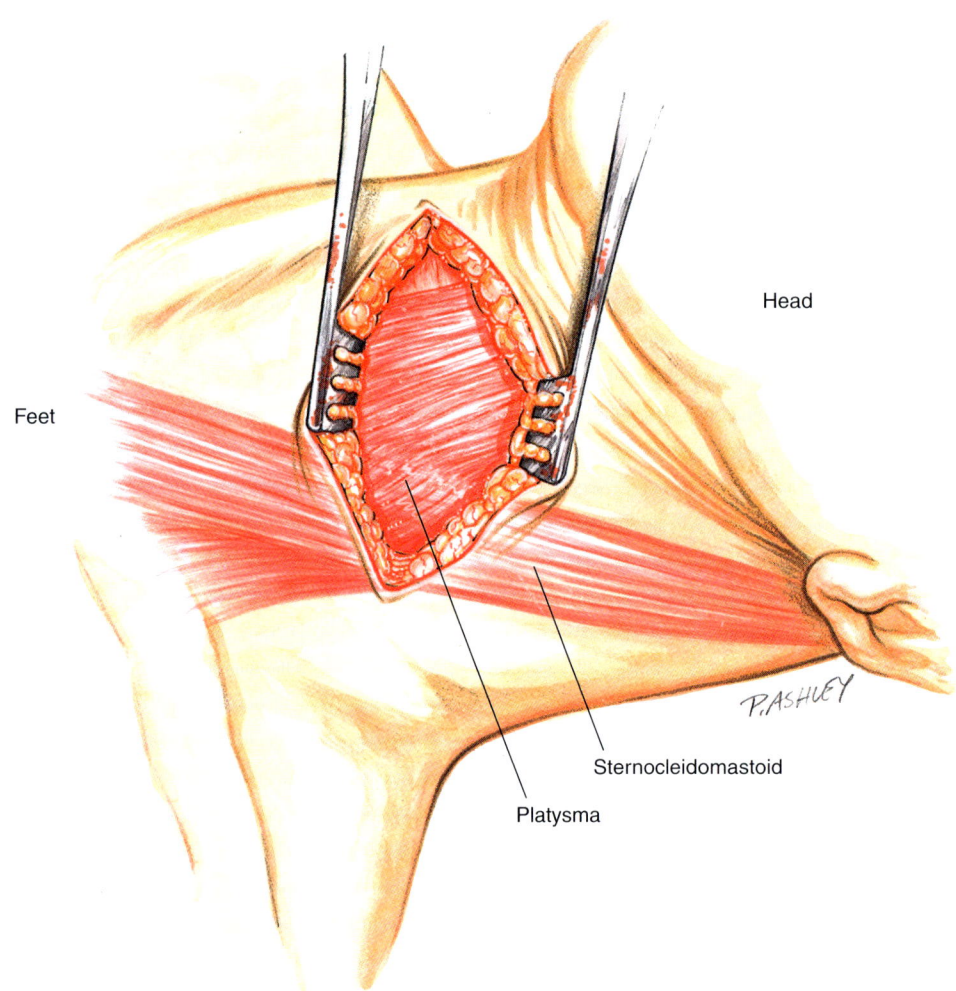

● **Figure 2–3.** After skin incision, the fat is wiped off the platysma before the platysma is sectioned. In this and all subsequent surgical views, the patient is lying in front of the surgeon and the surgeon is standing to the patient's left. The directions toward the head and feet are identified in each figure.

cause puckering of the skin after healing. Landmarks for the transverse incision include the cricoid cartilage at approximately C5-6, the thyroid cartilage at C4-5, and the hyoid just above C3-4 (see Figure 2–2). We prefer a left sided approach due to the reliable anatomy of the recurrent laryngeal nerve on the left.

The skin is infiltrated with local anesthetic and epinephrine, and the first knife cut is made to the subcutaneous fat (Figure 2–3). Gauze, is used to wipe the fat off the platysma to clearly delineate it, and the platysma is divided transversely and sharply to show the superficial layer of cervical fascia covering the strap muscles and the sternocleidomastoid laterally (Figure 2–4). The platysma is also rolled to the edges of the incision with a gauze sponge to make it easily accessible for later closure. With a fine-toothed forceps and Lincoln scissors the superficial fascia is divided transversely over the extent of the incision. Often encountered is the anterior jugular vein and the external jugular vein, which can be ligated for improved exposure (Figure 2–5). After complete dissection of the superficial fascia, longitudinal dissection is carried out along the sternocleidomastoid to expose the middle layer of the deep cervical fascia. The scissors is used in a vertical direction while pressure is applied to the sternocleidomastoid. Cushing vein retractors are used superiorly and inferiorly for longitudinal retraction above the sternocleidomastoid (Figure 2–6A). The release of the

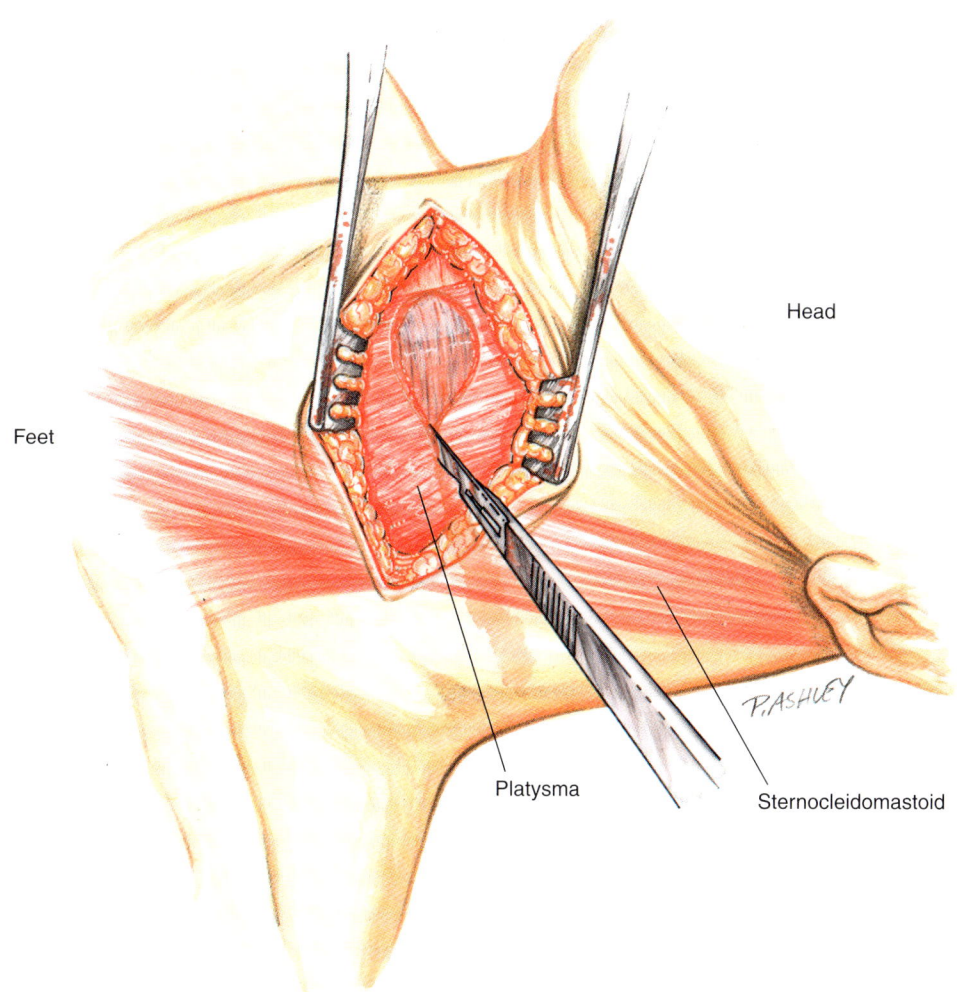

● **Figure 2-4.** The platysma is sectioned transversely and sharply for one or two disk levels or for three disk levels without instrumentation.

14 • SURGICAL APPROACHES TO THE SPINE

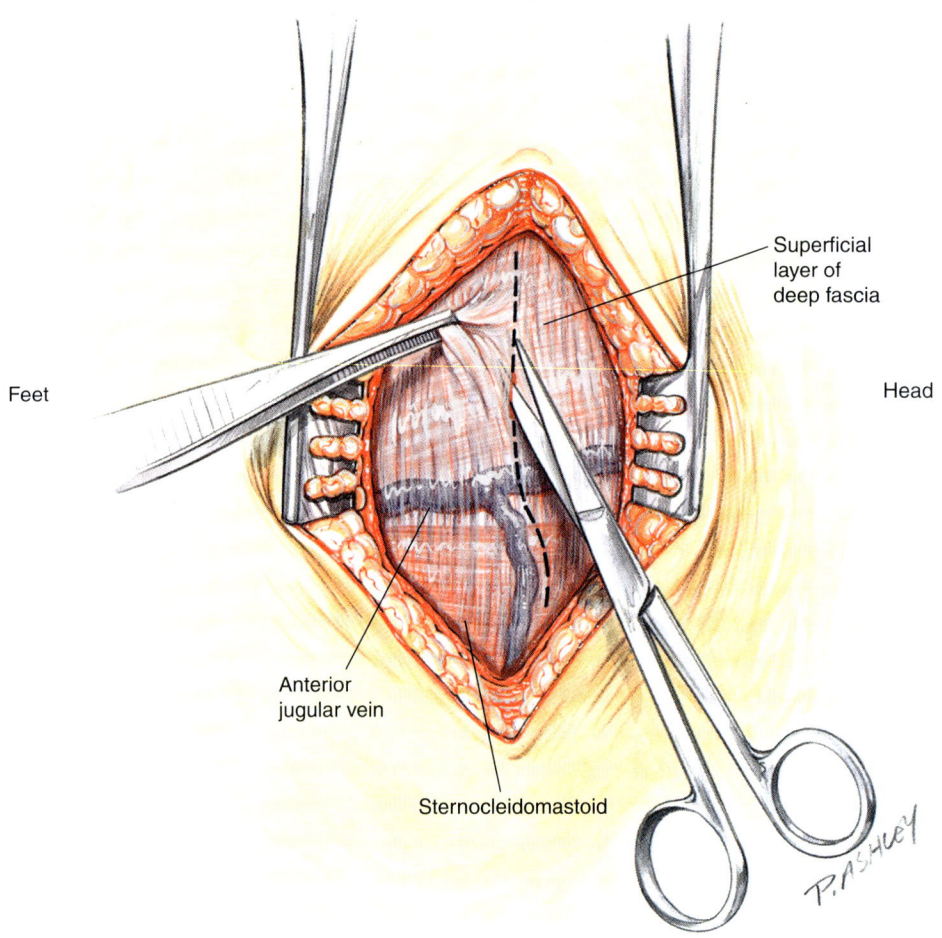

● **Figure 2-5.** The superficial fascia is divided with the scissors in a transverse direction to the sternocleidomastoid.

sternocleidomastoid is considered adequate if a finger can be placed into Burns' space and follow it distally until the head of the clavicle can be palpated. Superiorly as much dissection as necessary is done, depending on the level, to allow for a generous longitudinal exposure. Care is taken if encountering the superior thyroid artery in the area of C3, because injury to the superior laryngeal nerve can occur with vigorous dissection and retraction in this area. After the sternocleidomastoid muscle is released (see Figure 2–6B), the carotid artery is palpated with finger dissection and a Richardson appendiceal retractor is used to retract the medial structures. This usually exposes the middle layer of the cervical fascia, and in the area of C5-6 and C6-7 the omohyoid becomes visible. At this point, a peanut dissector can be used to bluntly expose the middle layer of fascia superiorly and inferiorly (keeping the dissection toward the carotid sheath to avoid harm to the recurrent laryngeal nerve). Usually the dissector causes a rent in the middle layer, allowing full longitudinal dissection and palpation of the anterior vertebral bodies. After this occurs it is much easier to retract the esophagus and trachea medially and the sternocleidomastoid laterally (Figure 2–7).

Once the release of the middle layer is completely performed with the dissector, appendical retractors are placed medially and laterally and the anterior longitudinal ligament is seen under the two deepest layers of cervical fascia (pretracheal/alar and prevertebral).

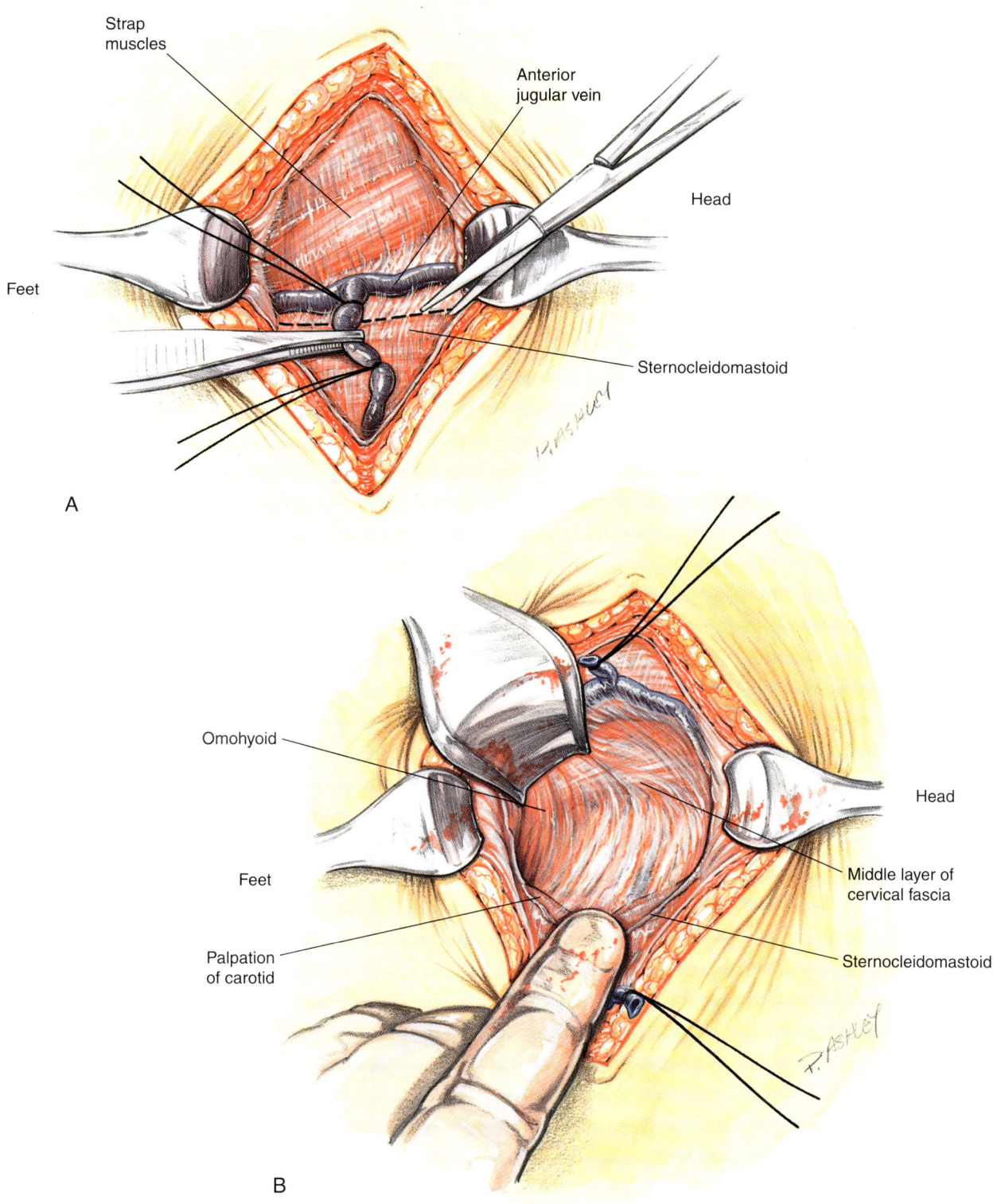

● **Figure 2-6.** *A*, Connecting veins between the internal and external jugular vein often need to be ligated. The vertical incision is in the fascia surrounding the sternocleidomastoid. Cushing vein retractors are used for superior and inferior retraction. *B*, The carotid is palpated after sternocleidomastoid release. An appendiceal retractor exposes the middle layer of the cervical fascia.

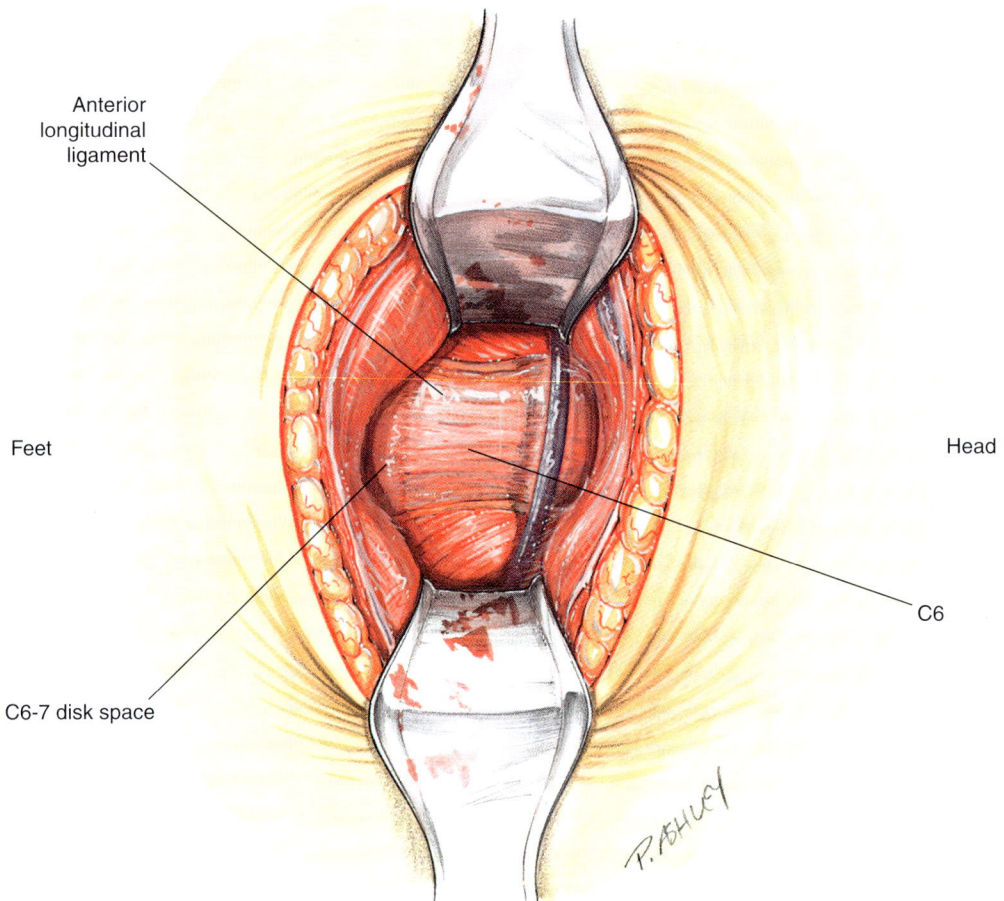

● **Figure 2-7.** After blunt dissection of the middle layer of the cervical fascia, the anterior longitudinal ligament and vertebral bodies come into view. After sectioning of the alar and prevertebral fascia, which are adherent, the self-retaining retractor exposes the longus colli and the vertebral body as well as the disk spaces. A radiograph is taken before further dissection.

The two deep fascial layers are easily and safely split or bluntly dissected. Identification of vertebral level becomes important at this time. Again palpation of Chassaignac's tubercle is helpful for identifying C6. A lateral radiograph is obtained with a bent 18-gauge spinal needle placed into the disk space to be operated on. This confirms the level. Two 90-degree bends in the tip of the needle are made so it cannot penetrate into the spinal canal. While the radiograph is being taken for one-, two-, or three-level interbody diskectomy and fusion procedures, the iliac crest is dissected and a bone graft is taken at this point.

Once the level is confirmed, with the use of hand-held retractors, the longus colli is elevated using a sucker as a retractor and cautery (Figure 2–8A). During elevation, venous sinusoids are often encountered on the lateral vertebral body that need to be cauterized or bone waxed. Care should be taken not to wander too far laterally because the vertebral artery could become endangered with the cautery at the disk space. At the level of the body, the bony anterior aspect of the foramen transfersarium (the transverse process) will protect

● **Figure 2-8.** *A*, Longus colli being elevated with cautery with hand held retractors in place. *B*, Division of the middle thyroid vein at the inferior aspect of the C5 vertebral body.

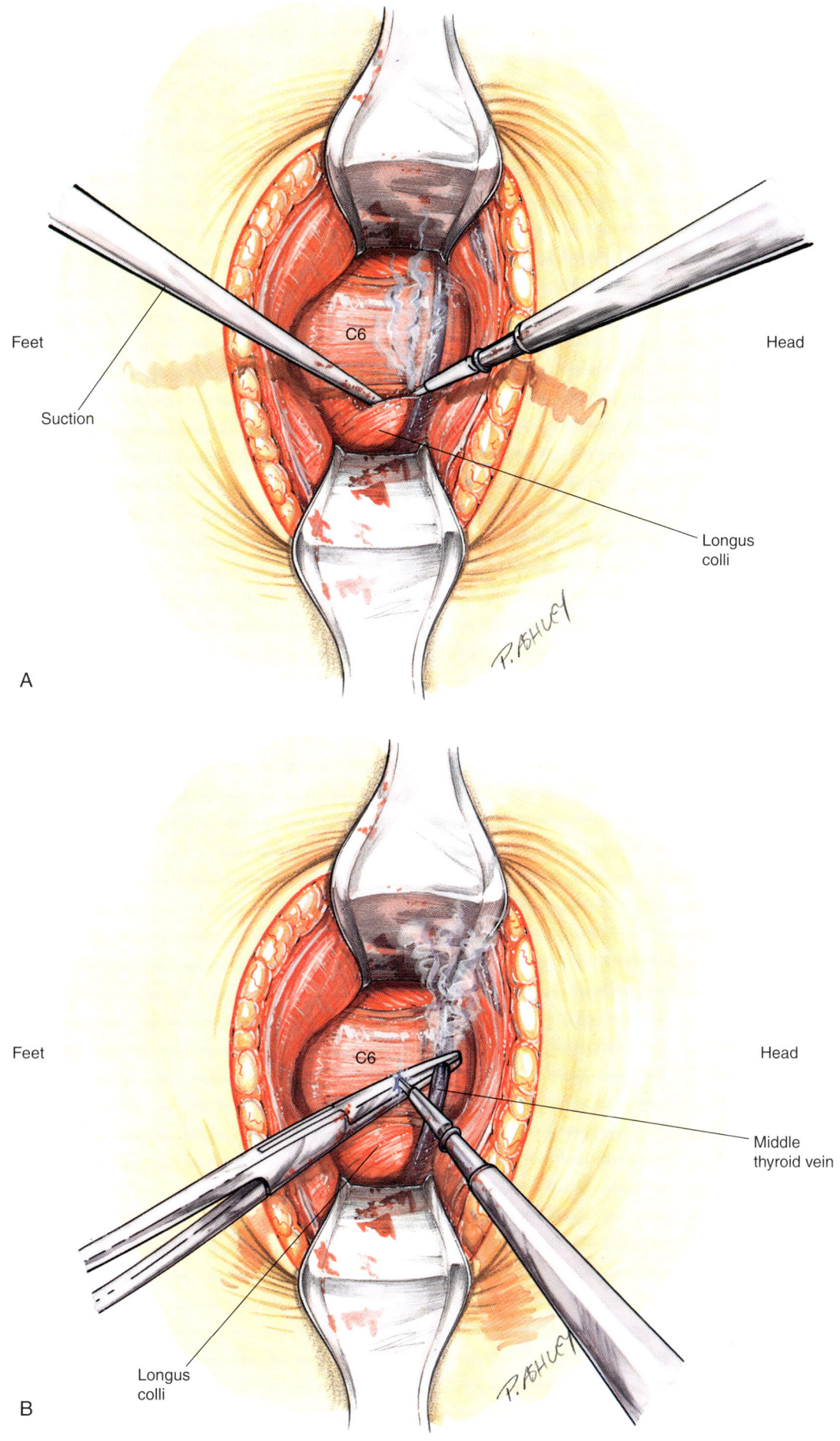

the vertebral artery from cautery. The object of elevating the longus colli is to widen the dissection but more importantly to protect the esophagus and carotid from retractor injury if retractors are placed under the longus colli. If a crossing vein is encountered during dissection, it is cauterized or ligated (see Figure 2–8B). After dissection of the longus colli, Cloward self-retaining retractors are placed into it. With self-retaining retractors the risk of injury to the esophagus and carotid is possible, so one must be meticulous in the placement of the retractors under the longus colli in the medial and lateral direction. Each retractor is placed individually under direct inspection into the longus colli on either side and then attached to the appropriate self-retaining articulation. Smooth retractors are used in an up/down fashion placed with a handle away from the operating surgeon (which is usually to the right side of the patient) (Figure 2–9). After retractor placement, intervertebral diskectomy is begun at the lowest level if more than one level is to be approached. This prevents any bleeding after diskectomy and grafting from interfering with the next level of the approach. To perform intervertebral diskectomy, the annulus is cauterized over the disk space and an annulotomy is performed with a No. 15 scalpel, taking care not to penetrate the blade too deeply. The annulus is removed with a pituitary or Leksell rongeur (Figure 2–10A). The disk space is cleared of all disk back to the posterior annulus with 1-0, 2-0, and 3-0 curets (see Figure 2–10B and 2–10C). Appropriate diskectomy includes exposure of both uncinate processes and the posterior annulus, with removal of the annulus back to the posterior longitudinal ligament (see Figure 2–11A).

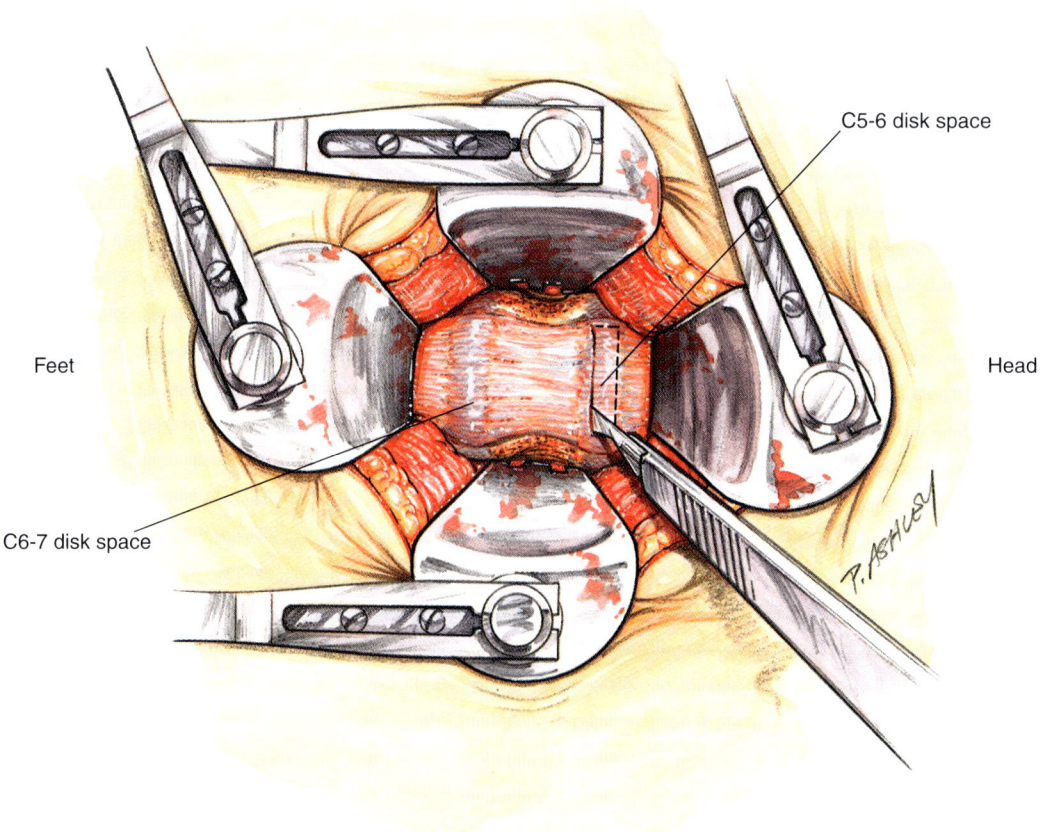

● **Figure 2–9.** Self-retaining Cloward retractors in place with toothed retractors under the longus colli in the medial lateral direction. The longitudinal retractors are smooth retractors. The toothed retractors are held down with a Kocher clamp fastened to the drape (*out of view of the picture*) on the esophageal side (usually the patient's right).

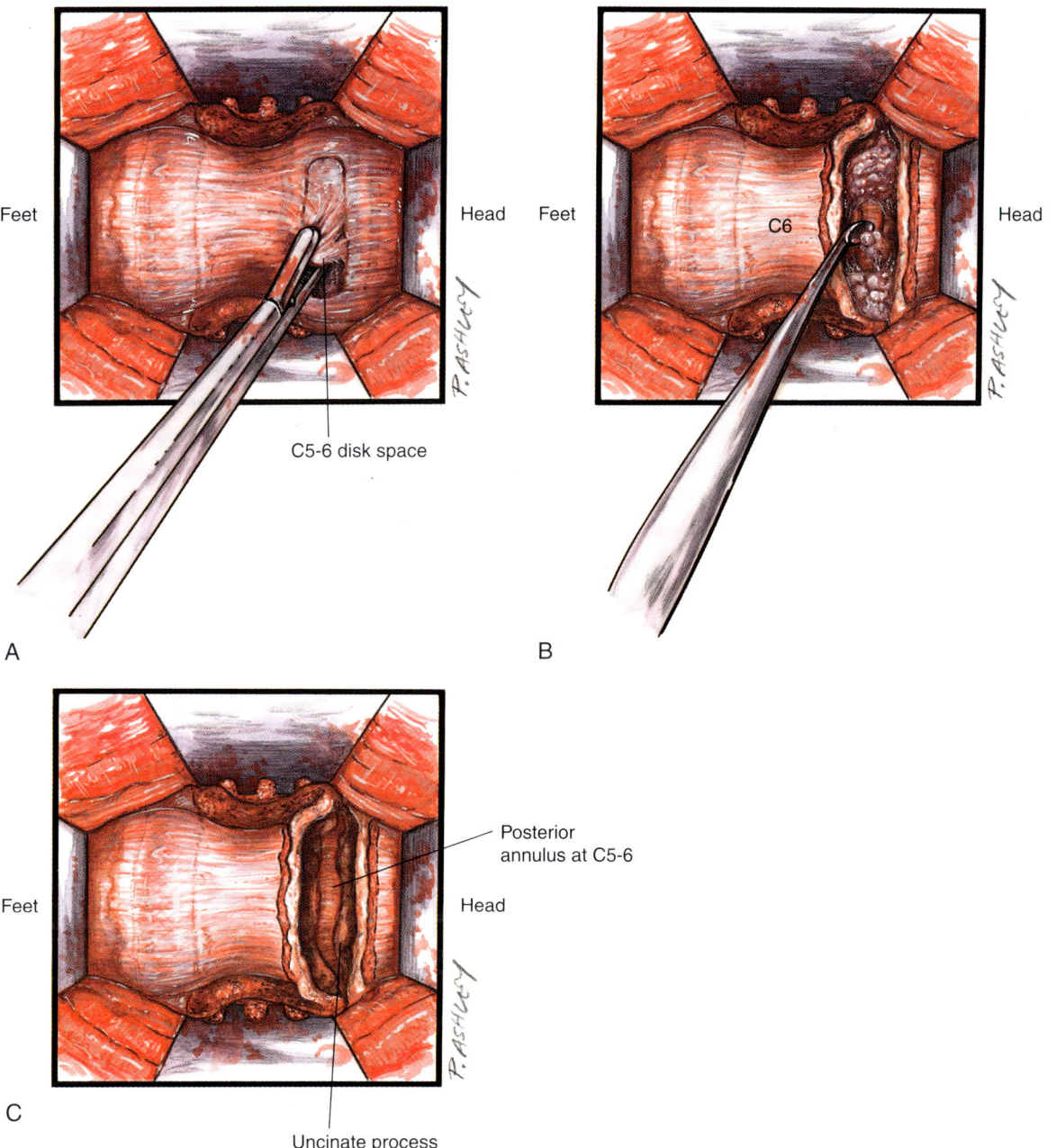

● **Figure 2-10.** *A*, After cauterization and annulotomy, the annulus is removed with a pituitary rongeur. *B*, Curettage of the disk material off the end plate with a goal of exposing both uncinate processes. *C*, After complete diskectomy, the uncinate processes are viewed, as is the posterior annulus.

For anterior foraminotomy, in the case of lateral disk herniation or stenosis, a 3-0 angled curet is used to puncture the foramen posterior to the vertebral body to clean the posterior annulus. The curet is then swept into the foramen superiorly and inferiorly (Figure 2–11*A*). One- and 2-mm Kerrison rongeurs are used to safely remove the hypertrophied uncinate process (see Figure 2–11*B*). This exposes the exiting nerve root with its vascular leash. Any bleeding is cauterized with bipolar cautery. The foramen can be checked with a

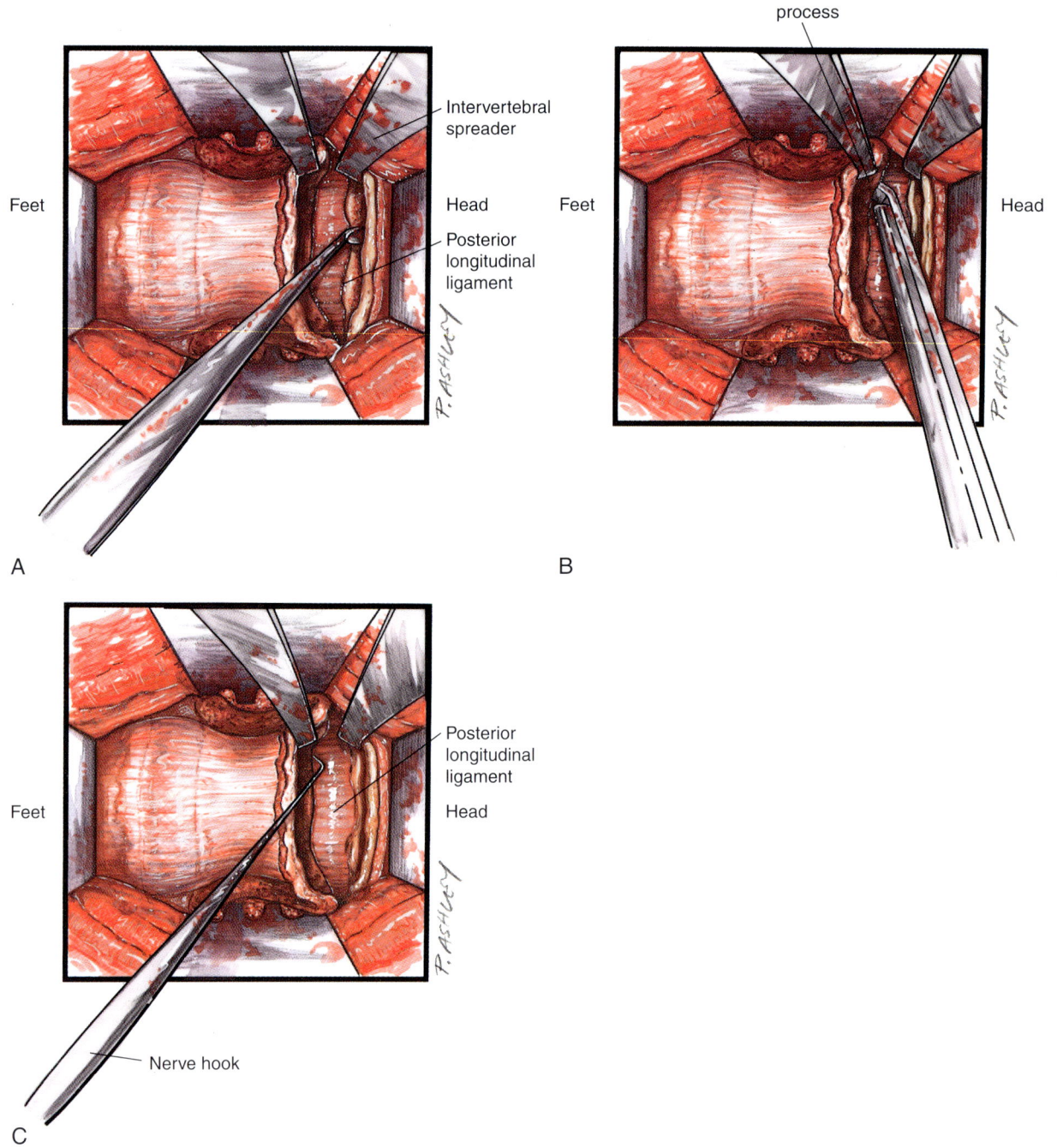

● **Figure 2-11.** *A*, The posterior annulus is removed and the foraminotomy is begun using a 3-0 angled curet to section the annulus. *B*, The foraminotomy is completed with 1- and 2-mm Kerrison punches, removing the osteophyte in a 180-degree fashion to expose the nerve root. *C*, The foramen is probed with a nerve hook to ensure that the nerve is free. Free disk fragments can often be brought into view using the nerve hook in a rotating fashion.

nerve hook (see Figure 2–11C). The osteophyte and uncinate process are removed until one is sure the exiting nerve root is free.

The procedure is made easier by intervertebral distraction with a Cloward intervertebral or Caspar distractor. An intervertebral distractor is held in place throughout the cleaning of the disk and foraminotomy. After initial diskectomy, a small Cobb elevator is placed into the disk space and twisted to fracture the posterior disk and annulus.

After complete resection of the disk and foraminotomy, a 4-mm bur is used to decorticate the end plate superiorly and inferiorly (Figure 2–12A). Next the height of the interspace is measured using a Cloward measuring device (see Figure 2–12B). The depth is measured using the Cloward depth gauge (see Figure 2–12C). The appropriate tricortical graft is shaped for height and depth. A depth of 3 to 5 mm is left for countersinking. The contoured graft is placed into the interspace, which is held under distraction either with an intervertebral spreader or a Caspar distractor, with screws in the adjacent vertebral bodies (Figure 2–12D). Using a tamp, the graft is gently tamped and countersunk into the disk space (see Figure 2–12E).

The same principles of exposure can be used for an extensile exposure of the cervical spine. For this, an oblique incision is made along the anterior border of the sternocleidomastoid (Figure 2–13). Division of the omohyoid is often necessary during this exposure for full visualization in the longitudinal manner. The same principles of dissection and division of fascial planes are used as are performed for transverse incision and a more limited approach.

Closure is over a small, round Jackson-Pratt (No. 7) drain, which is taken through the incision. Closure of the platysma layer is performed with interrupted absorbable sutures. The subcutaneous layer is closed with interrupted sutures. A pull-out Prolene suture is placed in the skin and removed on the second or third day postoperatively for best cosmetic effect.

Complications

One complication of the anterior cervical approach is injury to the vital neurovascular structures of the neck. Esophageal injury, if recognized, should be repaired immediately and nasogastric suction utilized until closure. Perforation of the esophagus can occur from retractor injury or overvigorous retraction as well as from sharp instruments or burs. Perforations that are overlooked can result in retropharyngeal abscess with fever and dysphagia. Radiopaque dye swallow is usually diagnostic. This complication can be prevented by using an orogastric tube that is pulled back and palpated in the neck and then flooded with 40 mL of diluted indigo carmine before closure. No leakage of dye represents an intact esophagus. This is done in every case.

Injury to the recurrent laryngeal nerve can lead to voice changes as well as difficulty with swallowing and potential aspiration. A left-sided approach is used in an attempt to decrease the chance of recurrent laryngeal nerve injury because its course is more constant on the left side of the neck.

The vertebral artery is at risk with overvigorous lateral deep dissection or when performing anterior foraminotomy if aggressive curettage or use of a Kerrison rongeur in the middle third of the vertebral body occurs. With vertebral artery injury, control must be obtained with packing. If control of bleeding cannot be accomplished, dissection of the vertebral artery above and below the injury is attempted, with clipping or ligation proximally and distally. The patient must be observed for a pseudoaneurysm if symptoms occur after packing stops the bleeding or in the long term after such an injury.

Horner's syndrome can occur if injury to Chassaignac's ganglion occurs in the lower cervical area. Subperiosteal dissection of the longest colli muscle usually prevents this occurrence. Damage to the external laryngeal nerve can result in hoarseness and can be avoided by respecting the area around the superior thyroid artery area where this nerve courses.

Injury to the thoracic duct can occur if dissection wanders laterally to the carotid sheath in the lower aspects of the neck on the left. Keeping dissection medial to the carotid artery and on the left side usually prevents this problem.

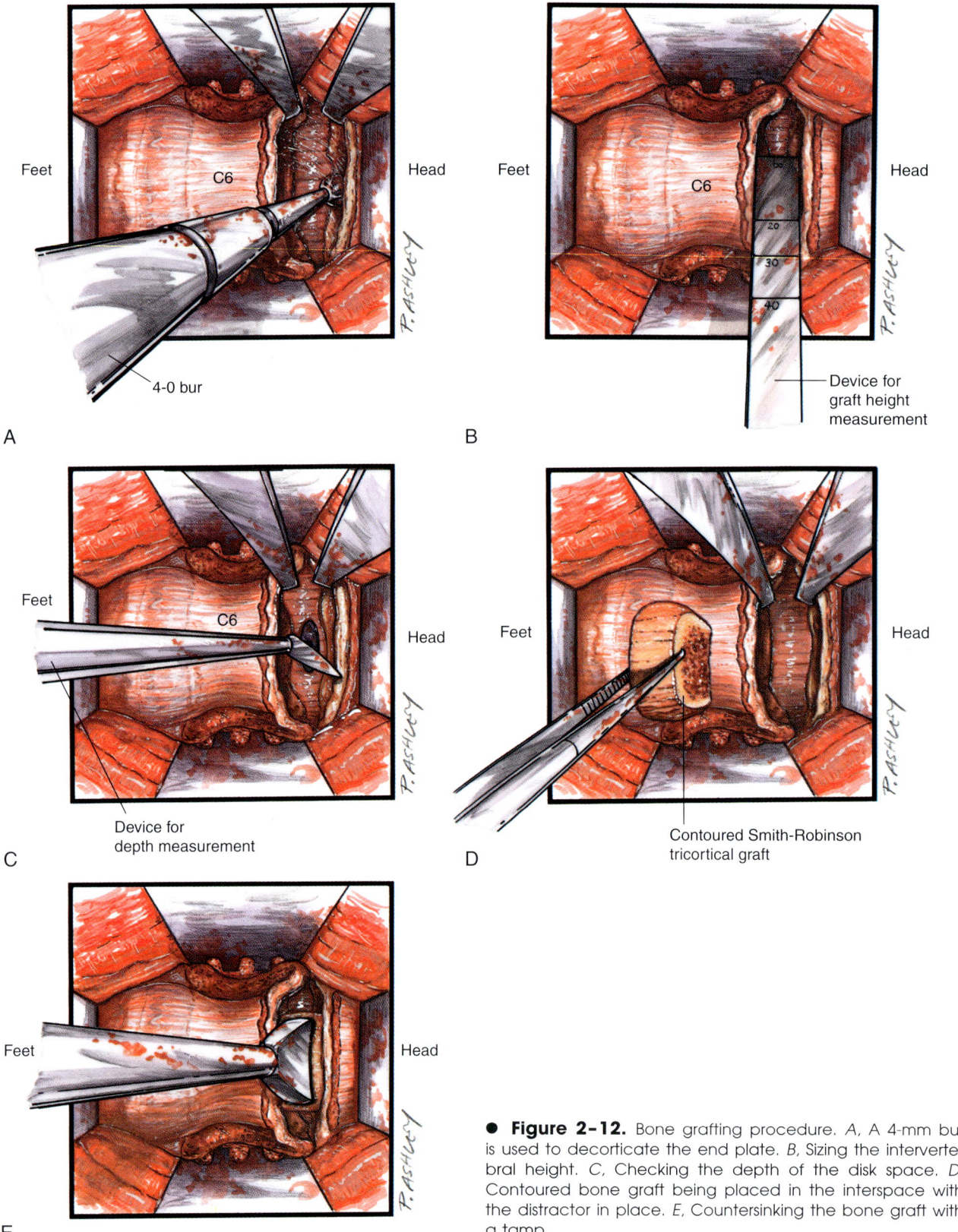

● **Figure 2-12.** Bone grafting procedure. *A,* A 4-mm bur is used to decorticate the end plate. *B,* Sizing the intervertebral height. *C,* Checking the depth of the disk space. *D,* Contoured bone graft being placed in the interspace with the distractor in place. *E,* Countersinking the bone graft with a tamp.

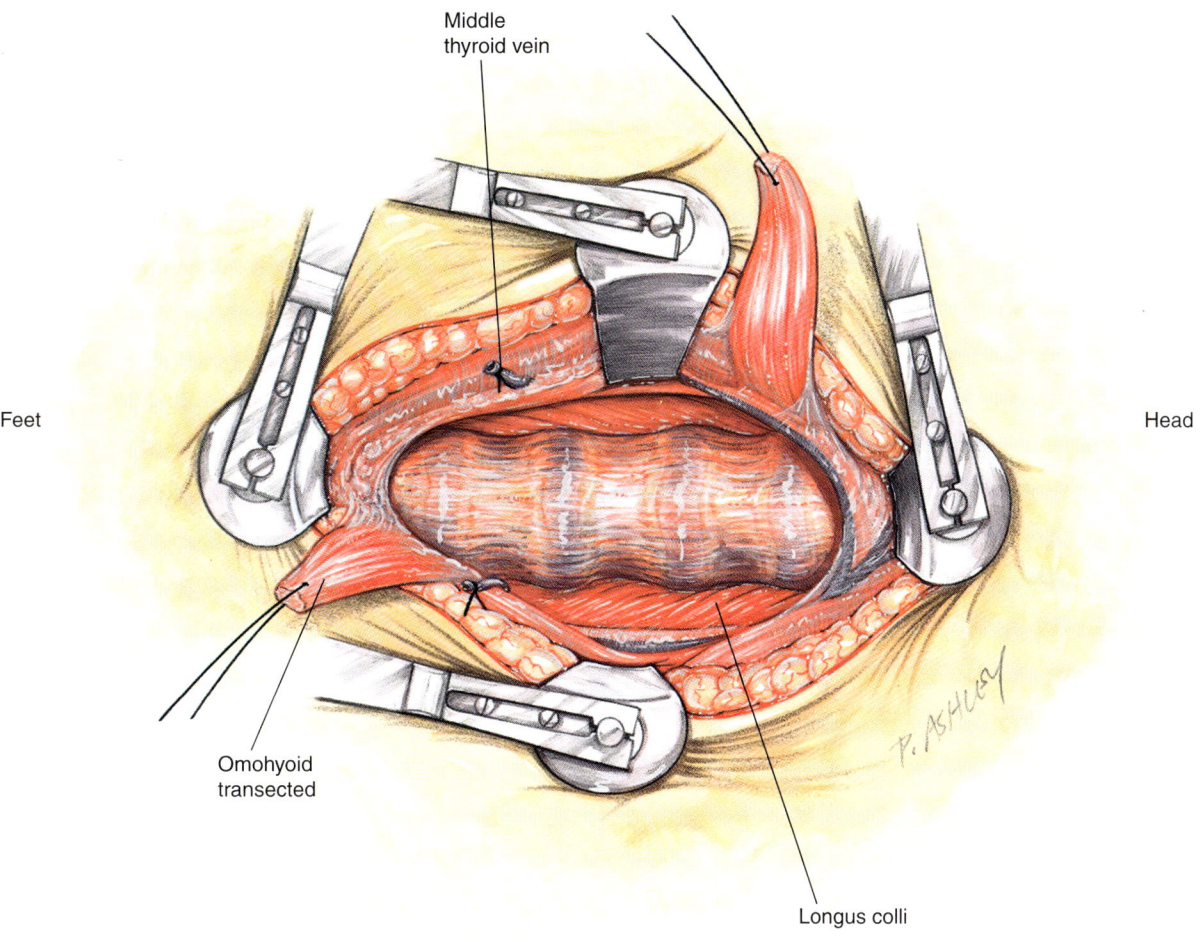

● **Figure 2-13.** Extensile exposure of the cervical spine with omohyoid sectioned.

In the short term, after the operation, patients often complain of swallowing problems or hoarseness from retraction with high cervical approaches. After very high cervical approaches and excessive submandibular retraction, the patient is usually left intubated for at least 24 hours after surgery. The airway is inspected endoscopically before extubation.

Conclusion

The anterior cervical approach is atraumatic, usually bloodless, and provides excellent access to the anterior vertebrae and disks of the cervical spine. It allows for direct decompression of degenerative, traumatic, infectious, or tumorous conditions. It also allows for stable constructs to be created with structural bone grafting in the anterior and middle column of the cervical spine.

BIBLIOGRAPHY

1. Bailey RW, Badgeley CE: Stablization of the cervical spine by anterior fusion. *J Bone Joint Surg Am* 42:565, 1960.

2. Henry AK: Extensile Exposure, pp 53–80. New York, Churchill Livingstone, 1957.
3. McAfee PC, Bohlman HH, Riley LH, et al: The anterior pharyngeal approach to the upper part of the cervical spine. *J Bone Joint Surg Am* 69:1371, 1987.
4. Robinson RA, Smith GW: Anterolateral cervical disc removal and interbody fusions for cervical disk syndrome. *Bull Johns Hopkins Hosp* 96:223, 1955.
5. Robinson RA: Fusions of the cervical spine. *J Bone Joint Surg Am* 41:1, 1959.
6. Robinson RA, Southwick WO: Indications and techniques for early stabilization in the neck and fractures and dislocation of the cervical spine. *South Med J* 53:565, 1960.
7. Robinson RA, Southwick WO: Surgical approaches to the cervical spine. Instr Course Lect 17:299, 1960.
8. Robinson RA, Bailey LH: Techniques of exposure and fusion of the cervical spine. Clin Orthop 109:78, 1975.
9. Southwick WO, Robinson, RA: Recent advances in surgery of the cervical spine. *Surg Clin North Am* 41:1661, 1961.
10. Verbiest H: Anterolateral operations for fractures and dislocations in the middle and lower parts of the cervical spine. *J Bone Joint Surg Am* 51:1489, 1969.
11. Whitecloud TS, LaRocca H: Fibular strut graft and reconstructive surgery of the cervical spine. Spine 1:33, 1976.

CHAPTER 3

ANTERIOR UPPER CERVICAL EXPOSURES

Marc R. Rosen, M.D.
William M. Keane, M.D.
David Rosen, M.D.

The complex anatomy of the anterior neck, makes safe exposure of the high cervical spine a challenging surgical procedure. The extensive neural pathways in the neck coupled with the tracheoesophageal complex often place the patient at risk for temporary and occasionally permanent morbidity involving speech and swallowing functions. The patient and surgeon must be aware of these risks, especially in the elderly, in whom they may more commonly occur due to preexisting weakness and disease. Different exposure techniques are required depending on the level of the pathologic process. The high cervical spine can be approached transorally, transcervically, or through a combined approach. There are five basic techniques for high cervical exposure:

1. Transoral
2. Transoral with lip split and mandibulotomy
3. Transoral with lip split, mandibulotomy, and tongue split
4. Transoral with combined extrapharyngeal exposure
5. High cervical and retropharyngeal exposure

Transoral approaches are useful for atlantoaxial pathologic processes, including tumors and bony compression. The amount of exposure necessary dictates the extent of the approach. For more limited problems, which require only small exposure, a simple transoral approach suffices. A transoral approach with lip split and mandibulotomy allows more inferior exposure. The most extensive exposure can be obtained with the transoral lip split, mandibulotomy, and tongue split approach.

Transoral Approach

Surgical Technique

The transoral exposure is relatively straightforward. Fiberoptic awake nasal intubation or oral intubation is accomplished based on the stability of the cervical spine. If there is extensive retraction or manipulation of the tongue and palate, tracheotomy should be considered. The uvula is retracted with a nasogastric tube, and an oral retractor is inserted. The nasotracheal tube is retracted laterally, and exposure of the posterior pharyngeal wall is accomplished (Figures 3–1 through 3–4). A vertical incision is made in the posterior pharyngeal mucosa and carried through the constrictor muscles and longus colli. The bony anatomy can be further delineated with subperiosteal retraction. Slightly more superior exposure can be obtained by splitting the uvula and soft palate in the midline. A portion of the hard palate can also be rongeured as necessary for exposure.

Complications

There are relatively few complications from the straight transoral approach. Wound infection has been reported as a complication. Despite the high bacterial level of the oral cavity, infection has not been a significant problem in our experience. Perioperative antibiotics are used routinely for prophylaxis, accounting for mouth flora.

Transoral Approach with Lip Split and Mandibulotomy

Surgical Technique

If more exposure is required than the simple transoral route can provide (if exposure to C3-4 is also needed), a lip split approach with mandibulotomy can be used. The limiting factor in

Text continued on page 31

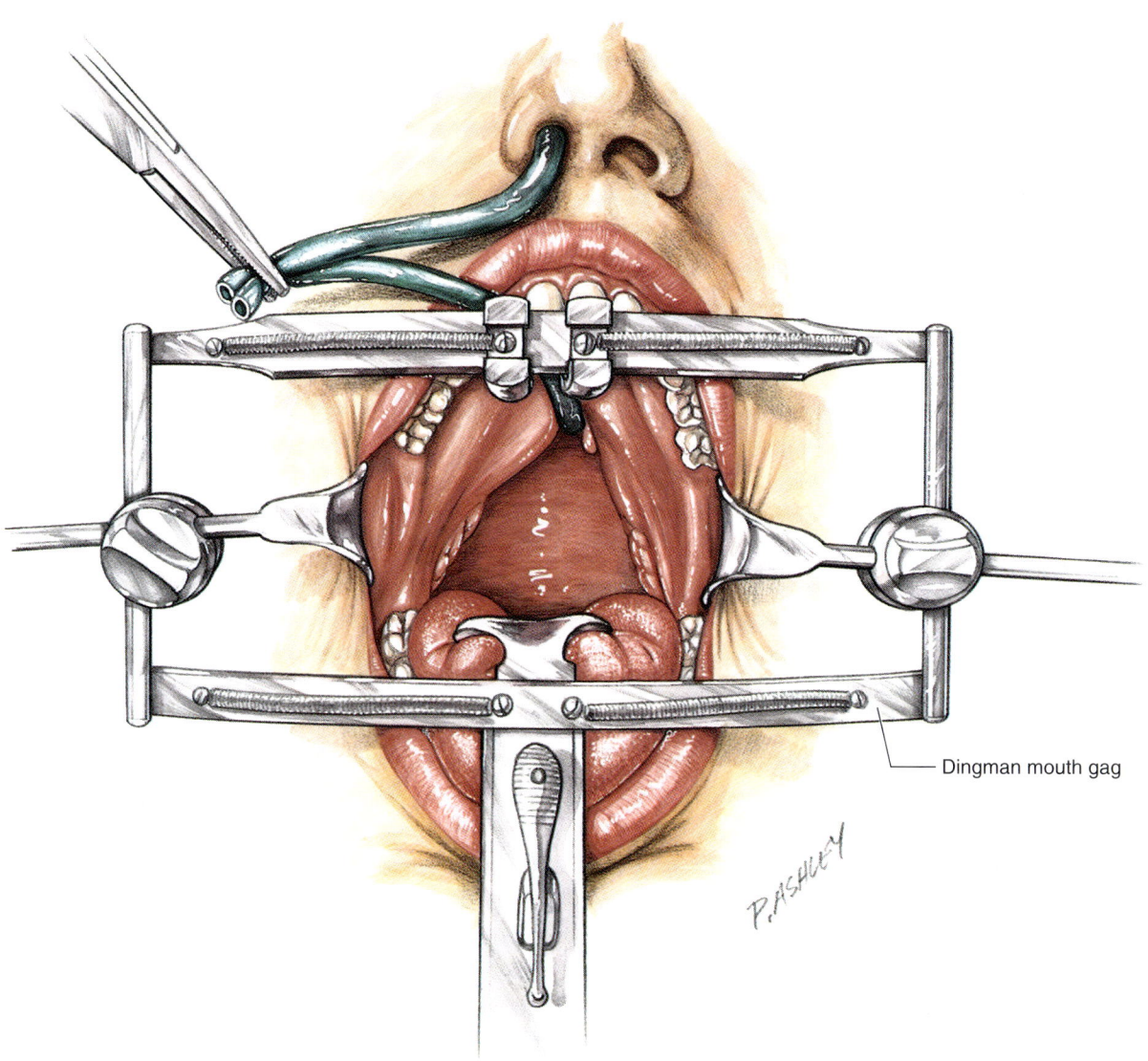

● **Figure 3-1.** Simple transoral exposure with Dingman mouth gag.

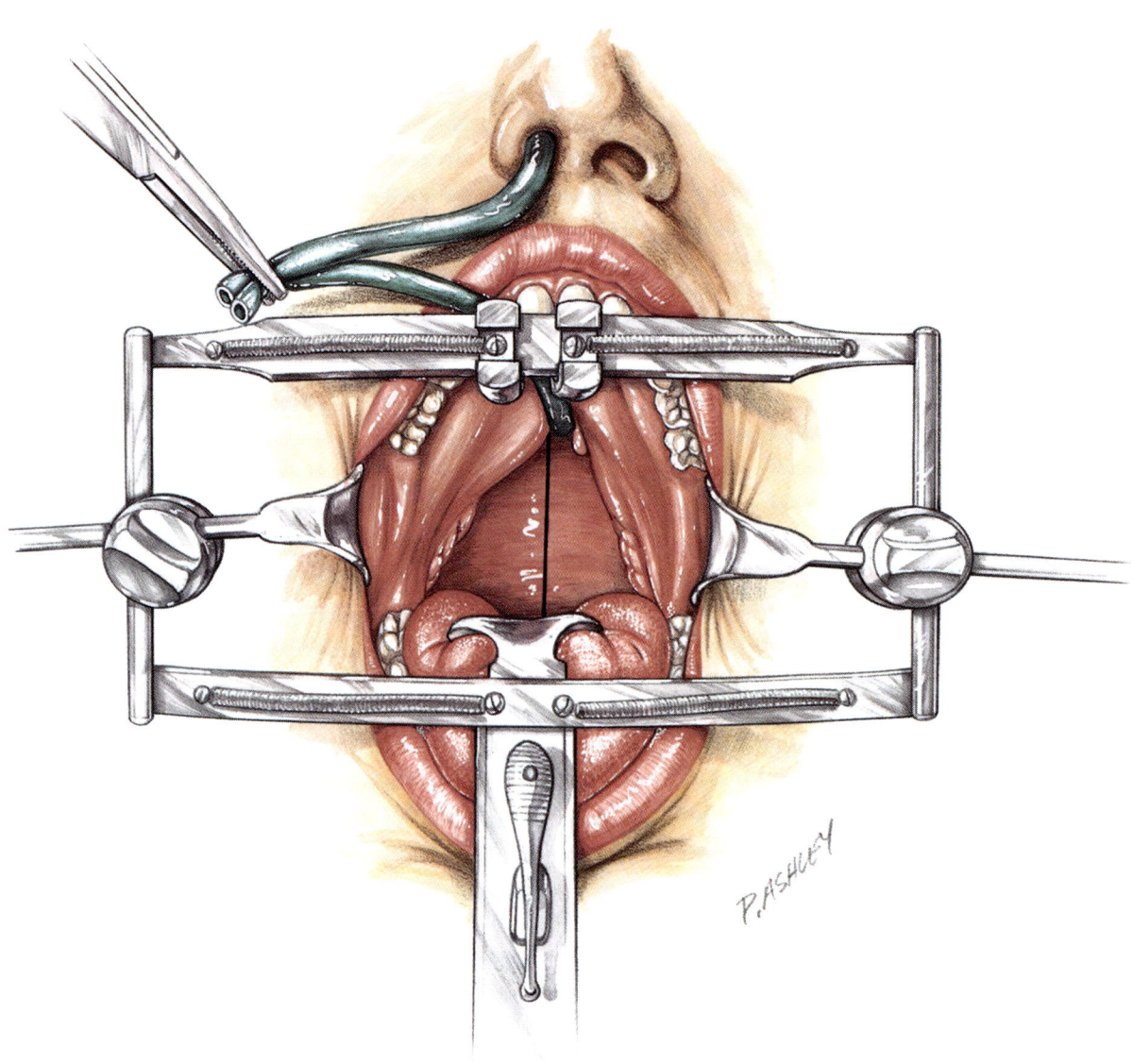

● **Figure 3-2.** Vertical incision through posterior pharyngeal mucosa.

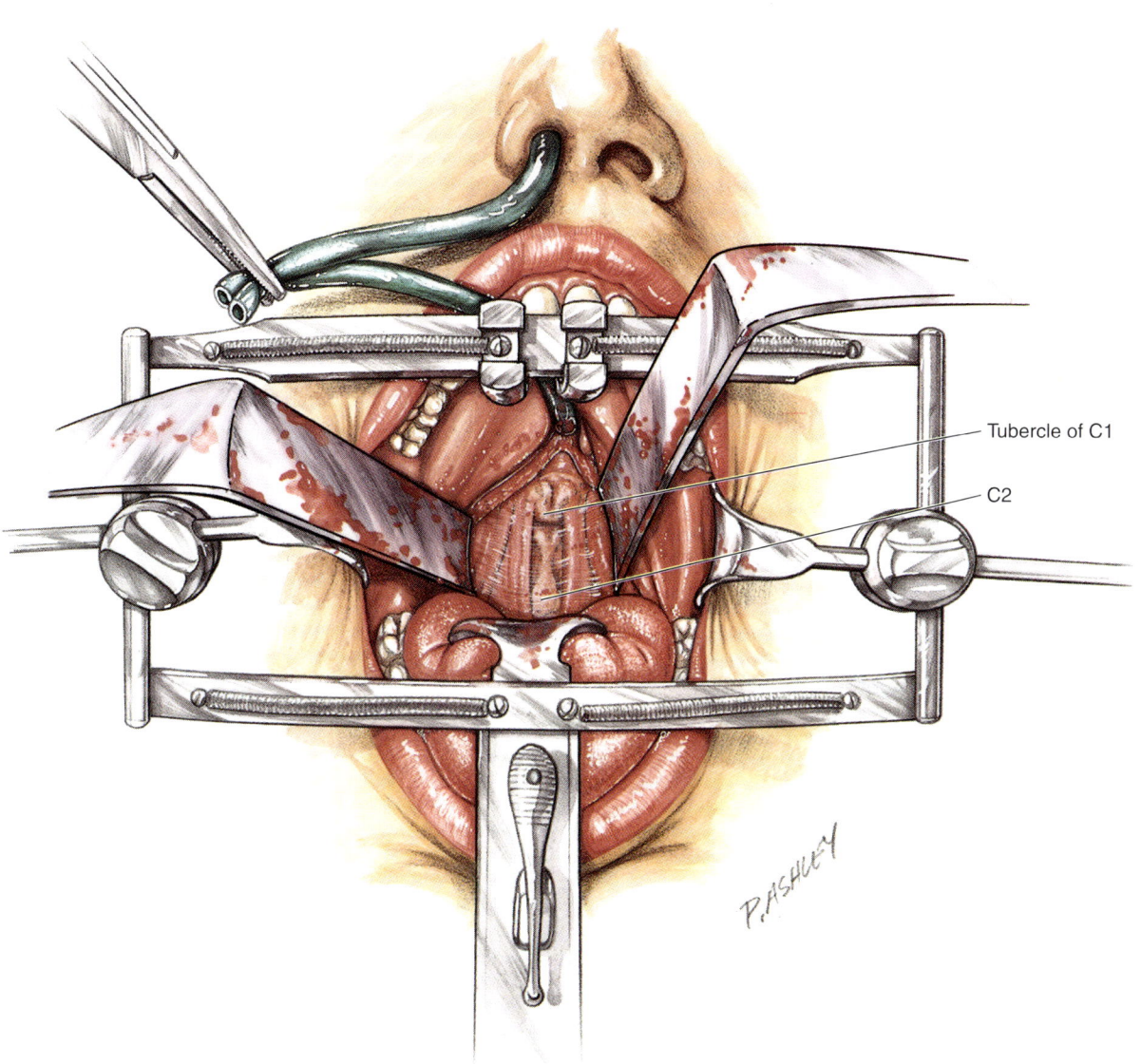

● **Figure 3-3.** Subperiosteal dissection exposing atlantoaxial complex.

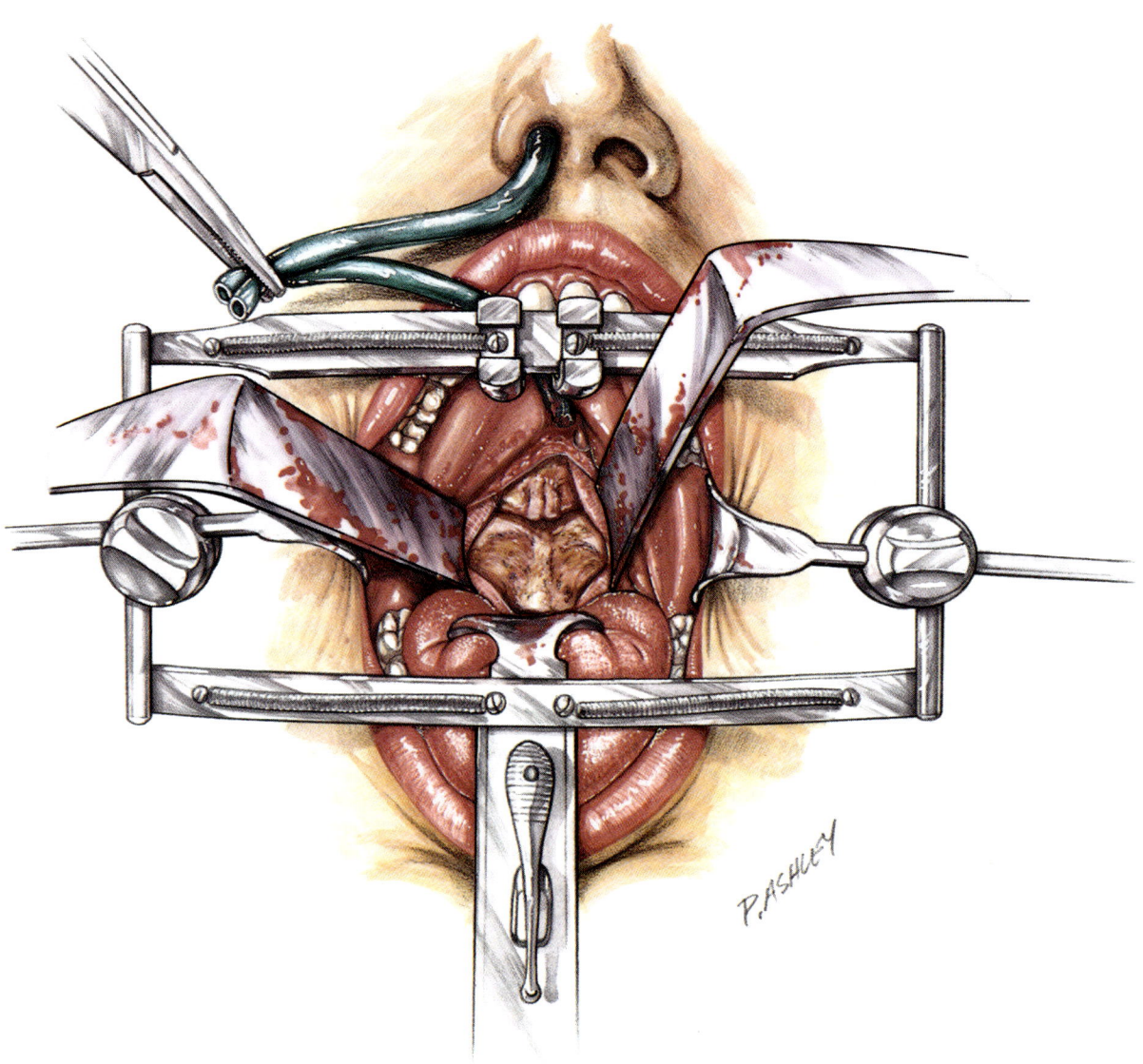

● **Figure 3-4.** Longus colli retracted.

the simple transoral approach is the amount that the oral cavity can be opened by the retractors. By splitting the mandible, a significant increase in exposure can be obtained with little increase in morbidity. An incision is made from the midline of the lower lip around the chin in a C-shaped fashion and then straight down to the hyoid bone (Figure 3–5). The incision is carried down to the mandibular periosteum both lingually and cervically (Figure 3–6). The periosteum is elevated approximately 3 cm on either side of the midline (Figure 3–7). A titanium reconstruction plate with a minimum of two holes on either side of the mandibulotomy, but preferably three holes, is bent to shape (Figure 3–8). The holes are drilled for later reconstruction (Figure 3–9). Care should be taken to keep the plate low on the mandible to avoid injuring the dental roots with the drill holes. The mandible is then divided between the central incisors, avoiding the tooth roots in a stairstep or, as is our preference, a triangular fashion (Figures 3–10 through 3–12). Once the mandible is divided, extended exposure is accomplished (Figure 3–13). The mucosa lingually should be divided between Wharton's duct to the root of the tongue (Figure 3–14). This affords extended exposure using the same retractors that are used in the simple transoral approach (Figure 3–15).

If additional exposure is required, the tongue can be divided in the midline back to the epiglottis, taking care not to injure the epiglottis. If the tongue is split, a tracheotomy should be performed. Closure is accomplished by using Vicryl sutures for the deep layers of the tongue and chromic sutures for the mucosal surfaces. The previously bent plate is then secured with screws (Figure 3–16), and the deep layers of the chin and neck are closed with Vicryl. We prefer a 6-0 fast-absorbing gut suture for the lip and skin closure. For better cosmesis, it is essential that the vermilion border be accurately aligned.

Text continued on page 43

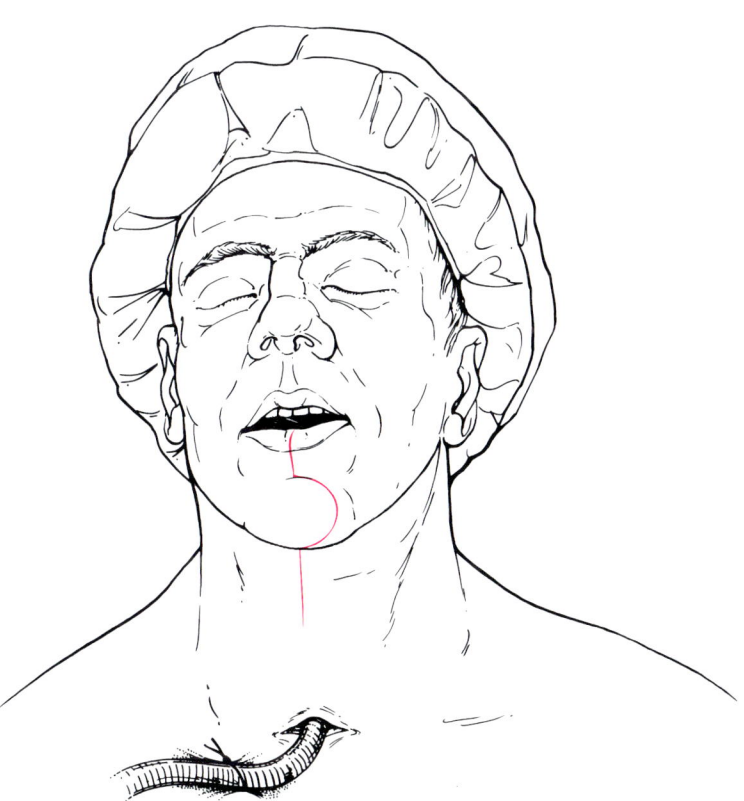

● **Figure 3–5.** Skin incision for mandibulotomy; note tracheotomy tube.

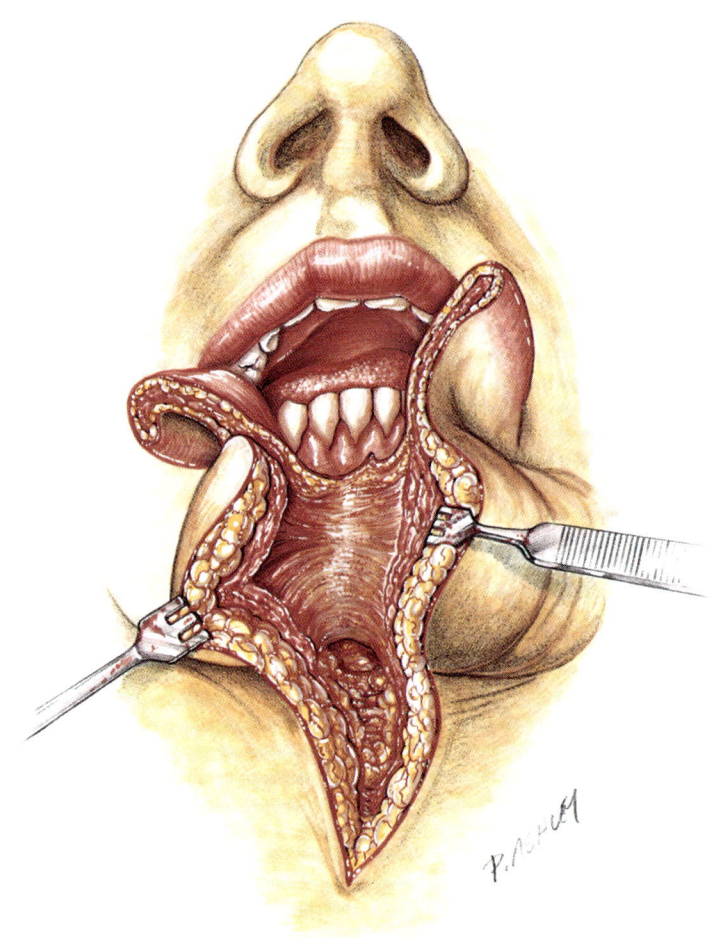

● **Figure 3-6.** Divison of skin and subcutaneous tissue to expose mandible.

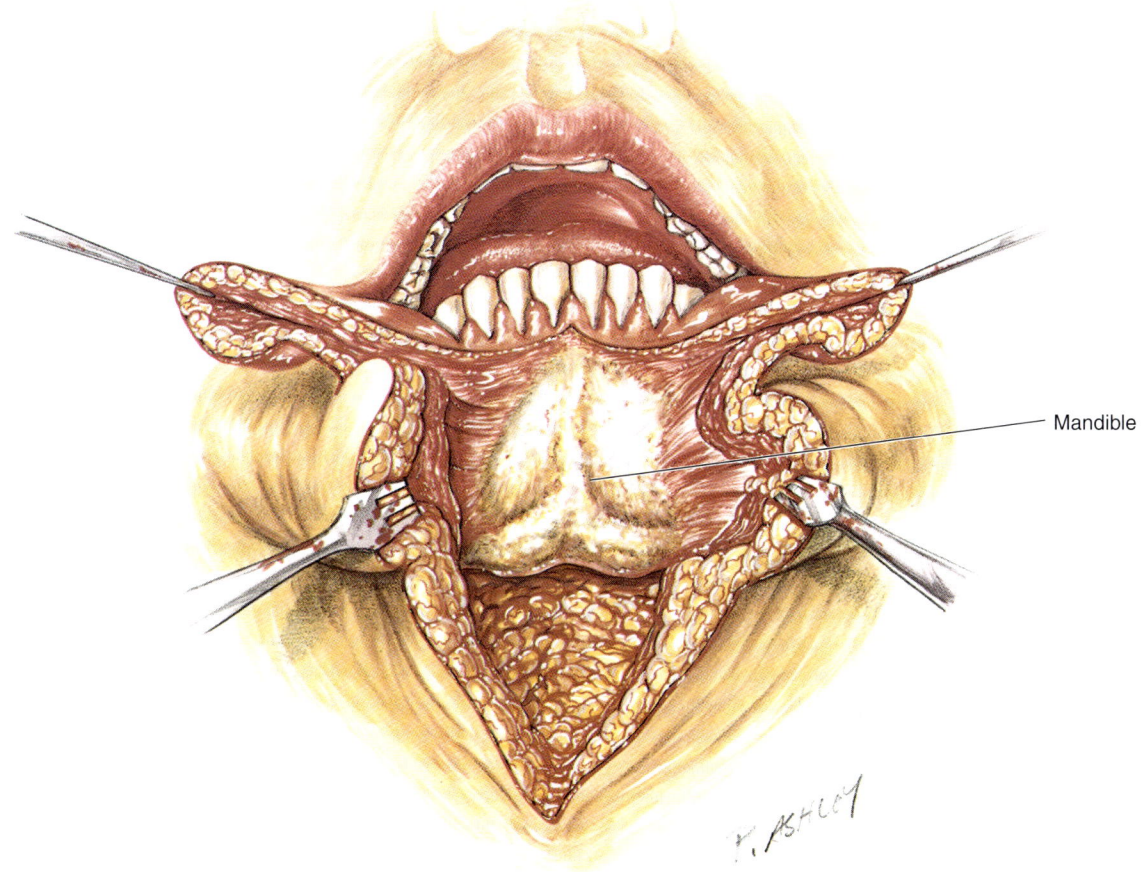

● **Figure 3-7.** Mandible exposed and periosteum elevated both lingually and cervically.

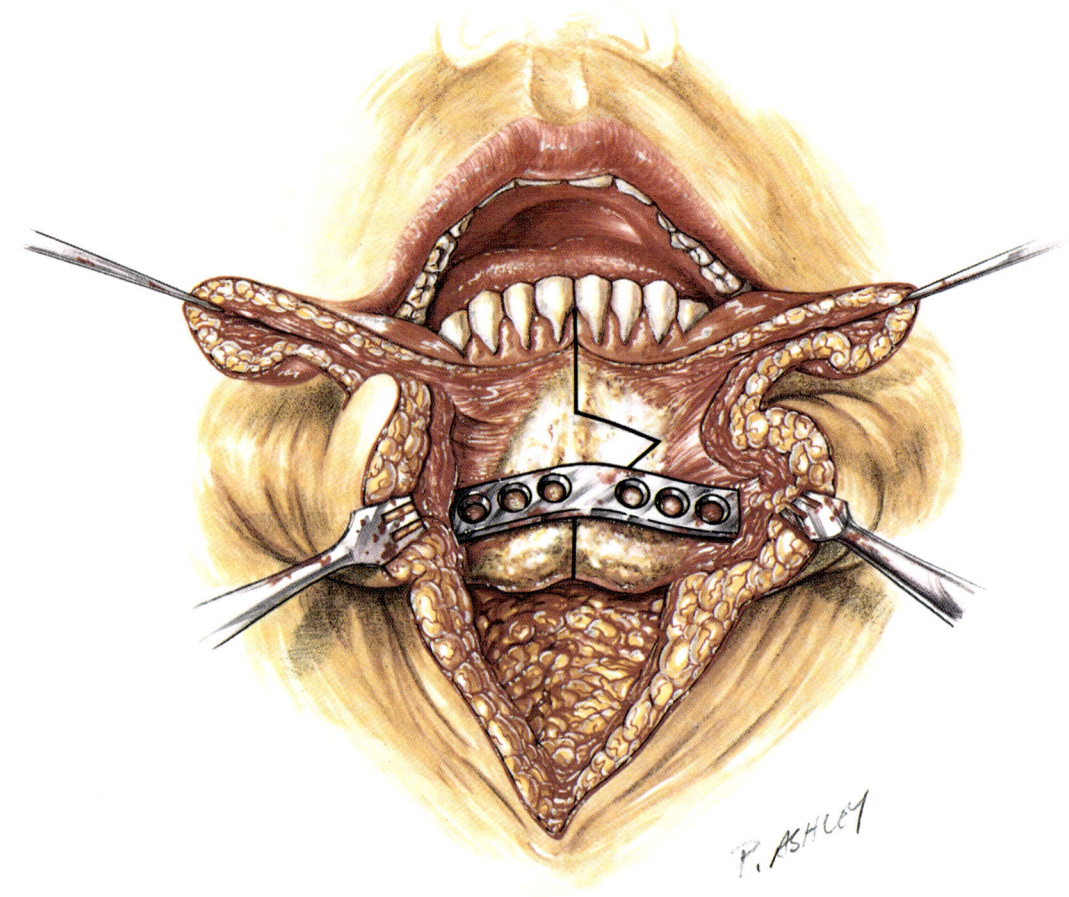

● **Figure 3-8.** Reconstruction plate is prebent to conform to mandibular contour.

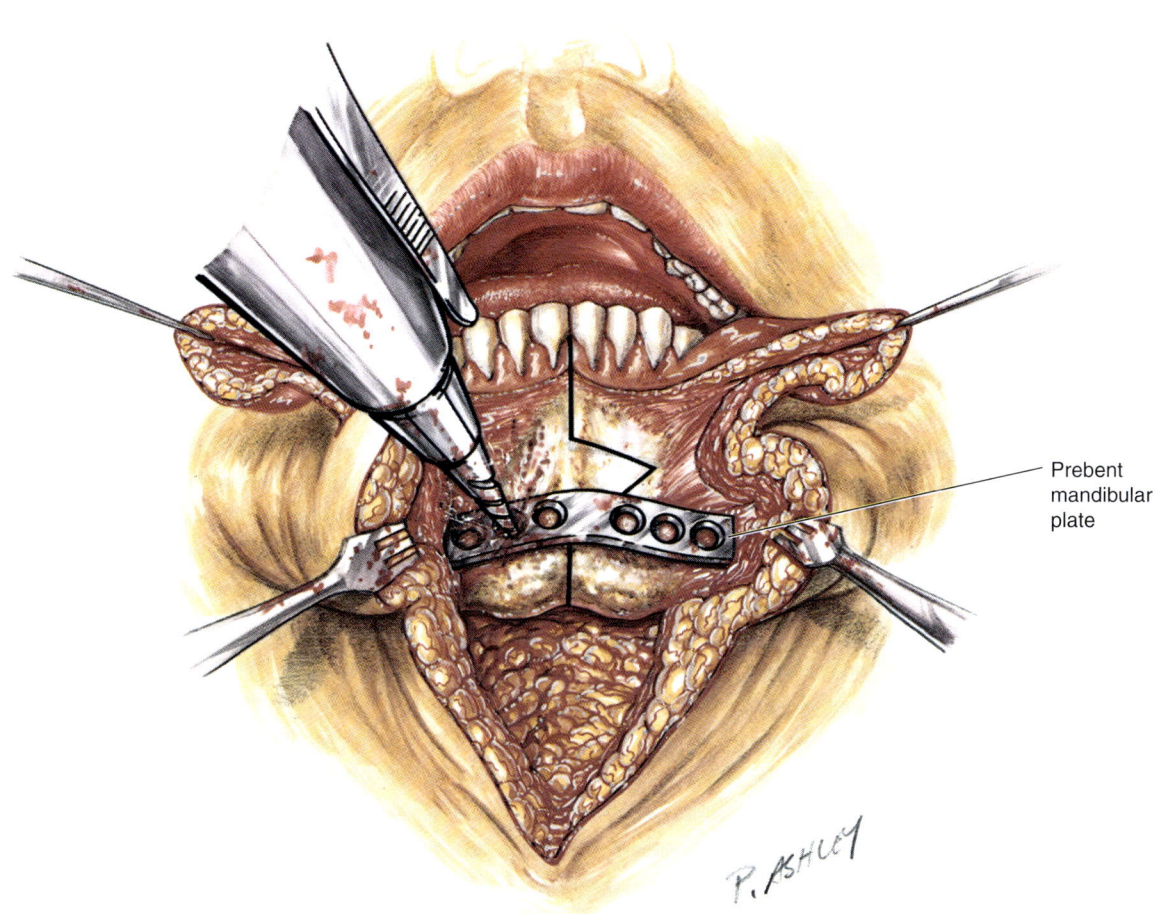

● **Figure 3-9.** Holes are predrilled before mandibulotomy to aid in final reconstruction.

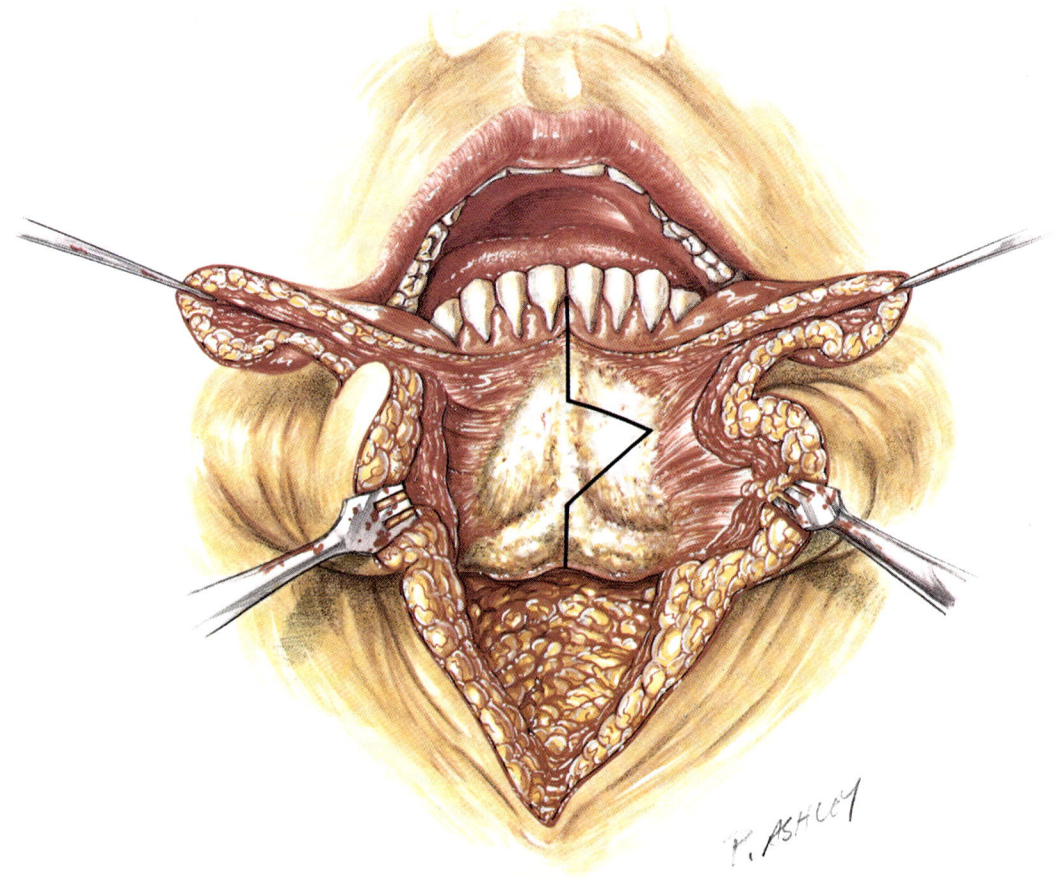

● **Figure 3-10.** Incision outlined on mandible in a triangular fashion.

ANTERIOR UPPER CERVICAL EXPOSURES • 37

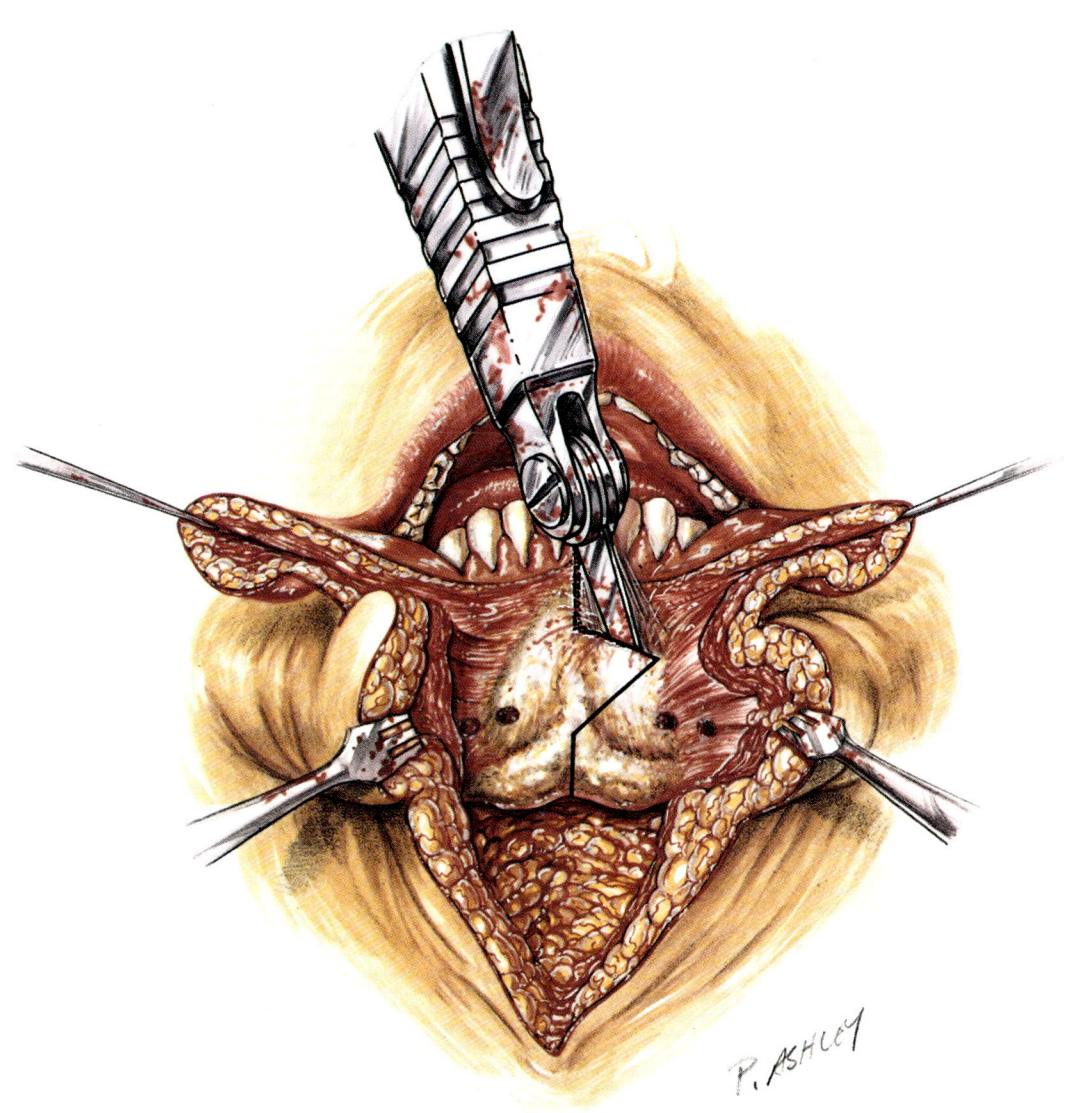

● **Figure 3-11.** Mandibulotomy accomplished with sagittal saw.

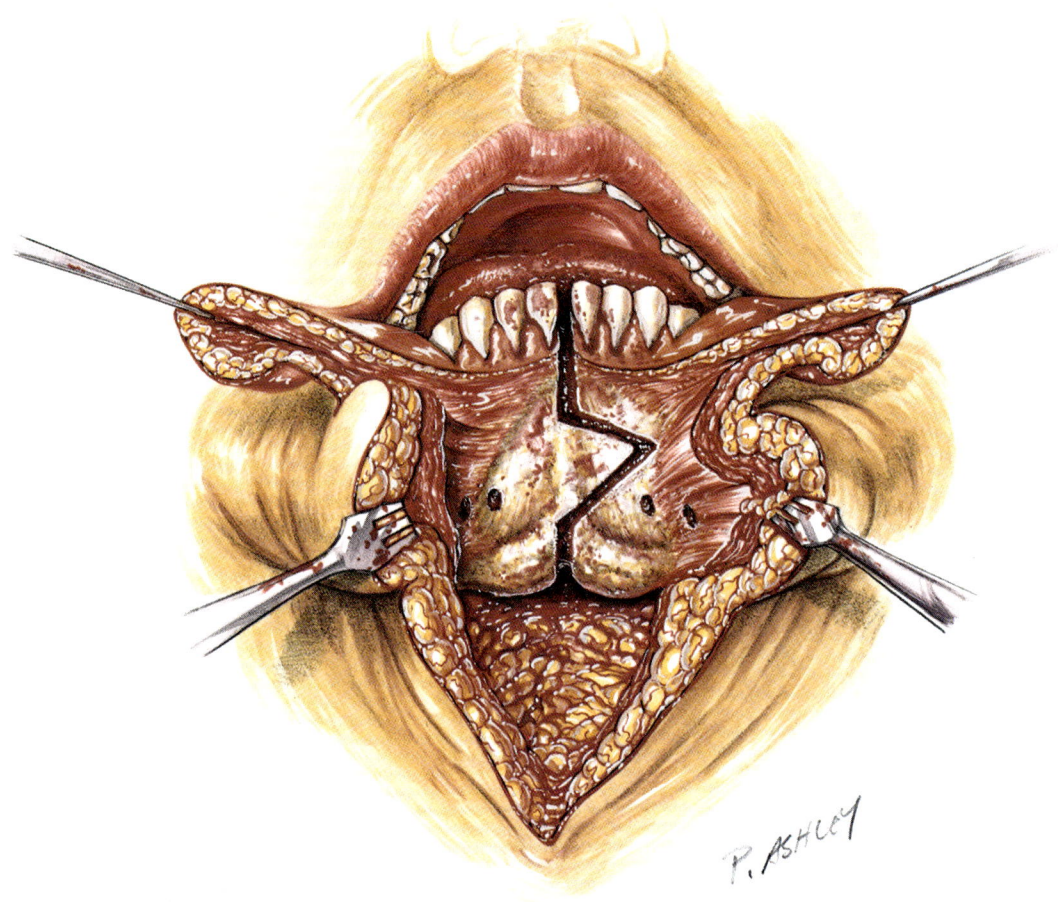

● **Figure 3-12.** Soft tissue divided and incision carried between Wharton's duct.

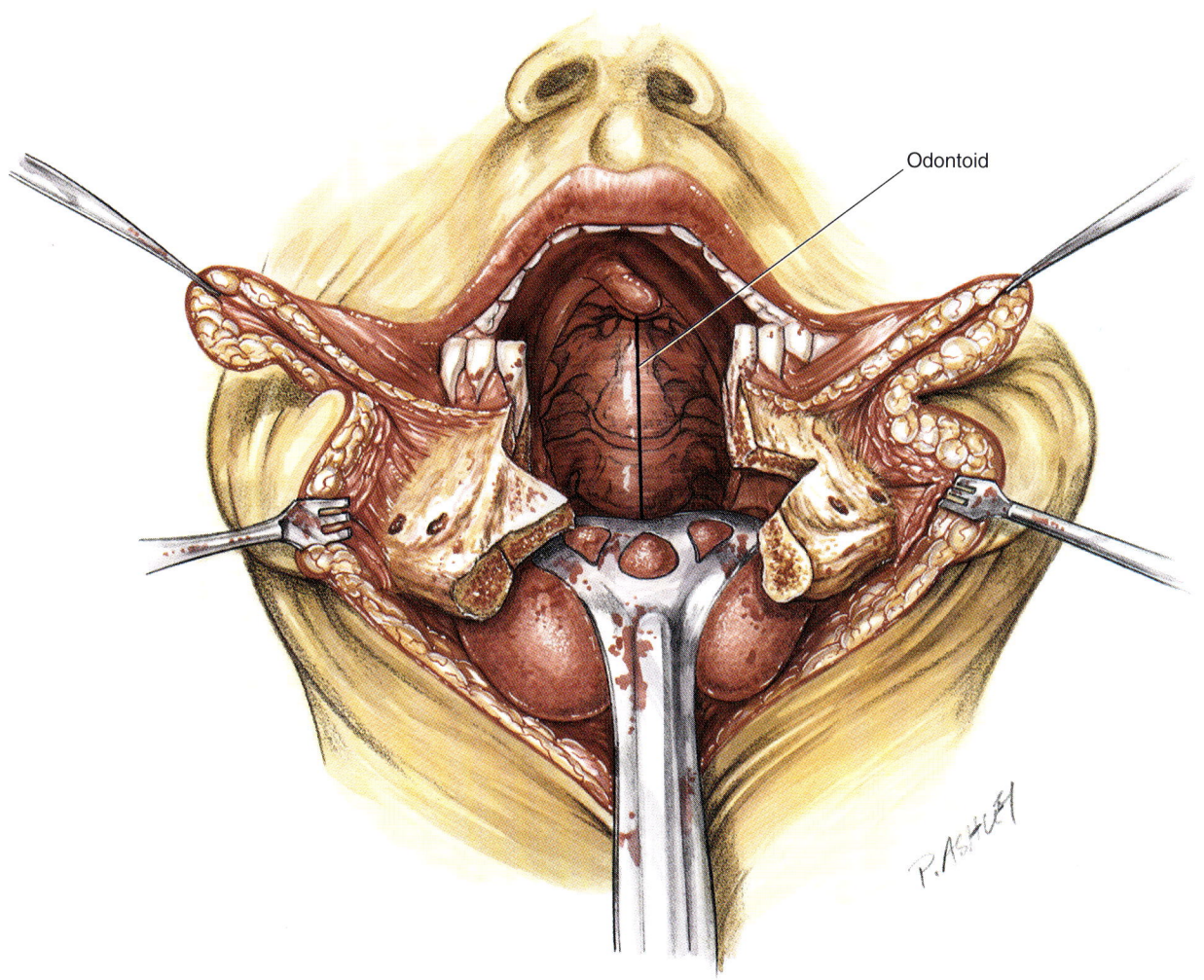

● **Figure 3-13.** Final exposure of lip split with mandibulotomy.

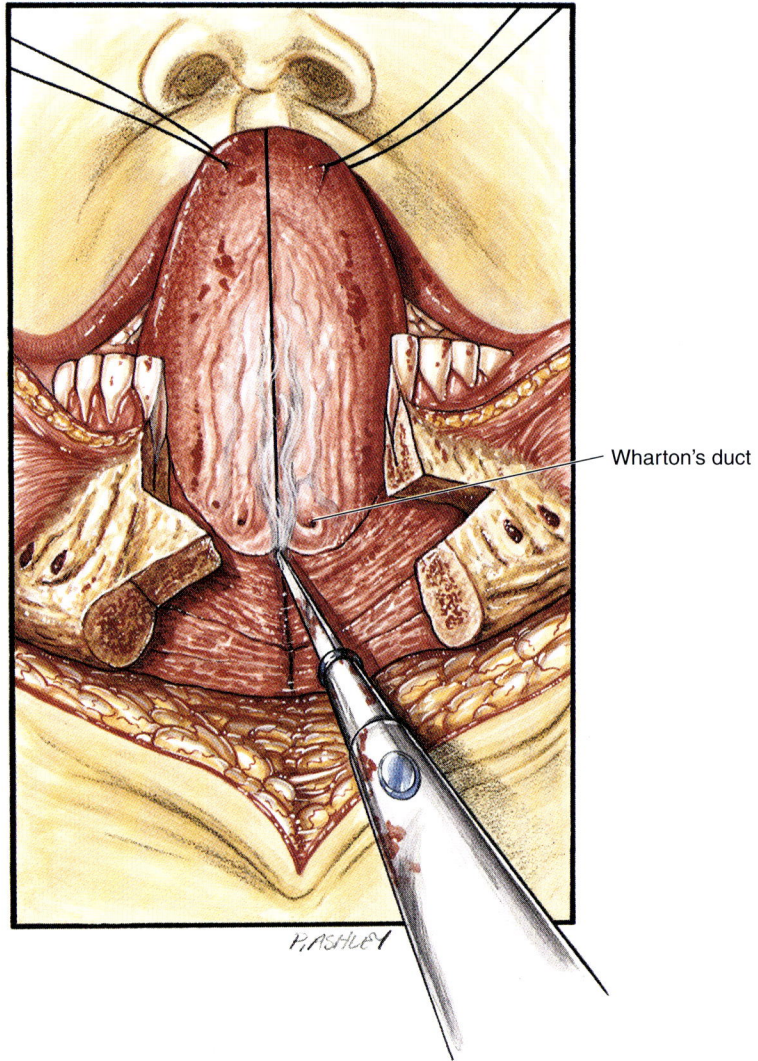

● **Figure 3-14.** Tongue is divided between Wharton's duct and down midline.

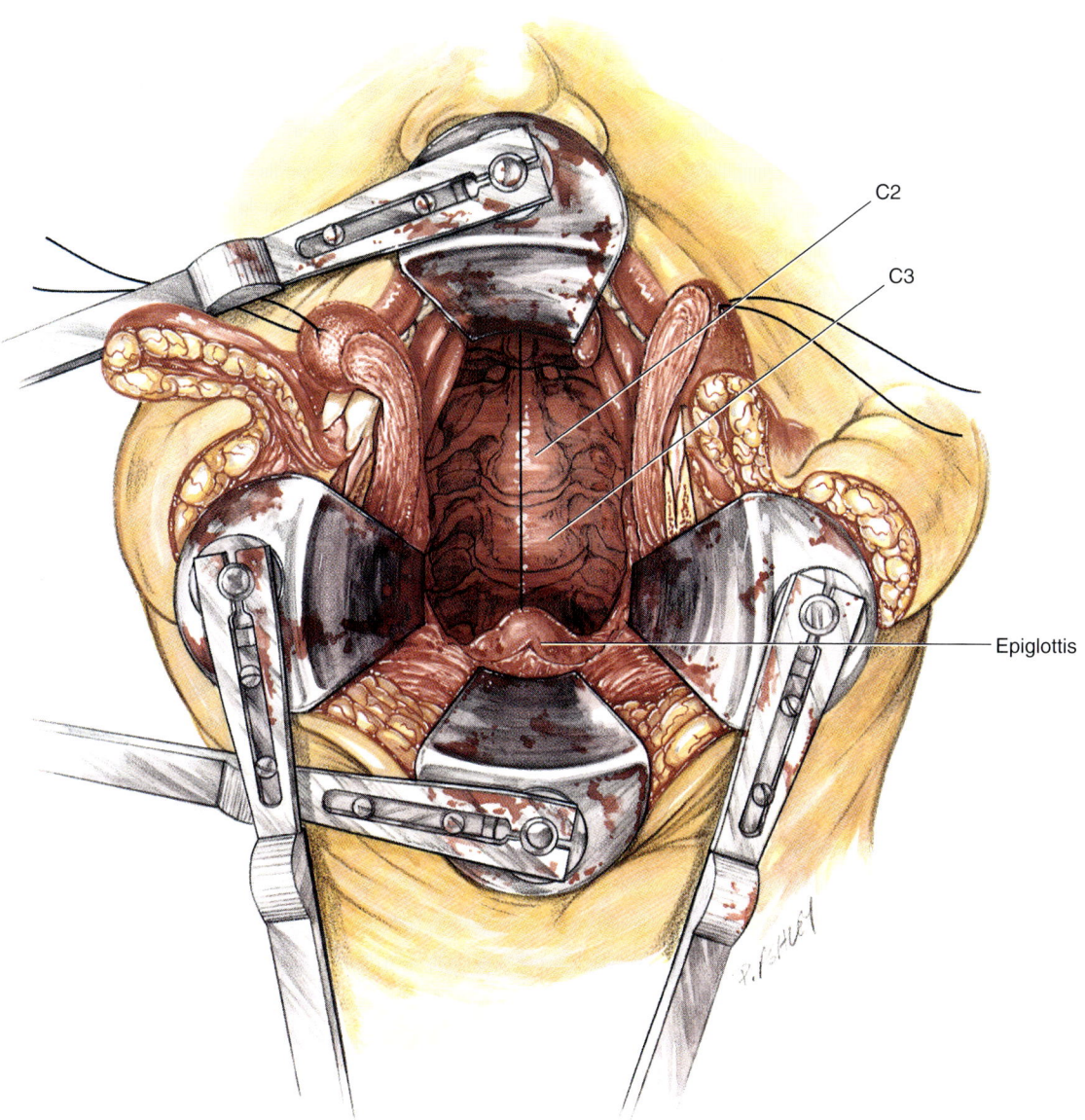

● **Figure 3-15.** Final exposure of mandibulotomy with tongue split.

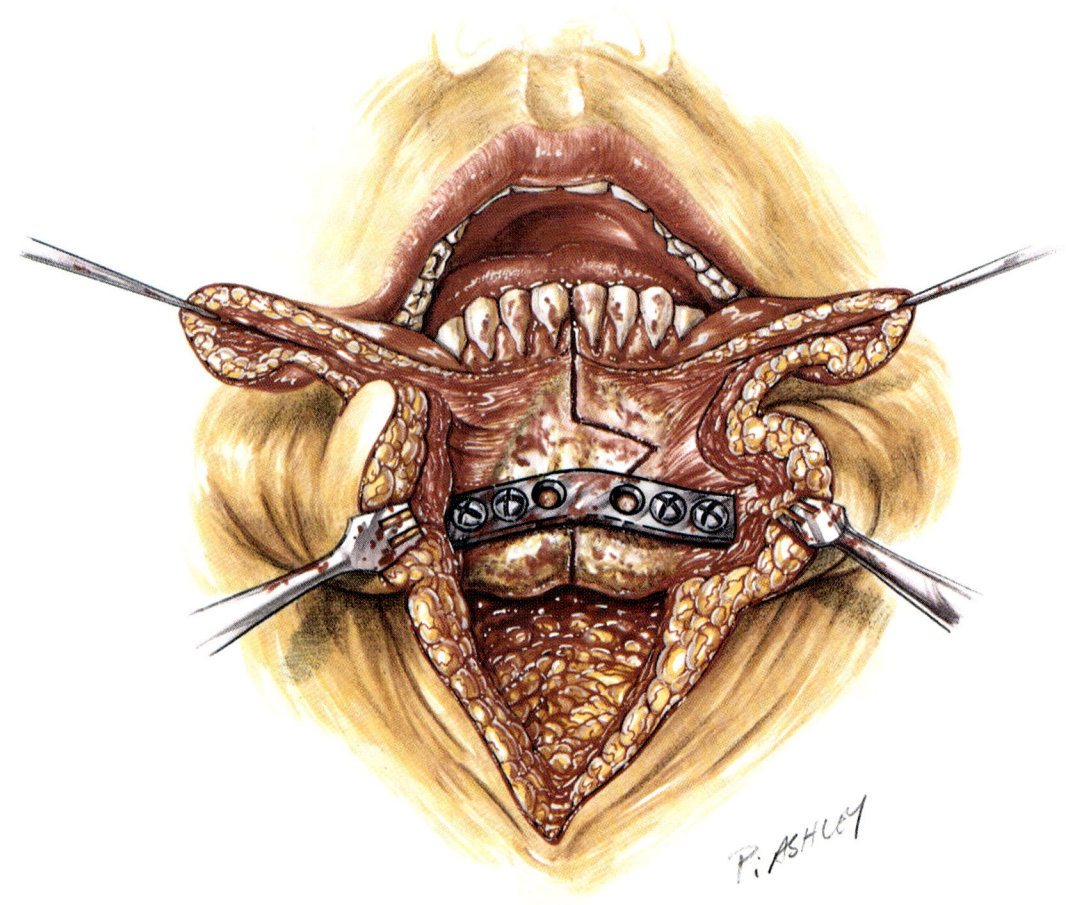

● **Figure 3-16.** Reconstruction of mandibulotomy with plate.

Complications

Complications of the approach include malocclusion, malunion of the mandible, and cosmetic deformity. With the use of perioperative antibiotics and plate fixation, malunion is rare. Cosmetic deformity is usually not significant if the skin edges are approximated meticulously.

Transoral Approach with Combined Extrapharyngeal Exposure

If extended exposure is required or if more superior exposure is necessary (i.e., central nervous system tumors) a combined approach can be employed. We believe that this approach affords improved exposure with less morbidity compared with the extended maxillotomy.

Surgical Technique

An incision similar to the lip-splitting incision is made but carried laterally at least 4 cm below the angle of mandible (to avoid damage to the marginal mandibular branch of the facial nerve) and then up toward the mastoid tip (Figures 3–17 and 3–18). This approach is

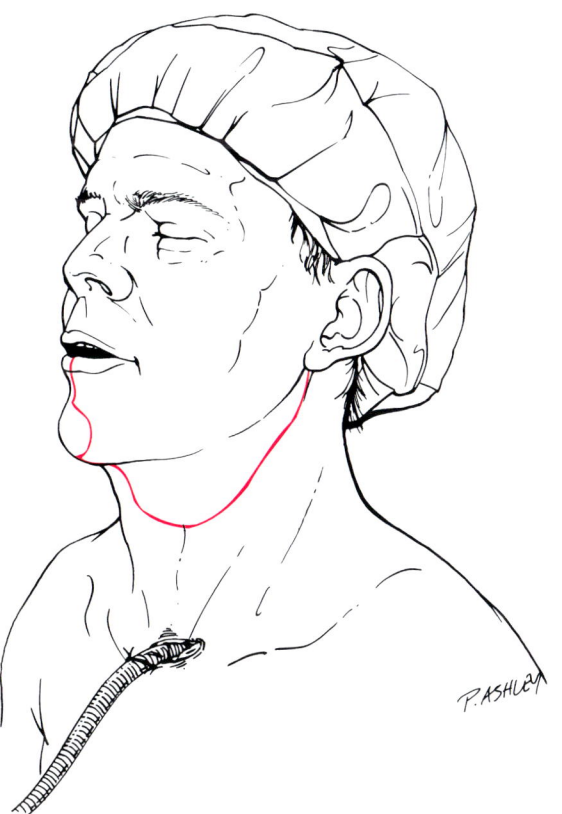

● **Figure 3-17.** Cervical incision for transoral approach with combined extrapharyngeal exposure.

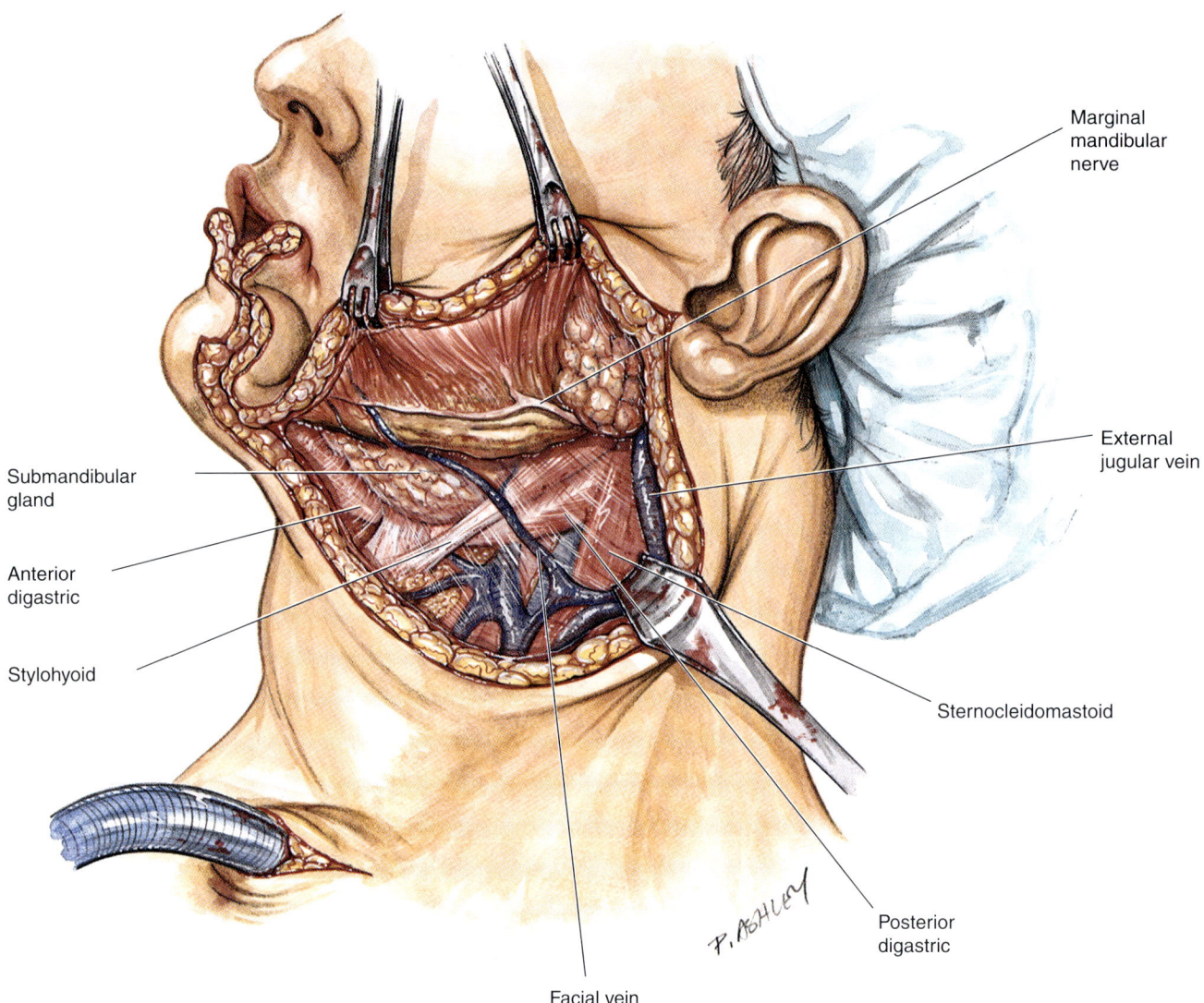

● **Figure 3-18.** Elevation of subplatysmal flap after skin incision completed.

routine for most head and neck surgeons, and there is little morbidity. The platysma is divided, and subplatysmal flaps are elevated. The facial vein is divided and used to help preserve the marginal mandibular nerve (the nerve is located between the platysma and the vein) (Figure 3–19). The submandibular gland is elevated, and the digastric and stylohyoid muscles are divided. The mandible is divided as previously described; and the internal carotid artery, internal jugular vein, and 10th, 11th, and 12th nerves are identified and protected (Figures 3–20 and 3–21). Attention is then paid intraorally, and again the floor of the mouth is divided between Wharton's duct. However, in this case the incision is carried laterally along the floor of the mouth toward the anterior tonsillar pillar (Figure 3–22). The lingual nerve is identified and preserved. Postganglionic fibers to the submandibular ganglion

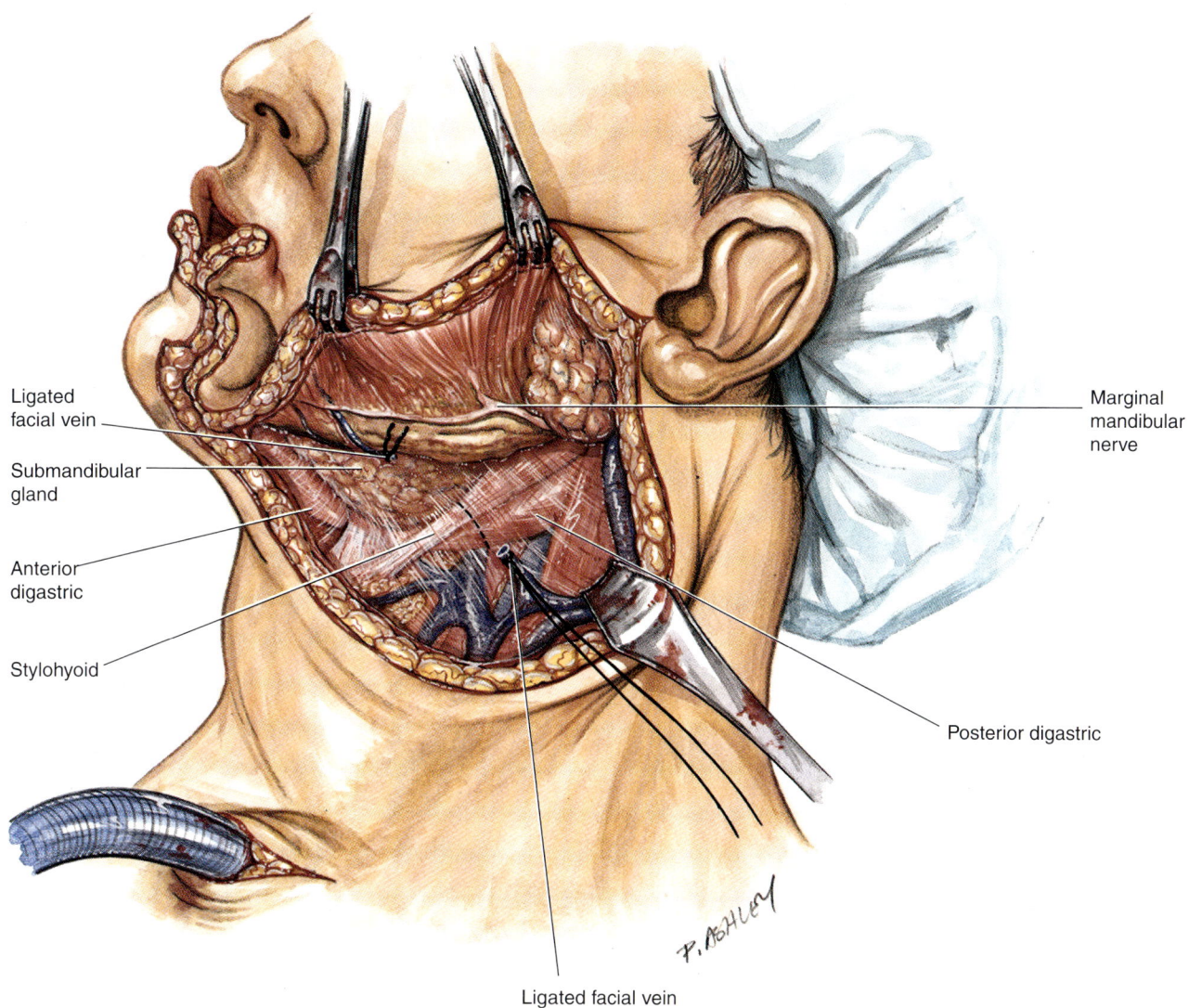

● **Figure 3-19.** Facial vein divided and retracted superiorly to protect marginal mandibular nerve.

can be divided at this point (Figure 3–23). Branches of the external carotid artery can be divided as necessary for exposure. The oral and extrapharyngeal approaches are connected, providing extensive exposure. If necessary, the incision can be carried to the palate and portions of the hard palate removed as necessary. Closure intraorally is similar to that for the previously described transoral approach with split lip and mandibulotomy. The platysma is approximated with Vicryl sutures, and the skin is closed with fast-absorbing gut sutures. A suction drain is essential in this approach.

Complications

Complications are usually no more significant than those of the mandibulotomy as described previously. There is potential for injury to the cranial nerves, most commonly the hypoglos-

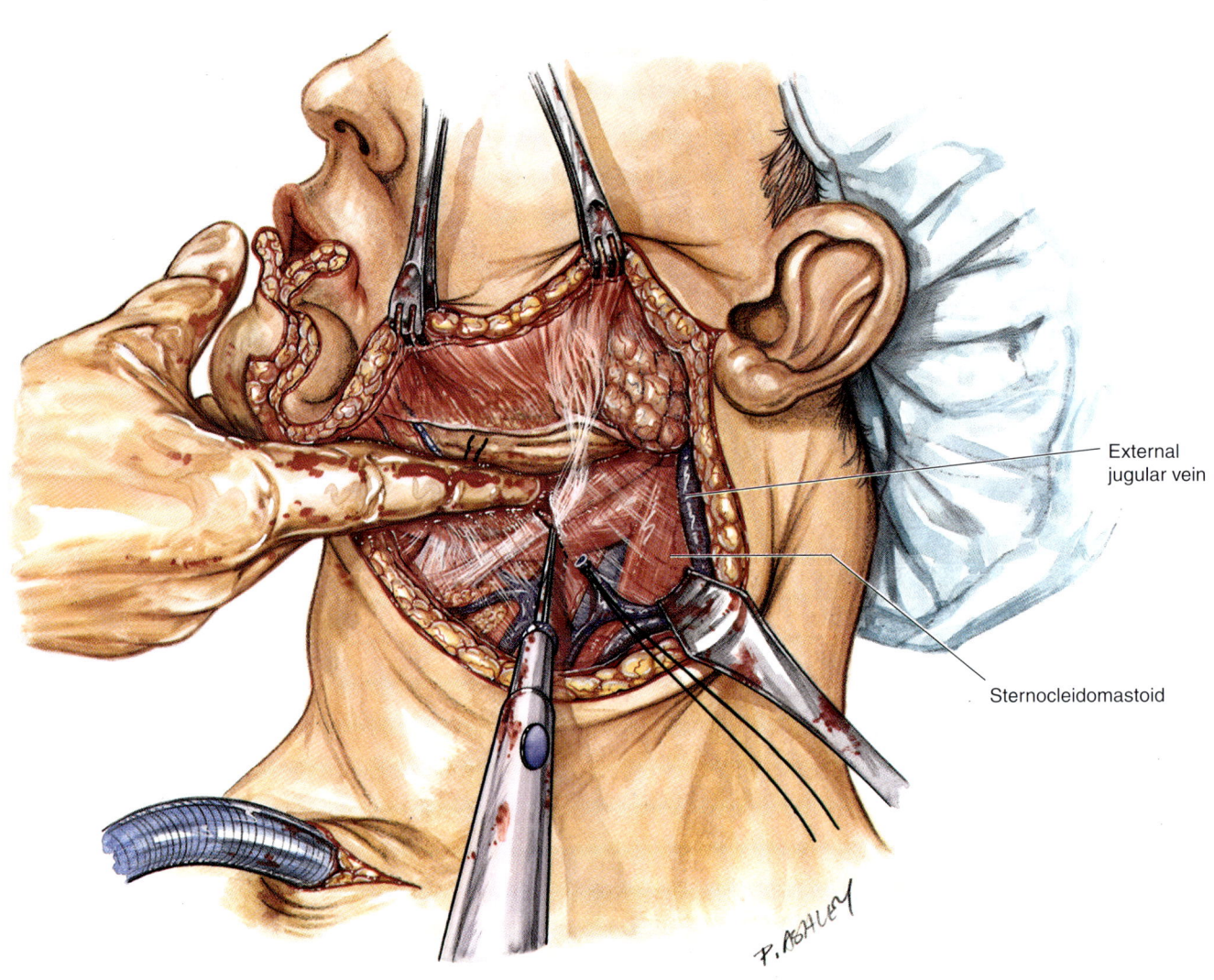

● **Figure 3-20.** Division of stylohyoid and posterior belly of digastric muscles.

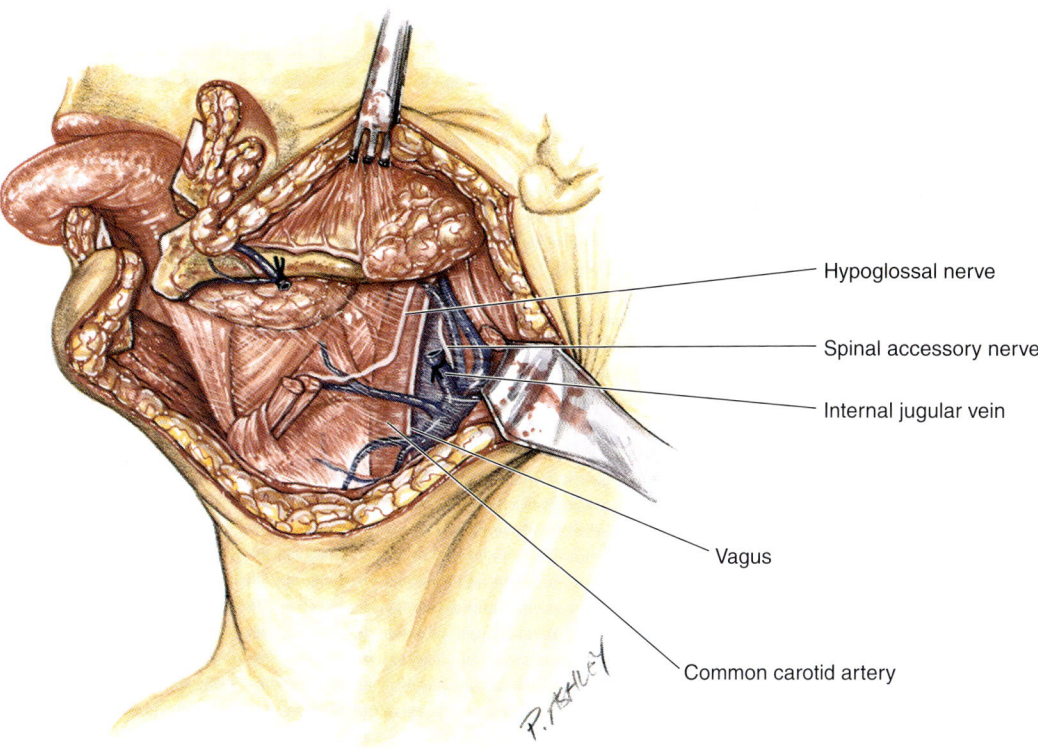

● **Figure 3-21.** Exposure of hypoglossal nerve, vagus nerve, and spinal accessory nerve.

sal, which results in weakness of the tongue. With careful mobilization this has been an unusual complication of this approach.

High Cervical and Retropharyngeal Exposure

Access to the upper cervical spine, although not technically demanding, carries significant risks of morbidity to the cranial motor nerves, which must be mobilized to gain exposure. Often the only way to obtain the necessary exposure is to place a significant amount of traction on these nerves. Nerve palsy is often seen as a result of this; and although most of these palsies are temporary, some may be permanent. In addition, because the exposure also requires mobilization of the trachea and the esophagus off the spine, these palsies are often magnified by the resultant esophageal edema that typically occurs. A period of swallowing therapy is often required postoperatively, especially in the elderly, and occasionally a feeding tube may be required.

Surgical Technique

The patient is routinely intubated awake through the nasotracheal route, and general anesthesia is induced. If possible, nerve paralysis is avoided until exposure of the cervical

48 • SURGICAL APPROACHES TO THE SPINE

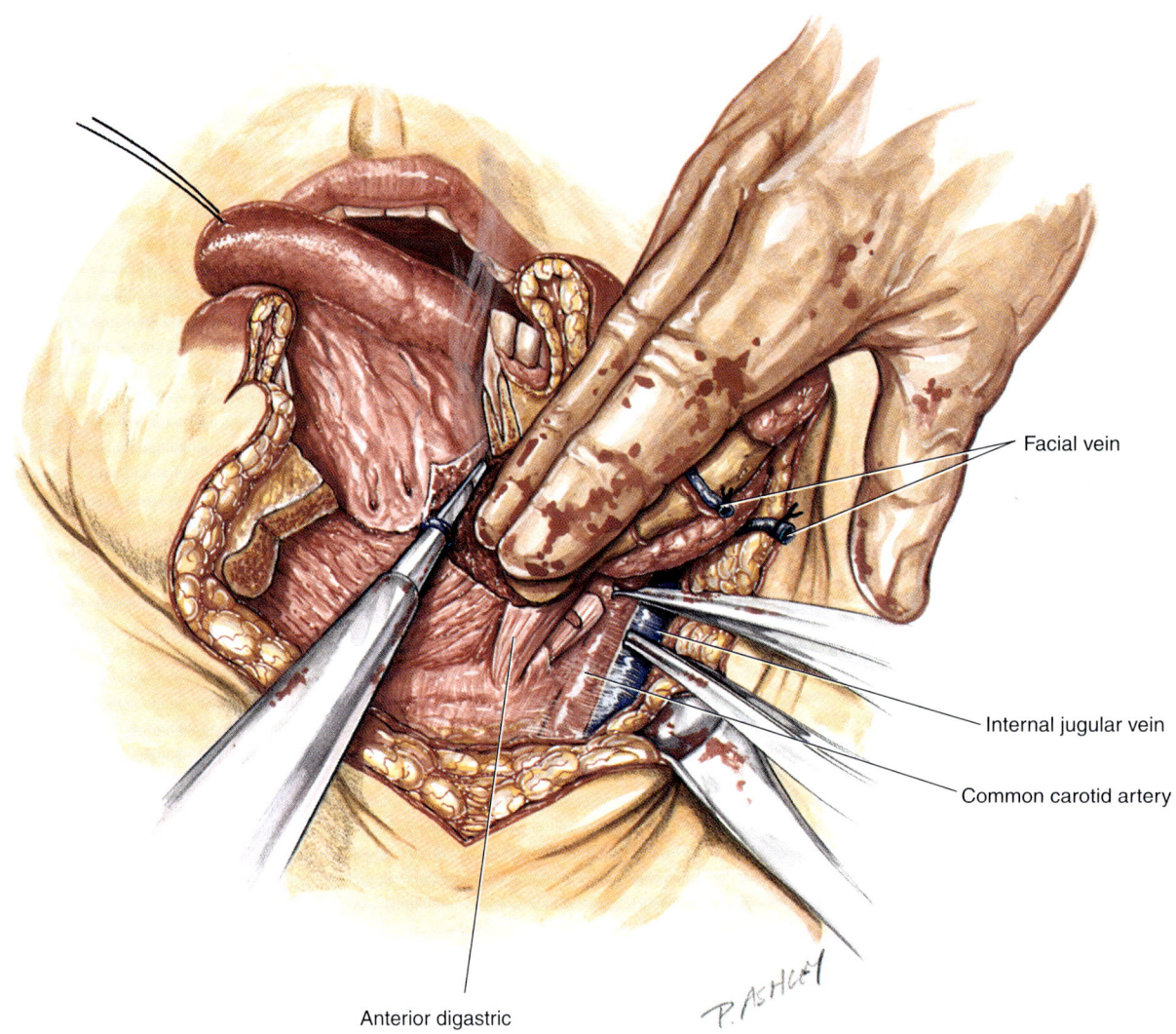

● **Figure 3-22.** Division of floor of mouth between Wharton's duct. Incision is then carried laterally along the floor of mouth to the tonsillar pillar.

spine to help in identification of the cranial motor nerves at risk. An incision is made in a natural skin crease, usually on the left side. The incision is placed approximately 4 cm below the angle of the mandible and extends from the midportion of the sternocleidomastoid muscle to the midline (Figure 3-24). Some authors place the incision more superiorly along the mandible, but we believe the risk to the marginal mandibular nerve is too great with this incision, although access is slightly easier.

Subplatysmal flaps are elevated, and the great auricular nerve is identified lying over the sternocleidomastoid muscle and preserved. Again, the facial vein is identified and divided, and dissection is continued deep to this vein to preserve the marginal mandibular nerve. The digastric and omohyoid muscles are identified. Both of these muscles may be divided if necessary for exposure. Only the digastric muscle needs to be reapproximated. The majority of the dissection from this point should be blunt and should take advantage of natural fascial planes. The hypoglossal nerve is identified deep to the digastric muscle and

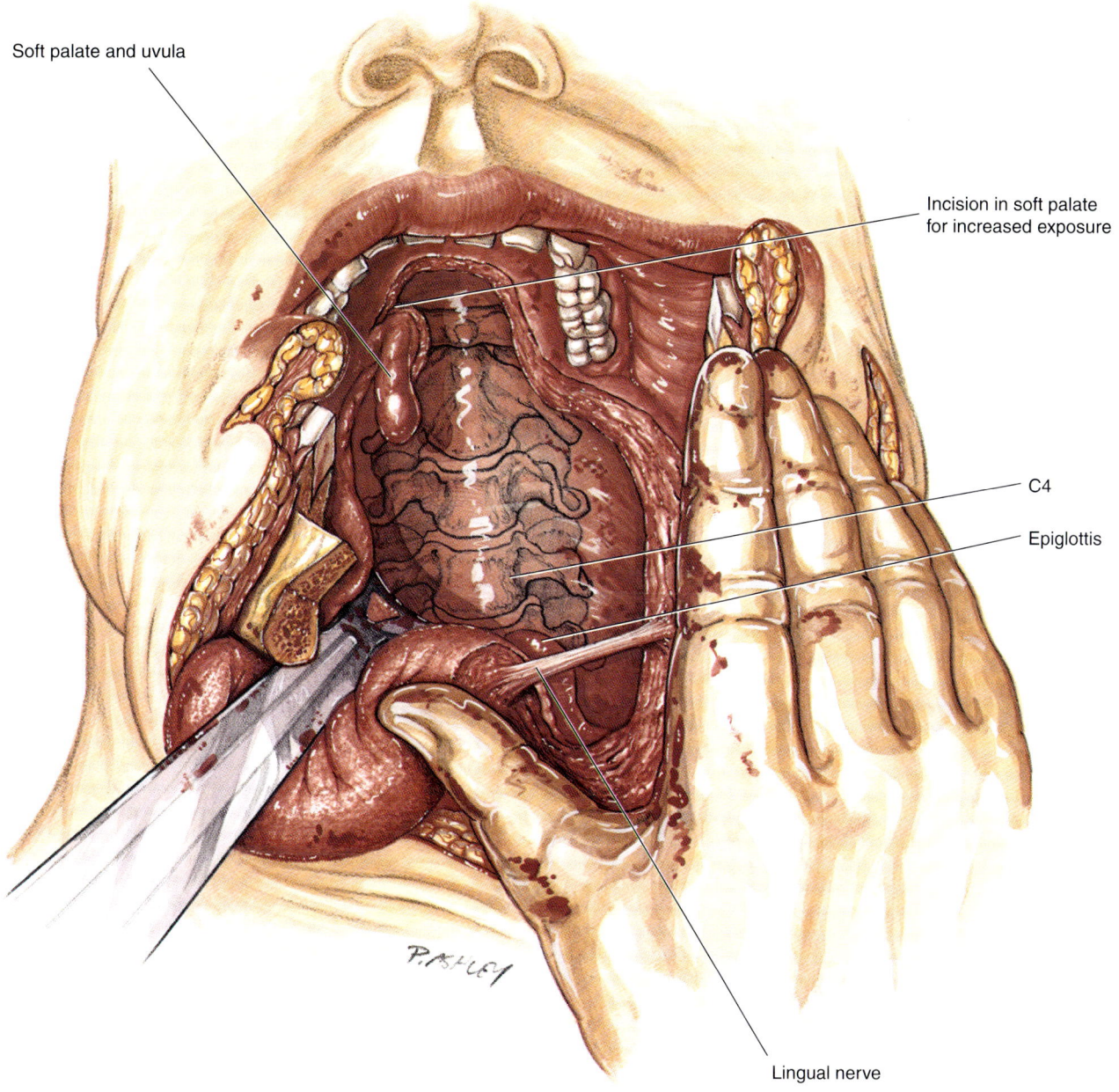

● **Figure 3-23.** Exposure and mobilization of lingual nerve.

lies superiorly and medially. We usually retract the hypoglossal nerve superiorly, although others prefer to approach the spine above the hypoglossal nerve. We find that this requires too much retraction of the nerve. The anterior border of the sternocleidomastoid muscle is followed until the carotid sheath is identified. The carotid sheath is retracted laterally, and branches of the internal jugular vein and external carotid artery are divided as necessary. The superior laryngeal vessels are mobilized along with the superior laryngeal nerve. Vessels often must be divided for exposure and the superior laryngeal nerve mobilized from the vagus nerve at its entry into the larynx through the thyrohyoid membrane. The difficulty in this exposure as compared with the lower cervical exposure is that both the hypoglossal and

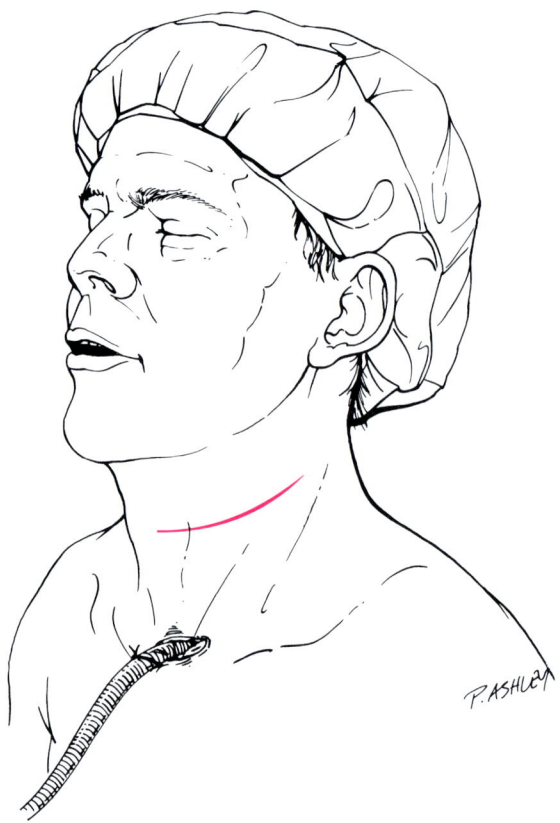

● **Figure 3-24.** Incision for His retropharyngeal approach.

superior laryngeal nerves course horizontally across the field whereas in the lower approach the recurrent laryngeal nerve crosses vertically and is more easily retracted. Once the superior laryngeal nerve and the hypoglossal nerve are mobilized, blunt dissection is used to expose the prevertebral fascia (Figure 3–25). It is essential to gain access to this space bluntly and laterally. Once this space is identified, it can be bluntly separated, reducing the risk of esophageal injury. The laryngoesophageal complex is then mobilized off the vertebrae and retractors are placed after the longus colli is subperiosteally elevated, as described for lower cervical exposures. Closure is accomplished with Vicryl sutures for the platysma and subcuticular pullout sutures for the skin.

Complications

Primary complications from this approach are injury to cranial nerves and penetration into the hypopharynx and cervical esophagus. The hypoglossal nerve is most at risk from this procedure; however, meticulous dissection and gentle retraction can usually prevent this injury. Isolated hypoglossal nerve injury results in loss of motor function to the ipsilateral side of the tongue. This injury on its own can usually be compensated for by the patient. However, if it is combined with other cranial nerve injuries, it can become a significant source of morbidity, both in swallowing and speech. Injury to the superior laryngeal nerve results in loss of sensation to the superior portion of the larynx and loss of motor function to the cricothyroid muscle. The cricothyroid muscle usually functions to tense the vocal cords and, unless the patient is a professional singer, this injury is rarely noticed. In the elderly, the loss of sensation can lead to a mild degree of aspiration. Injury to the hypopharynx or

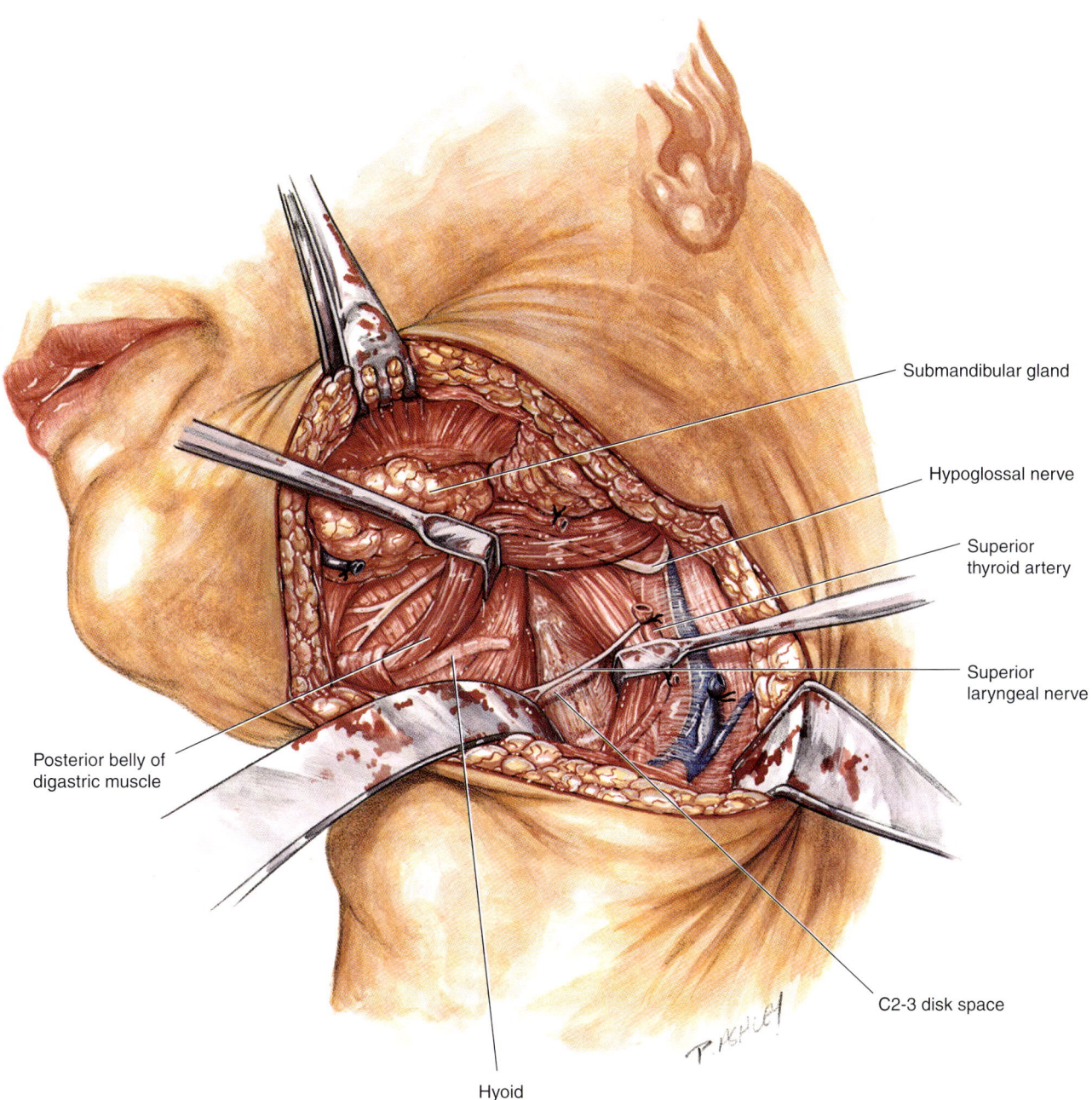

● **Figure 3-25.** High retropharyngeal approach after dissection.

esophagus needs to be recognized immediately and repaired. Suction drainage should be placed at the time of injury, and the patient observed closely postoperatively for development of a fistula.

Conclusion

Access to the upper cervical spine and craniocervical junction is a challenging technical exercise. Respect for the complex anatomy of this region is required. Meticulous exposure of the neural structures and gentle retraction should prevent complications. Choice of exposure depends on the pathologic process to be treated and the levels over which the process or necessary reconstruction spans.

BIBLIOGRAPHY

Arbit E, Patterson RH Jr.: Combined transoral and median labiomandibular glossotomy approach to the upper cervical spine. Neurosurgery 8(6):672–674, 1981.

Ashraf J, Crockard HA: Transoral fusion for high cervical fractures. J Bone Joint Surg Br 72:76, 1990.

Crockard HA: Midline ventral approaches to the cervical spine. In Sherk HH (ed): The Cervical Spine: An Atlas of Surgical Procedures, pp 93–112, Philadelphia, JB Lippincott, 1993.

Hadley MN, Sonntag VK: Cervical disc herniations. The anterior approach to symptomatic interspace pathology. Neurosurg Clin North Am 4:45, 1993.

Hadley MN, Spetzler RF, Sonntag VK: The transoral approach to the superior cervical spine. A review of 53 cases of extradural cervicomedullary compression. J Neurosurg 71:16, 1989.

Komisar A, Tabaddor K: Extrapharyngeal (anterolateral) approach to the cervical spine. Head Neck Surg 6:600, 1983.

Krespi YP, Har-El G: The transmandibular-transcervical approach to the skull base. In Sekhar LN, Janecka IP: *Surgery of Cranial Base Tumors,* 261–265. New York, Raven, 1993.

Krespi YP, Har-El G: Surgery of the clivus and anterior cervical spine. Arch Otolaryngol Head Neck Surg 114:73, 1988.

McAfee PC: Anterior surgical approaches to the lower and upper cervical spine. In Sherk HH (ed): The Cervical Spine: An Atlas of Surgical Procedures, pp 37–70. Philadelphia, JB Lippincott, 1993.

McAfee PC, Bohlman HH, Riley LH Jr., et al.: The anterior retropharyngeal approach to the upper part of the cervical spine. J Bone Joint Surg 69A:1371, 1987.

Menezes AH: Complications of surgery at the craniovertebral junction—avoidance and management. Pediatr Neurosurg 17:254, 1992.

Menezes AH, Van Gilder JC: Transoral-transpharyngeal approach to the anterior craniocervical junction. Ten-year experience with 72 patients. J Neurosurg 69:895, 1988.

Merwin GE, Post JC, Sypert GW: Transoral approach to the upper cervical spine. Laryngoscope 101(7 pt 1): 780, 1991.

Nachlas NE, McAfee PC, Johns ME: Anterior extraoral approach to the atlas and axis. Laryngoscope, 97(7 pt 1): 814, 1987.

Shaha AR, Johnson R, Miller J, Milhorat T: Transoral-transpharyngeal approach to the upper cervical vertebrae. AM J Surg 166:336, 1993.

Stauffer ES: Open-mouth and transmandibular approaches to the cervical spine. In Sherk HH (ed): The Cervical Spine: An Atlas of Surgical Procedures, pp 79–91. Philadelphia, JB Lippincott, 1993.

CHAPTER 4

LATERAL RETROPHARYNGEAL APPROACH TO THE UPPER CERVICAL SPINE (THE WHITESIDES APPROACH)

Todd J. Albert, M.D.
Thomas Whitesides, M.D.

The lateral approach to the upper cervical spine (lateral to the carotid sheath) was first described by Whitesides and Kelly in 1966. The advantages of this approach, as opposed to a transpharyngeal approach, include low risk of infection and few neural structures at risk during dissection. The disadvantage of the approach is that it places the surgeon more lateral than the medial retropharyngeal approach or the transoral approach with mandibular split. This approach is indicated for the excision of tumors at C1-2, certain instability problems, a failure of prior fusion attempts, the need for anterior placement of screws, and the treatment of infection.

Relevant Anatomy

The relevant anatomy has been described in Chapter 1. Of utmost importance is an appreciation of the carotid sheath and the sternocleidomastoid. This approach usually requires detachment of the sternocleidomastoid from its insertion on the mastoid tip. During dissection, the greater auricular nerve is encountered (Figure 4–1).

Surgical Technique

Patients requiring the lateral retropharyngeal approach are often being treated for instability or potential instability created by resection. The ideal position to perform this surgery is with the patient in the supine position with the head turned away from the side of the approach. Nasotracheal intubation opposite to the side of incision is preferred. Often the patient is in a halo ring with traction or a vest attachment at the time of surgery and has to be positioned with the restraints imposed by these devices. Before the patient is positioned, the lobe of the ear is usually sewn anteriorly to give access to the skin posterior to the ear. The skin inside and outside the ear is prepared with povidone-iodine (Betadine). After usual draping techniques, the incision is carried out beginning posterior to the earlobe and running

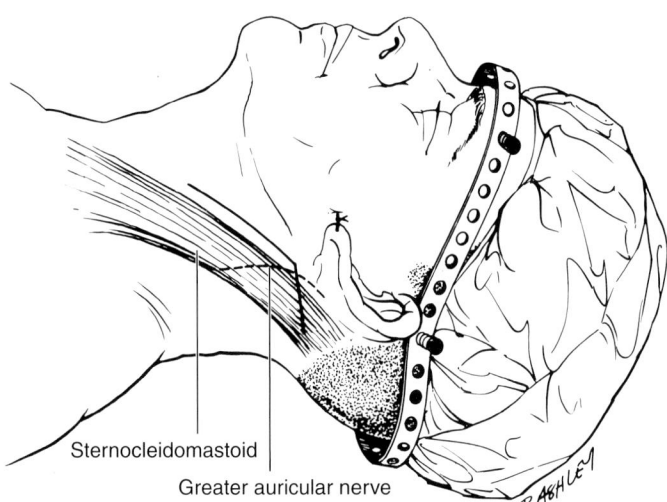

● **Figure 4-1.** The patient is in a supine position with halo ring in place. A "hockey stick" incision is outlined. The ear is sewn anteriorly. The greater auricular nerve is shadowed in. In rare circumstances, the greater auricular nerve needs to be sacrificed, producing a small insensate area that is not disabling to the patient.

anteriorly transversely across the tip of the mastoid process. It is then carried longitudinally and distally along the anterior border of the sternocleidomastoid. The incision looks like a hockey stick (see Figure 4–1). The plane of dissection that will be used is shown in Figure 4–2. One can readily see that the carotid sheath, as well as its contents, and the parotid gland are anterior to the dissection high in the neck. The first palpable bony prominence is the lateral process of the ring of C1.

After skin incision is completed, the greater auricular nerve is identified when it is dissected in the subcutaneous tissue. Dissection bidirectionally allows the nerve to be retracted in either a cranial or caudal direction. In rare instances, the nerve is in the way of dissection and must be resected, which does result in a small patch of sensory deficit (see Figure 4–1).

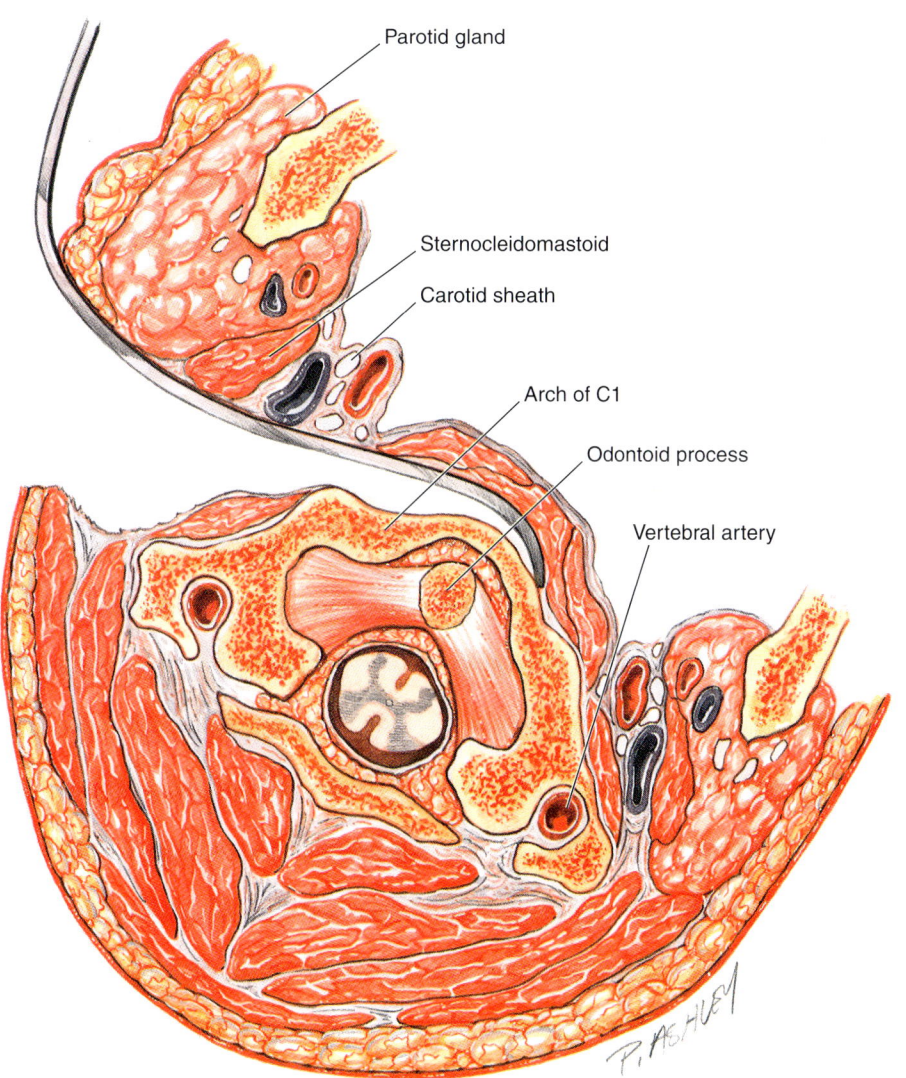

● **Figure 4–2.** Cross-sectional reference at the C1 arch showing plane of dissection. A bent malleable retractor is levered against the contralateral anterior portion of the atlas to retract the parotid gland, sternocleidomastoid, and contents of the carotid sheath, as well as the esophagus. This plane of dissection does not place at risk the vertebral arteries because they are posterior and encased in bone at this level.

The sternocleidomastoid is prominent after an incision is made through the subcutaneous levels. In most cases, the sternocleidomastoid is detached from the mastoid process. If the patient is small and the muscles are not of significant bulk, the sternocleidomastoid attachment can be preserved if only limited exposure is planned for. The spinal accessory nerve enters the sternocleidomastoid approximately 3 cm distal to the mastoid tip. This is identified and protected (Figure 4–3).

The cross-sectional anatomy of this dissection is viewed in Figure 4–2. Typically, a malleable retractor is bent to the appropriate curvature and levered on the contralateral side or transverse process at the appropriate vertebral body. This cross section shows the standard dissection at C1 posterior to the carotid sheath and sternocleidomastoid as well as the parotid gland.

If only the C1-2 level is approached (the limited exposure), the spinal accessory nerve can be retracted anteriorly along with the sternocleidomastoid and the contents of the carotid sheath. The dissection can be carried almost to the jugular foramen proximally for this exposure. When a more extensile approach is needed to the subaxial vertebral bodies, the spinal accessory nerve is dissected from the jugular foramen and retracted laterally and posteriorly after eversion of the sternocleidomastoid (Figure 4–4).

After eversion of the sternocleidomastoid, the lateral arch of C1 and other transverse processes of the subaxial vertebral bodies are easily palpable. The C1 transverse process is

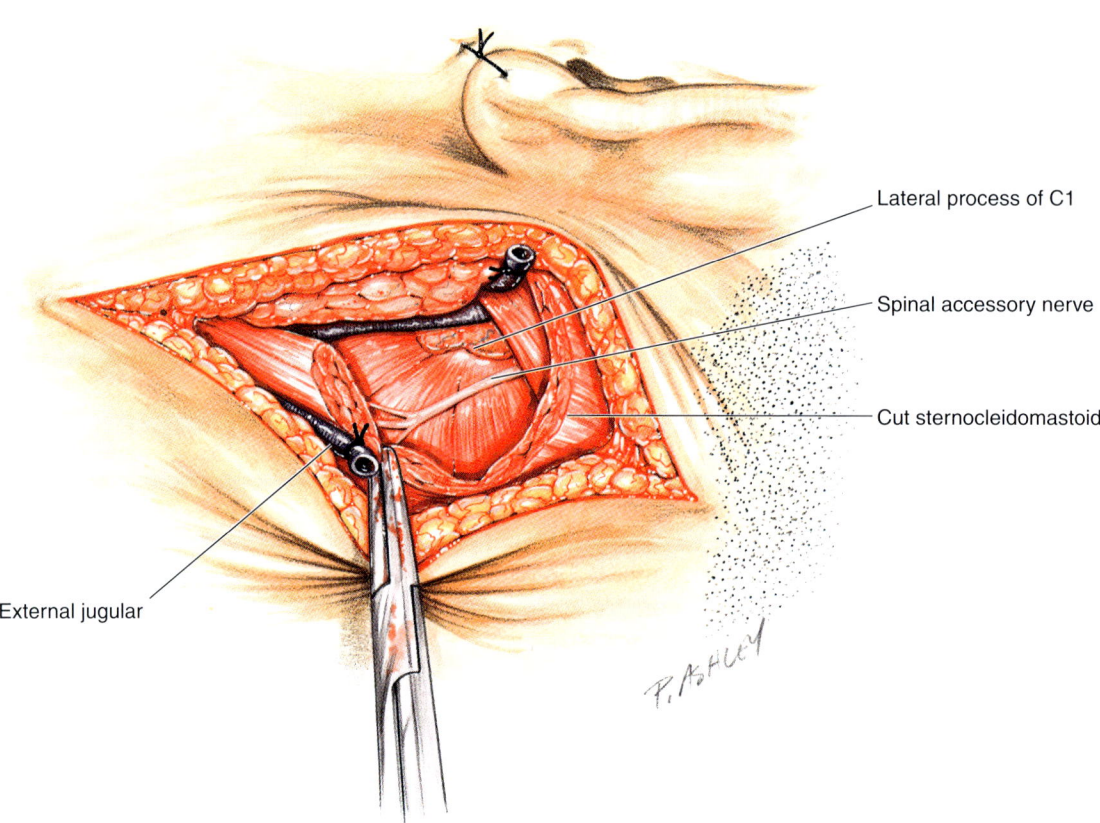

● **Figure 4-3.** After skin and subcutaneous dissection, the spinal accessory nerve is identified as it enters the sternocleidomastoid. The sternocleidomastoid has been cut proximally close to its insertion on the mastoid process.

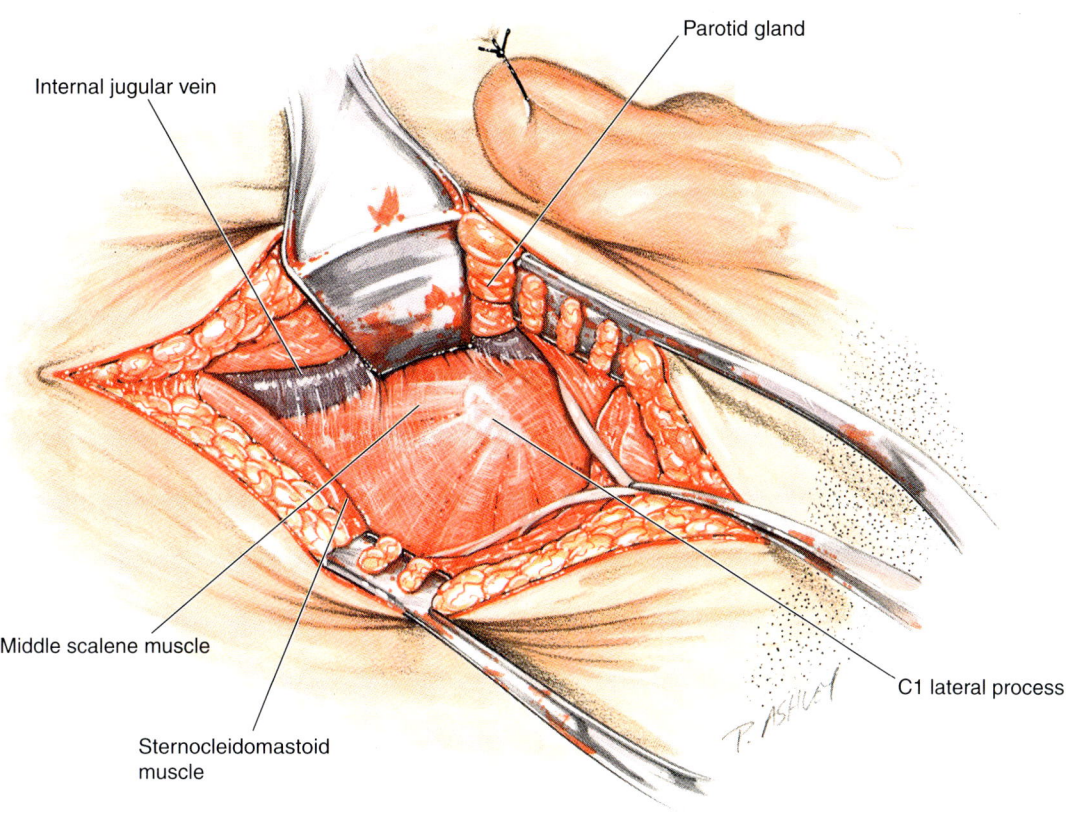

● **Figure 4-4.** After retraction of the spinal accessory nerve and removal of the large lymph nodes in the area including the jugular node, the lateral process of C1 becomes obvious and attachments to the middle scalenes are apparent. The carotid sheath contents and parotid gland are retracted medially.

most prominent laterally compared with the other vertebral bodies. Dissection medially often requires resection of the large lymph nodes in this area, including the jugular node. As the dissection proceeds medially, the fibers attaching the prevertebral fascia are dissected, creating a plane that allows the surgeon distal dissection if it is needed along the anterior longitudinal ligament to the subaxial vertebral bodies. The extensile approach to the neck utilizing the lateral retropharyngeal approach is carried out simply by dissecting posterior to the sternocleidomastoid and carotid sheath and utilizing the same plane of dissection demonstrated in Figure 4–3. As in the medial retropharyngeal approach, exposure of the more distal vertebral bodies often requires removal of the longus colli covering them from medial to lateral. As stated previously, a malleable retractor is bent posterior to the esophagus and levered on the opposing transverse process for exposure of the anterior vertebral bodies (Figure 4–5).

At the end of the procedure, a drain is placed deep in the neck and the sternocleidomastoid is repaired anatomically. Superficially, only the platysma and skin layers need to be approximated. External orthotic management is dependent on the indication for this surgery. As with all proximal anterior approaches, prolonged intubation is usually appropriate to allow the swelling of the retropharyngeal tissues to subside.

58 ● SURGICAL APPROACHES TO THE SPINE

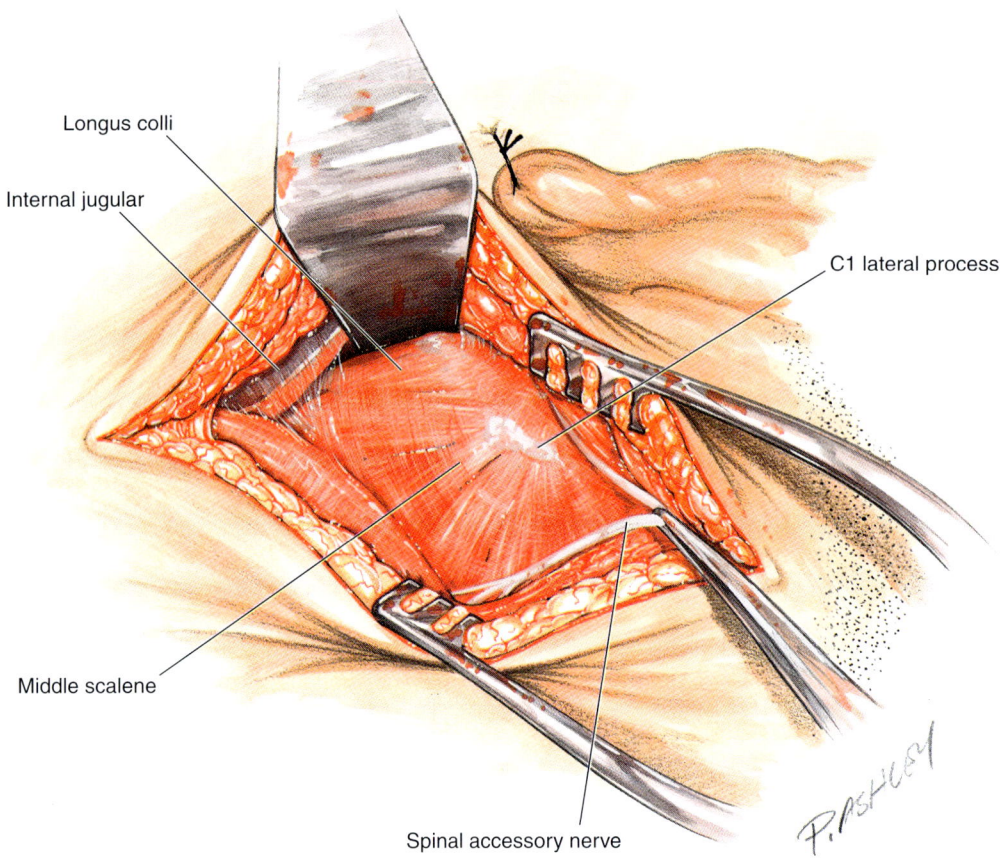

● **Figure 4-5.** Further delineation of the lateral process is carried out. The dissection can be made extensile by dissecting distally the same plane anterior to the vertebral bodies. The longus colli may need to be taken off the lateral aspect of the vertebral body to identify the disk spaces and vertebral bodies.

Complications

Obvious complications include injury to the spinal accessory nerve with consequent trapezial wasting and shoulder problems. Injury to the vessels in this area (internal jugular vein and carotid) is possible but unlikely with care taken during dissection. As with other cervical approaches, injury to the esophagus should be avoided and checked for at the time of surgery by flooding the esophagus with dilute indigo carmine. Risks to the vertebral arteries are minimal because the dissection is carried out anteriorly to these important structures.

Conclusion

The lateral retropharyngeal approach to the upper cervical spine is an important alternative to the transpharyngeal approaches. The infection rate is lower, and the risks to vital structures are less owing to the relative safety of dissection in this area. This approach should be part of the armamentarium of any surgeon practicing a significant amount of cervical surgery because of its utility in specific situations such as a tumor, an infection, and nonunion of atlantoaxial fusion.

BIBLIOGRAPHY

de Andrade Jr, McNab I: Anterior occipitocervical fusion using extrapharyngeal approach. J Bone Joint Surg Am 51:1621, 1969.

Fang HS, Ong GB: Direct anterior approach to the upper cervical spine. J Bone Joint Surg Am 44:1588, 1962.

Hall JE, Denis F, Murray J: Exposure of the upper cervical spine for spinal decompression by a mandible and tongue-splitting approach. J Bone Joint Surg Am 59:121, 1977.

Henry AK: Extensile Exposure, 2nd ed, p 53. Edinburgh, E & S Livingstone, 1957.

Simmons EH, DuToit G Jr: Lateral atlantoaxial arthrodesis. Orthop Clin North Am 9:1101, 1978.

Whitesides TE Jr, Kelly RP: Lateral approach to the upper cervical spine for anterior fusion. South Med J 59:879, 1966.

Whitesides TE Jr, McDonald P: Lateral retropharyngeal approach to the upper cervical spine. Orthop Clin North Am 9:115, 1978.

CHAPTER 5

ANTERIOR EXPOSURES OF THE CERVICOTHORACIC JUNCTION AND UPPER THORACIC SPINE

Lawrence T. Kurz, M.D.
Harry N. Herkowitz, M.D.

The overwhelming majority of pathologic entities occurring at the cervicothoracic junction or upper thoracic spine are located anteriorly in the vertebral body. Surgical accessibility is quite limited, mostly by the great vessels, sternum, and clavicle. Because the biomechanical forces acting around the cervicothoracic junction are very large, vertebral body collapse is not infrequent. The subsequent development of a spinal deformity hinders the access even more. Therefore, a surgical approach to the anterior aspect of the cervicothoracic junction and upper thoracic spine must account for these problems.

There are three approaches that attempt to address the issue of access: the modified anterior approach to the cervicothoracic junction, the sternal-splitting approach, and the transthoracic approach. Each has its own advantages and disadvantages, which, although limiting, may aid the surgeon in choosing the appropriate approach.

The modified anterior approach to the cervicothoracic junction is probably the best one to use for access to the cervicothoracic junction. It is not limited in offering good visualization of the anterior spinal structures from C4 to T4. It also provides adequate working room to perform resection of anterior pathologic processes, decompression of the spinal cord, correction of the spinal deformity, as well as reconstruction and even stabilization if necessary. Exposure is usually quite simple, and complications are rare. The only disadvantage is that the medial clavicle and sternoclavicular joint are resected.

Theoretically, postoperative weakness of the left shoulder girdle musculature could occur secondary to the joint resection.

The sternum-splitting approach, by itself, is inadequate for exposure of the upper thoracic spine. This is a significant disadvantage; this approach should not be used when addressing lesions at the cervicothoracic junction. However, the sternum-splitting approach may be combined with an anterior approach to the cervical spine. This extends the exposure into the neck up to C4 and down to T4 by facilitating retraction of the great vessels and removing hindrance by the sternum. The major disadvantages of the sternum-splitting approach relate to its limited exposure and the complications attendant to entering the pleural cavity.

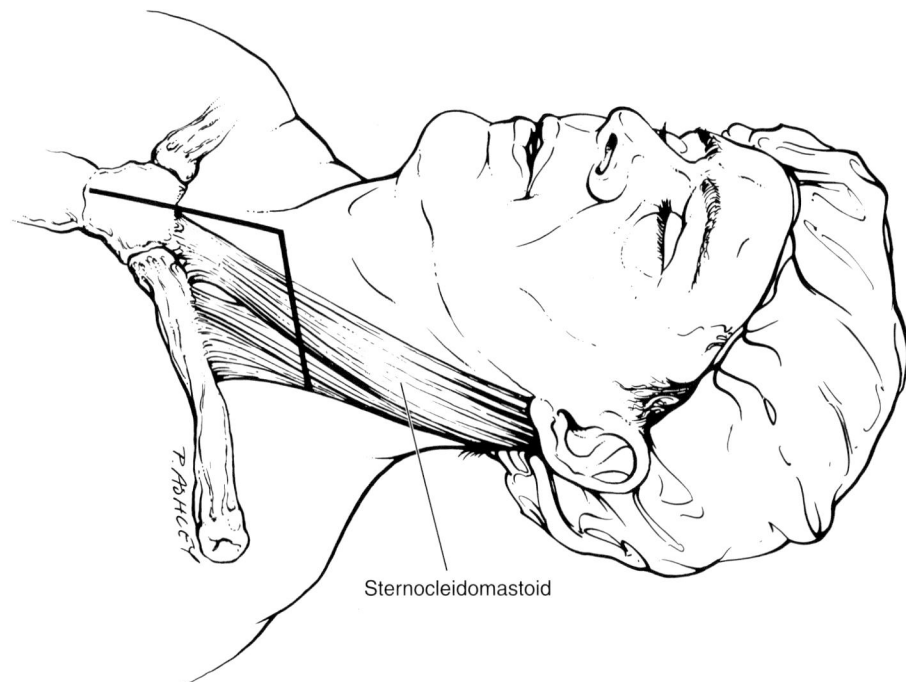

● **Figure 5-1.** Incision line for modified anterior cervicothoracic approach.

A proximal thoracotomy is an approach that allows exposure of the upper thoracic spine. There are even times when the C7 vertebral body may be visualized enough to actually receive a bone graft. However, in general, the working room in the very proximal thoracic spine, which is afforded by this approach, is limited. Hindrance is usually due to inability to retract the scapula and the cupula of the lung. Furthermore, as the surgeon works progressively from T3 to C7, the thoracic inlet significantly narrows and constricts the surgical field. The major disadvantage of this approach is its general inability to expose the cervical spine.

Anatomy of the Cervicothoracic Junction and Upper Thoracic Spine

The anatomy of the cervicothoracic junction includes the anatomy of the thoracic inlet. A complicated layering of arteries and veins brings blood from and returns blood to the heart. The top of the sternum (manubrium) articulates with the two clavicular heads. Immediately behind this area are the subclavian vein and artery. The sternocleidomastoid inserts with a

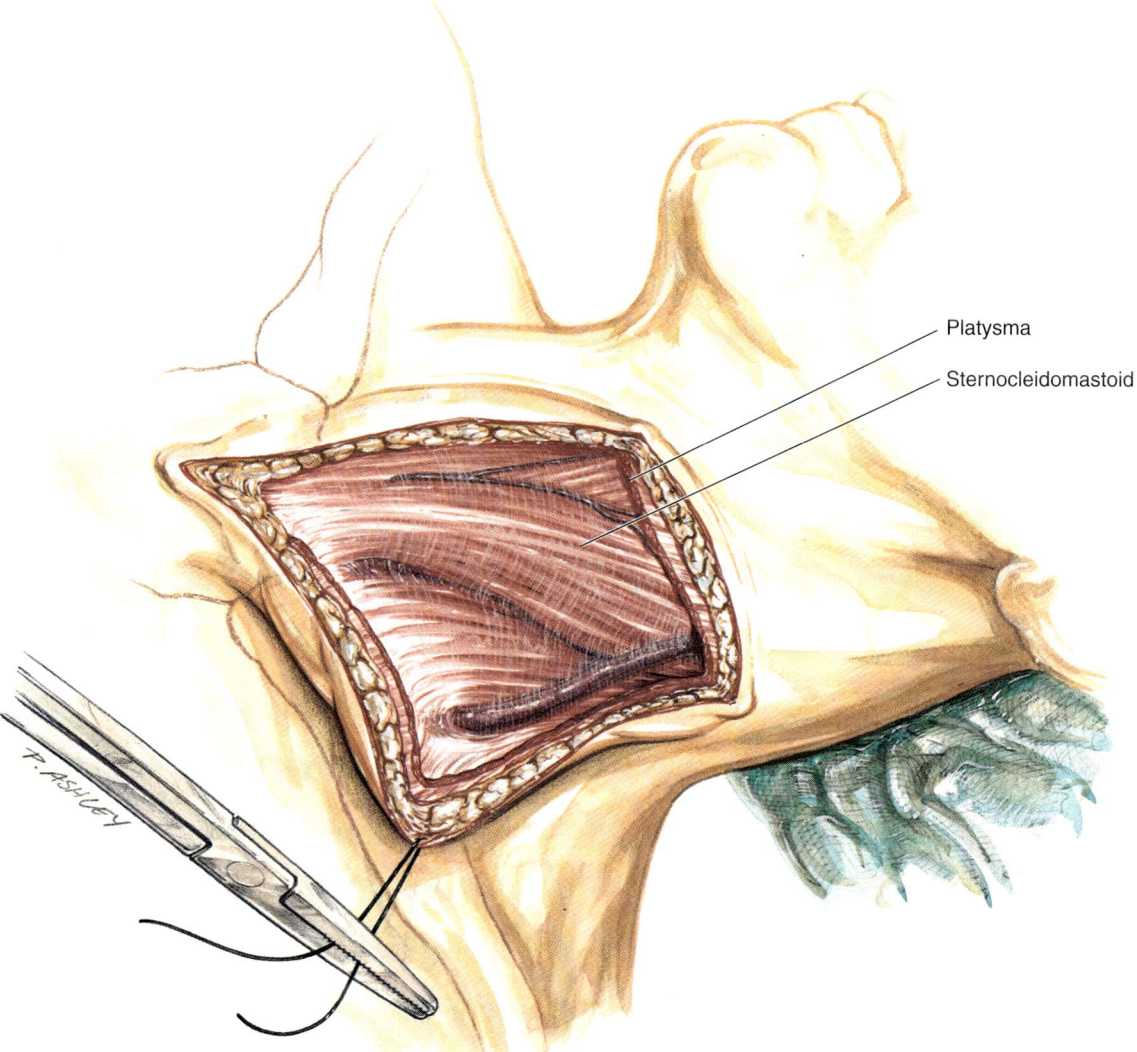

● **Figure 5-2.** After division of platysma and elevation of subcutaneous flaps.

sternal and a clavicular head. Posterior to the sternocleidomastoid, at the root of the neck, the junction of the internal jugular vein into the brachiocephalic vein on the left is apparent. The thoracic duct is at the cervicothoracic junction but lateral to the carotid system. Keeping dissection medial to the carotid system should avoid injury to the thoracic duct.

The left recurrent laryngeal nerve arises at the level of the aortic arch within the thorax, loops beneath the arch, and ascends between the trachea and esophagus. The right recurrent laryngeal nerve arises from the vagus nerve usually at the level of the subclavian artery and loops beneath the subclavian artery, ascending between the trachea and esophagus and protected by the visceral fascia. A potential space, known as Burns' space, lies between the sternocleidomastoid invested with its fascia and the carotid sheath and its fascia. Blunt finger dissection behind the sternocleidomastoid and in front of the carotid sheath delineates this space and protects the vessels of the inlet from injury. The cupula of the lung is adjacent inferiorly to the thoracic inlet on either side.

Modified Anterior Approach to the Cervicothoracic Junction

The patient should be positioned supine on the operating table with a rolled towel between the scapulae. The neck is thus hyperextended and rotated toward the patient's right side. If intraoperative traction is used, then skull tongs or a halo ring should be placed after induction of anesthesia. General endotracheal anesthesia is preferred. All areas must be well padded, and the patient's arms should be tucked into his or her sides. The anterior and lateral neck, the anterior and lateral chest to the midsternal level, and the left clavicle should all be prepared and draped in typical sterile manner.

The cervical spine is entered on the left side because of the constancy of the recurrent laryngeal nerve there. There is an unacceptable incidence of aberrant recurrent laryngeal nerves on the right side, which increases the risk of injury. An angled skin incision is made into the anterior portion of the left side of the neck (Figure 5–1). The transverse limb begins 1 to 2 inches proximal to the left clavicle, in the midsagittal plane of the body. It proceeds parallel to the left clavicle and extends laterally all the way to the lateral border of the left sternocleidomastoid muscle. The vertical limb is within the midsagittal plane, begins proximally at the medial aspect of the transverse incision, and extends distally to a point just past the junction of the manubrium and sternum.

After skin and subcutaneous tissue are incised, the platysma muscle is cleared and then incised in line with the skin incision. Although there is great variation in the thickness of the platysma muscle, it must not be confused with the strap or sternocleidomastoid muscles. Through undermining, subcutaneous flaps are developed and then the superficial anterior veins are cauterized. Although the medial supraclavicular nerve and the external jugular vein can usually be safely retracted, the external jugular vein can be sacrificed if necessary for exposure (Figure 5–2).

The clavicular and manubrial heads of the sternocleidomastoid muscle are subperiosteally elevated off their distal attachments to bone and then are retracted proximally and laterally (Figure 5–3). As a group, the strap muscles are cut deep to the clavicle and are elevated proximally and medially. The remaining periosteum is stripped from the medial third of the left clavicle and left half of the manubrium. A Gigli saw is then used to cut the clavicle at the junction of its middle and medial thirds (Figure 5–4A). Extra care must be taken to avoid injuring the left subclavian vein, which is closely apposed to the posteroinferior surface of the clavicle (see Figure 5–4B). The medial third of the clavicle is then disarticulated from the manubrium (Figure 5–5). In a few cases, just medial to this dissection, the inferior thyroid vein must be ligated for exposure.

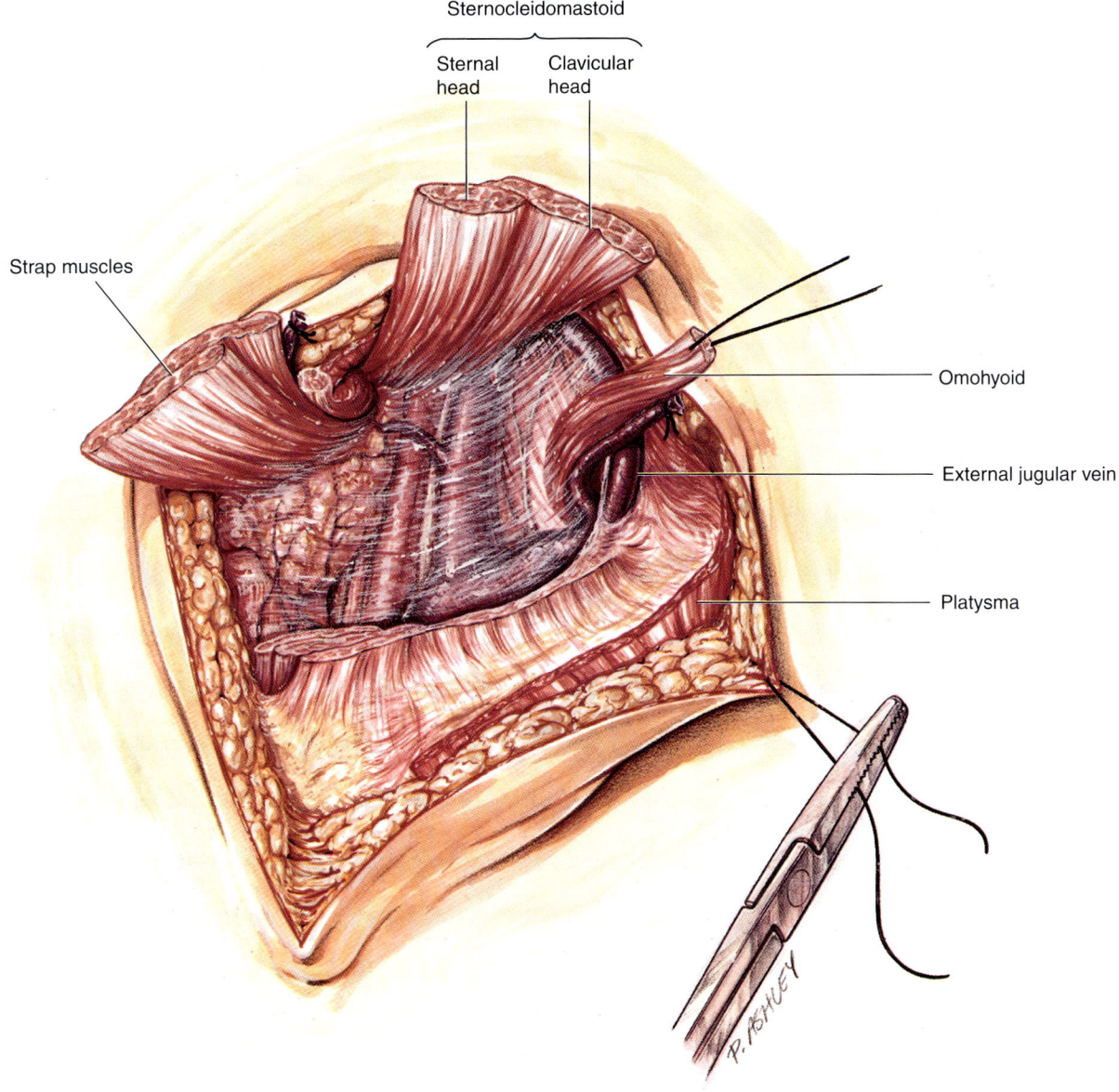

● **Figure 5-3.** After division of sternal and clavicular heads of sternocleidomastoid and division of strap muscles. Omohyoid is also seen divided.

Proximally, the fascia over the carotid sheath is dissected free, and an interval is found between the trachea and esophagus and the carotid sheath. The recurrent laryngeal nerve is usually constant in its location between the trachea and esophagus on the left side of the neck. It must be safely retracted medially, along with the strap muscles, esophagus, and trachea.

The sternocleidomastoid muscle and carotid sheath are then retracted laterally (Figure 5–6). Safe retraction of these structures is aided by hand-held Richardson retractors. These instruments have broad, smooth edges and are ideal for retraction of nerves, vessels, and hollow viscera. Self-retaining retractors are of no use because of the large field of exposure. Retractors with teeth should not be used.

At this point, the brachiocephalic vessels are seen in the most distal portion of the wound. Along with the esophagus and trachea, the right brachiocephalic artery and, even

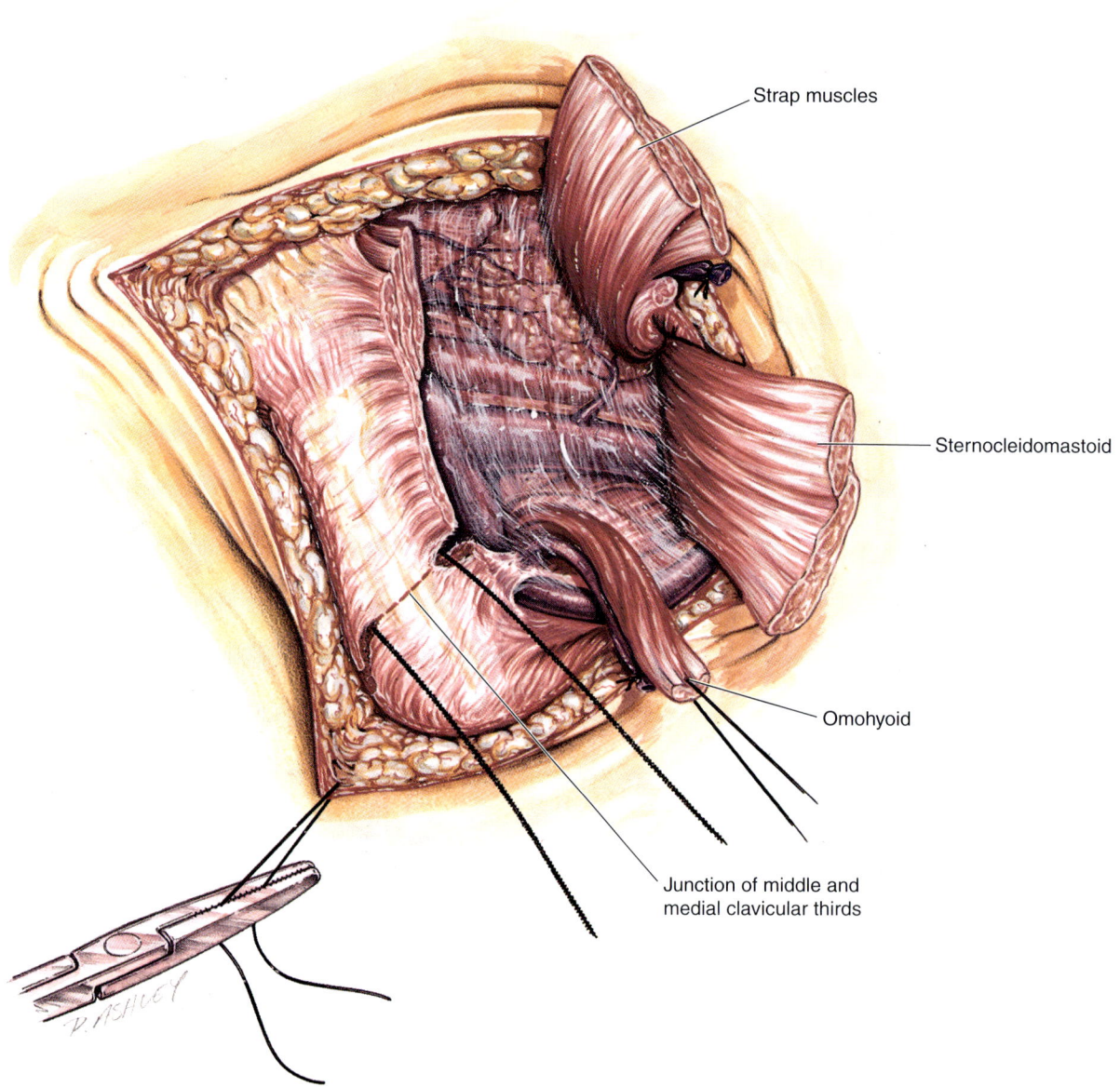

● **Figure 5-4.** *A* and *B*, Gigli saw is used to cut clavicle at the junction of the middle and medial thirds. Care is taken to avoid injury to the closely apposed subclavian vein.

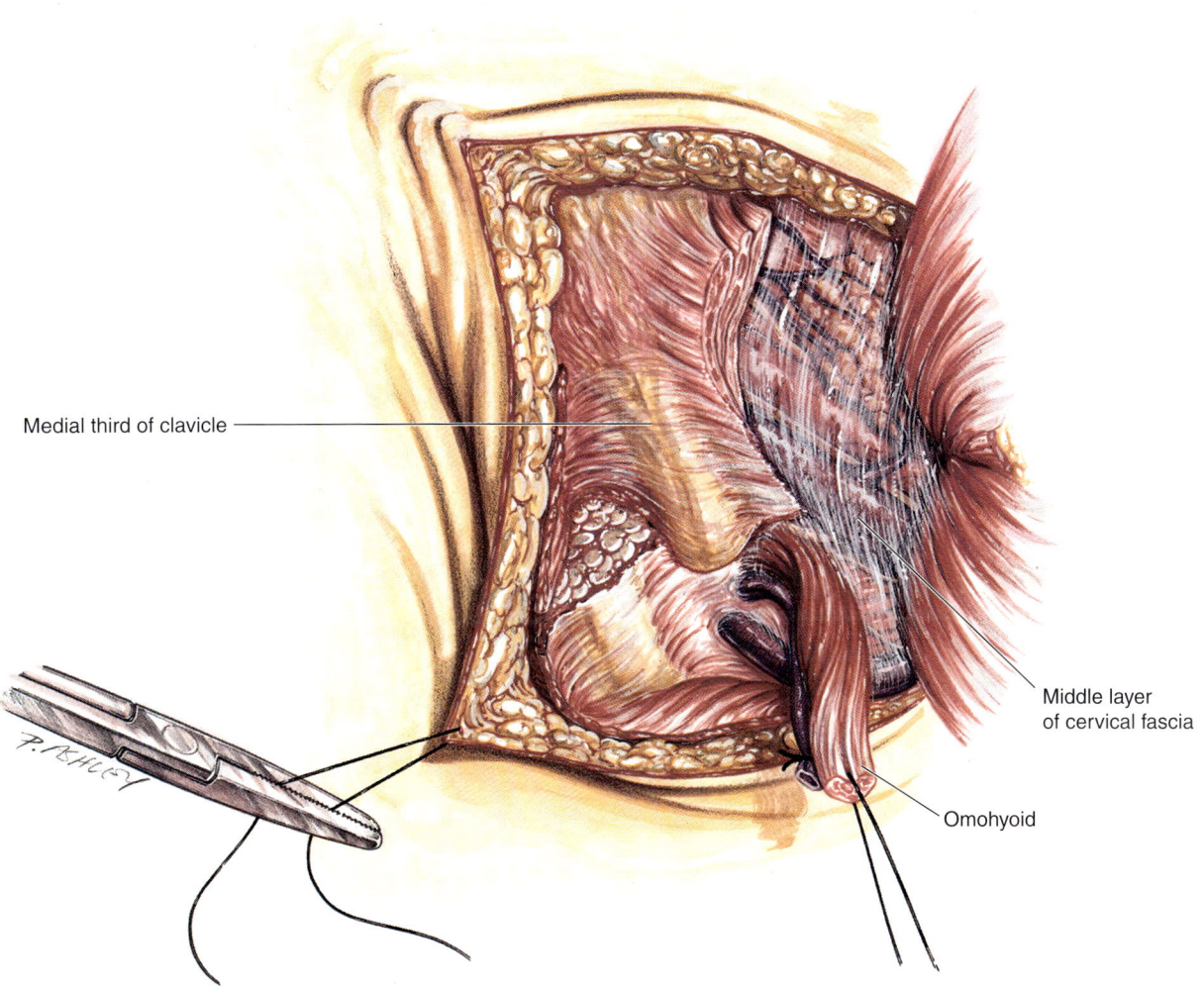

● **Figure 5-4.** Continued

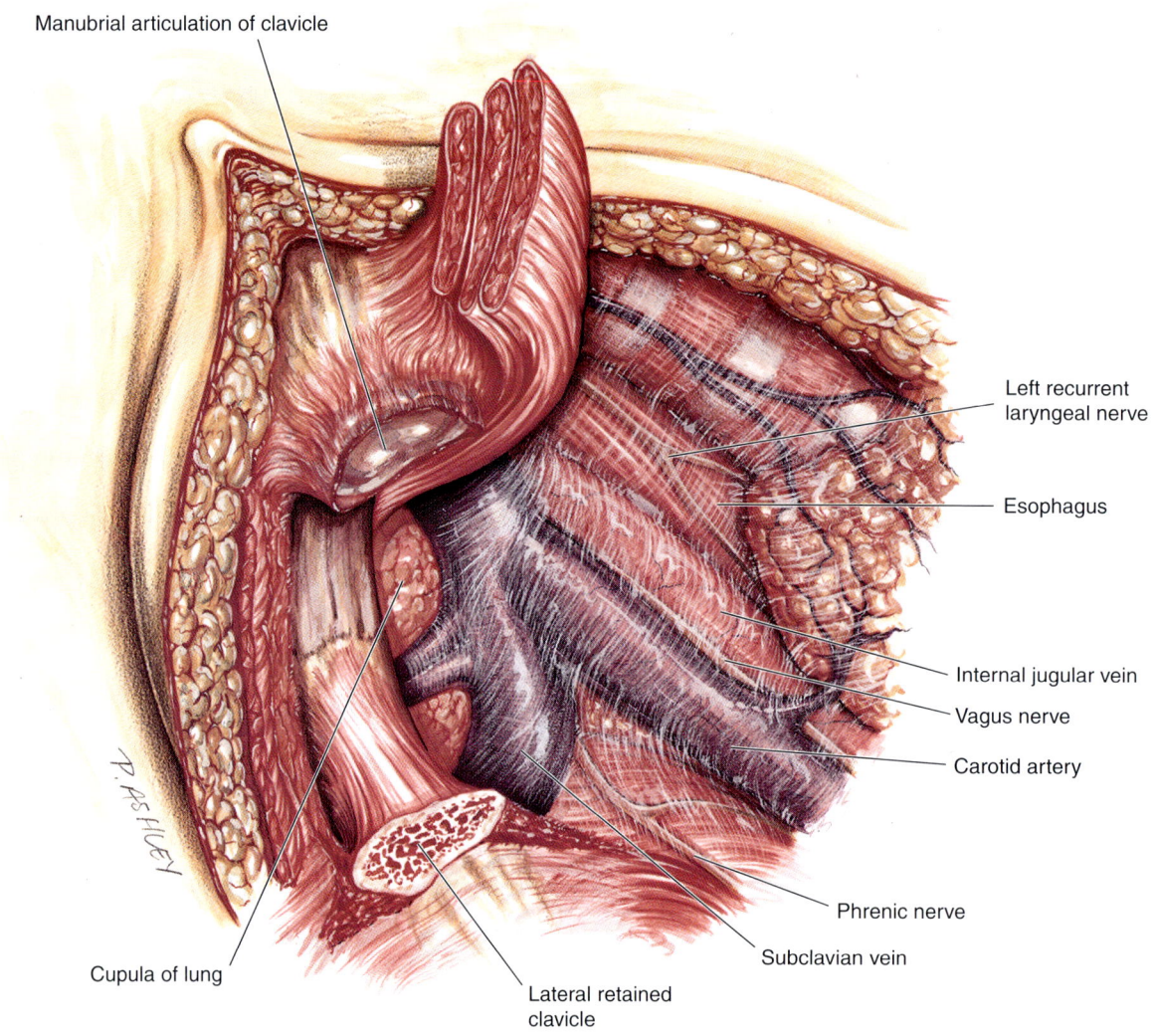

● **Figure 5-5.** Resected medial one third of clavicle reveals thoracic inlet, carotid sheath, and tracheoesophageal complex medially.

more laterally, the right brachiocephalic vein are retracted inferolaterally to the patient's right. Along with the left carotid sheath, the left brachiocephalic and subclavian veins are retracted inferolaterally to the patient's left. This brings the cervicothoracic junction into view. Once the prevertebral fascia is dissected free, the surgeon can usually view the vertebral bodies of C4 to T4. Visualization and identification of the anterior vertebral structures are aided by the constancy of distal insertions of the longus colli muscles into the lateral aspects of the T1, T2, and T3 vertebral bodies.

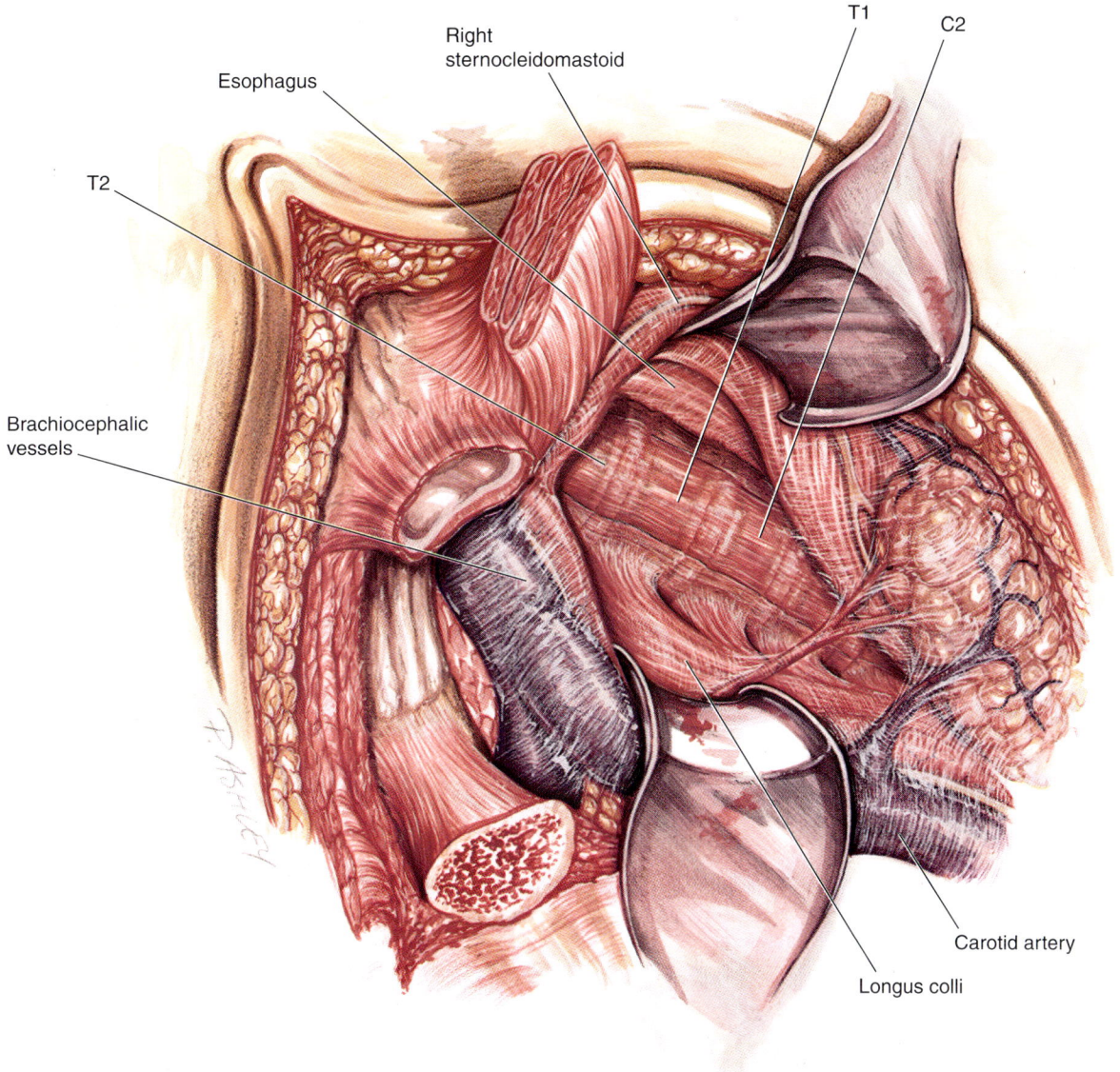

● **Figure 5-6.** After dissection of deep layers of cervical fascia, exposure of the cervicothoracic junction is facilitated with Richardson retractors. Self-retaining retractors should not be used.

Proximal Thoracotomy

After induction of general endotracheal anesthesia, the patient is placed on the operating table in the left lateral decubitus position and then rolled 30 degrees toward the supine position. Although all areas must be well padded, it is especially important to place a large padded roll in the left axilla to prevent neurovascular compromise of the left upper extremity. The right arm is padded out of the way of the operative field in the direction of the jaw. This leaves the right back, right chest, and right lateral rib area to be prepared and draped in typical sterile manner (Figure 5–7). The right side of the chest is preferred for entry because of the proximity of the heart and great vessels on the left side.

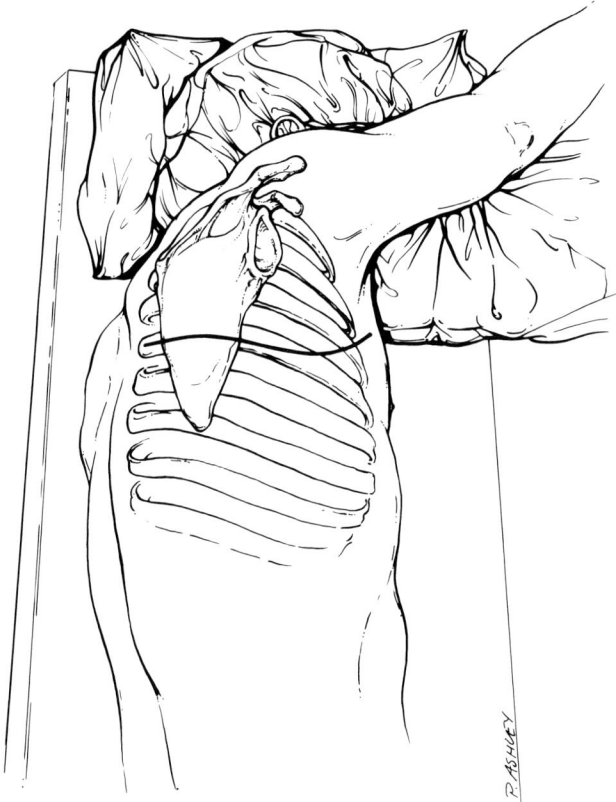

● **Figure 5-7.** Incision for proximal thoracotomy after positioning in 30 degrees off the left lateral decubitus position with an axillary roll and incising over the third or fourth rib.

The thoracotomy is usually performed either by removing the third or fourth rib or simply by spreading the intercostal space between those two ribs. Surgical exposure is much greater with rib resection when compared with spreading of the intercostal space. The shorter first and second ribs are not used for entry because their removal or separation limits the exposure and the scapula interferes posteriorly at this very proximal level.

A skin incision is made over the right third or fourth rib beginning at the anterior axillary line and extending laterally and posteriorly to the lateral border of the right paraspinal muscles (Figure 5–8). The skin and subcutaneous tissue are incised, and the latissimus dorsi and trapezius muscles are sectioned and then retracted (Figure 5–9). Muscular retraction allows easy identification of the rib cage, as well as the subscapular space (Figure 5–10). The right scapula is then retracted (usually with a Love or Sweetheart retractor), and the surgeon can palpate and identify the third or four right rib by counting down from the thoracic inlet. Some slips of the serratus anterior may cover the ribs and may need to be divided.

Sharp subperiosteal dissection of the appropriate rib is performed. Rib resection may be carried out by cutting the rib as far anteriorly and posteriorly as possible. Care must be taken to protect the intercostal artery, vein, and nerve during rib sectioning. This serves two purposes: It allows maximum exposure and yields the largest possible piece of autogenous bone graft if needed. A rib cage spreader is placed, and then a wet towel is used to cover the right lung before it is retracted anteriorly (Figure 5–11). Lung retraction allows visualization of the upper thoracic vertebra. The parietal pleura, which overlies the vertebral bodies, should be incised to allow identification of the segmental vessels (Figure 5–12). These arteries and veins are ligated at appropriate levels, and the pleura is stripped back (Figure 5–13). This completes the exposure of the upper thoracic disks and vertebral bodies.

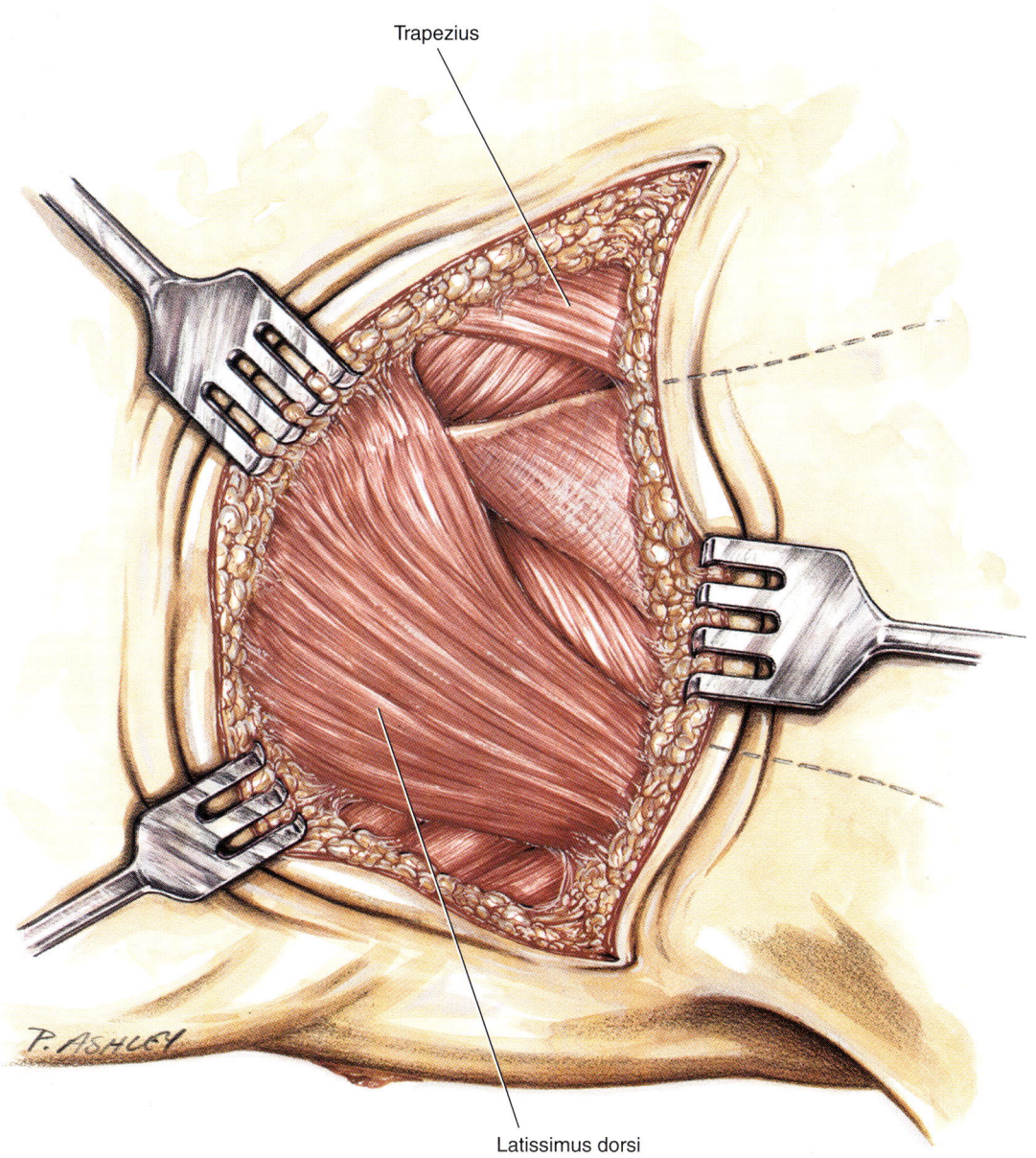

● **Figure 5-8.** After subcutaneous exposure from the anterior axillary line to the lateral border of the paraspinal muscles, the latissimus dorsi muscle and trapezius are sectioned.

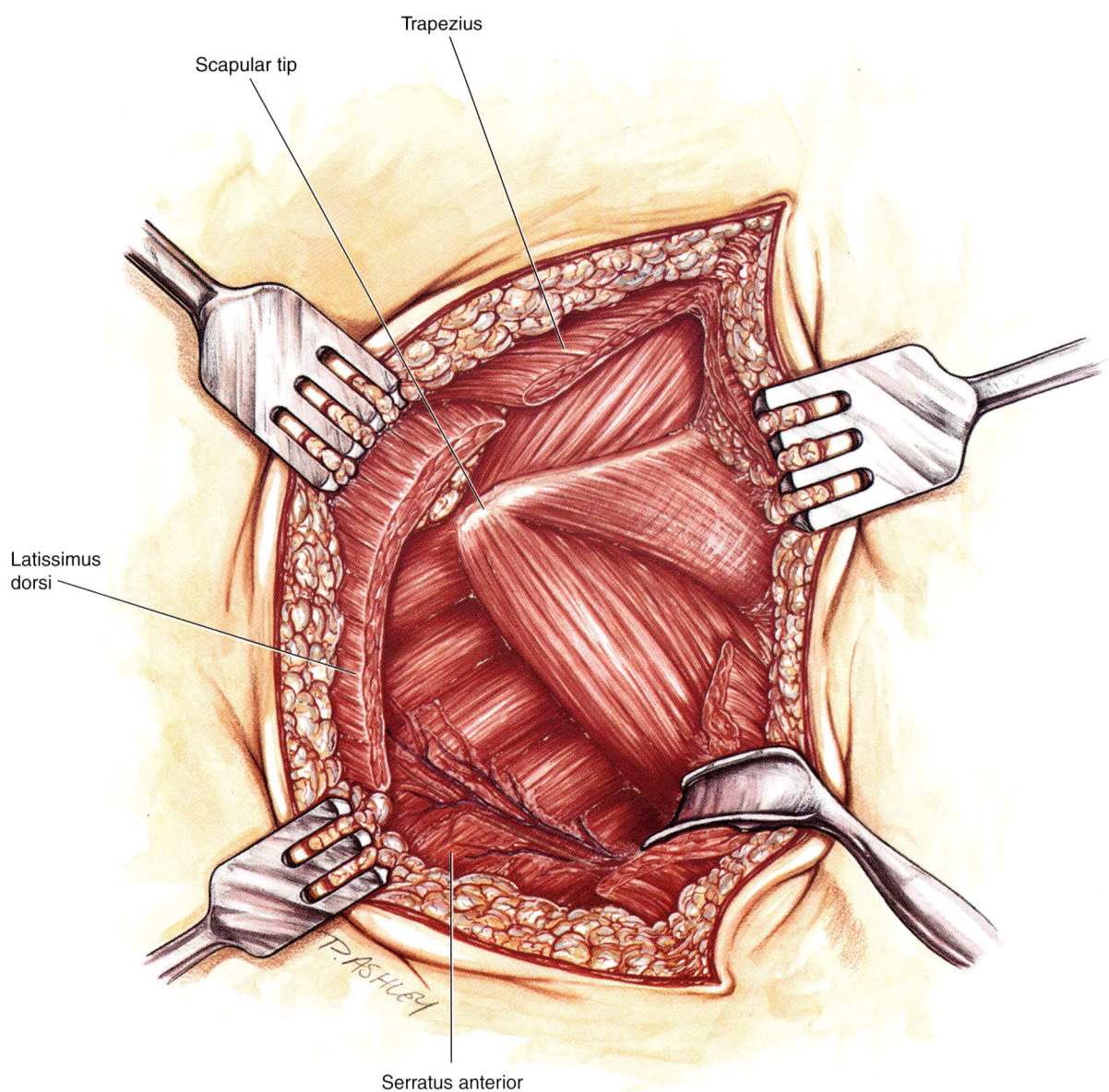

● **Figure 5-9.** Sectioning of latissimus dorsi and trapezius exposes the scapular tip.

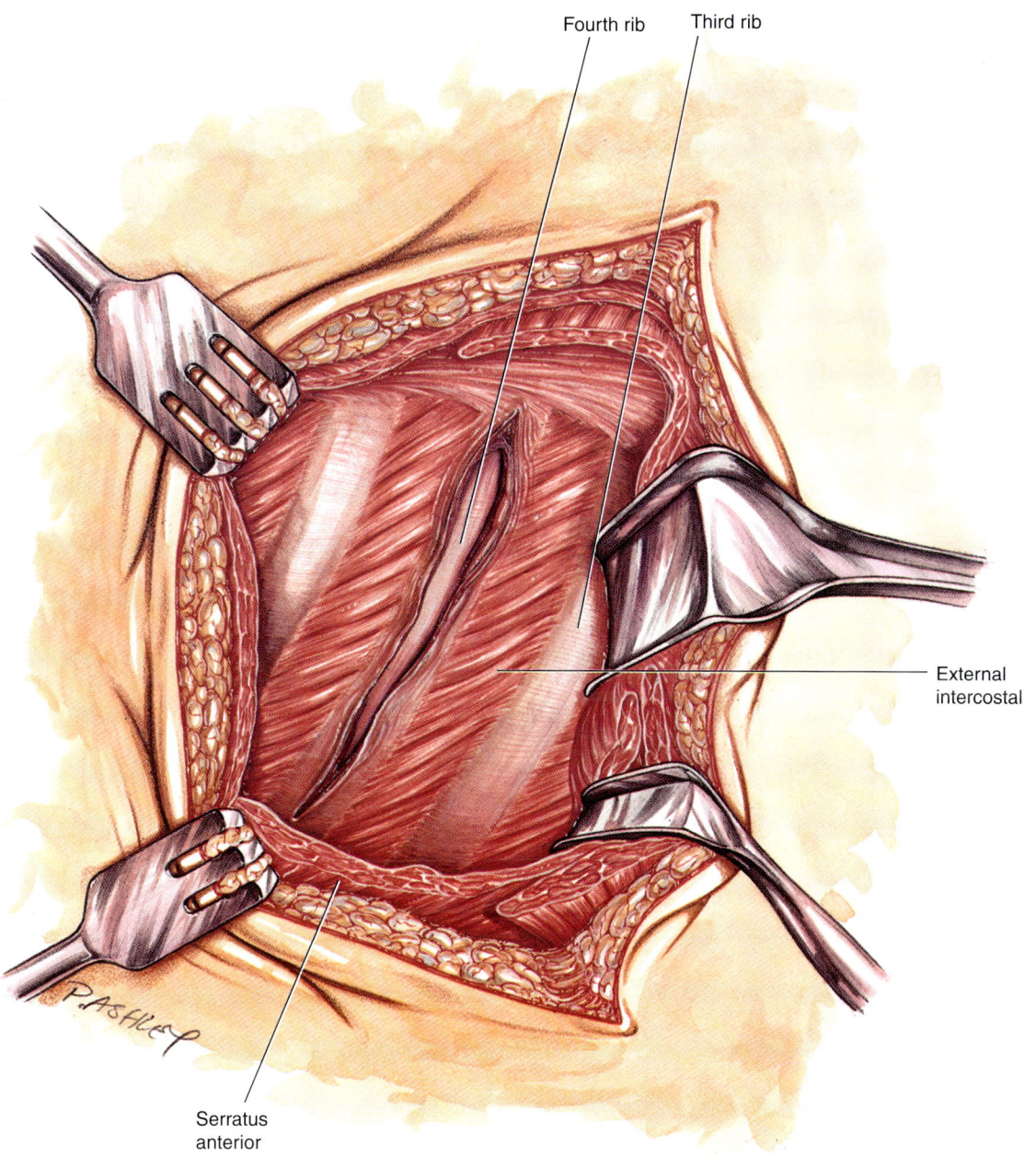

● **Figure 5-10.** Retraction of the scapula allows dissection of the third or fourth rib subperiosteally.

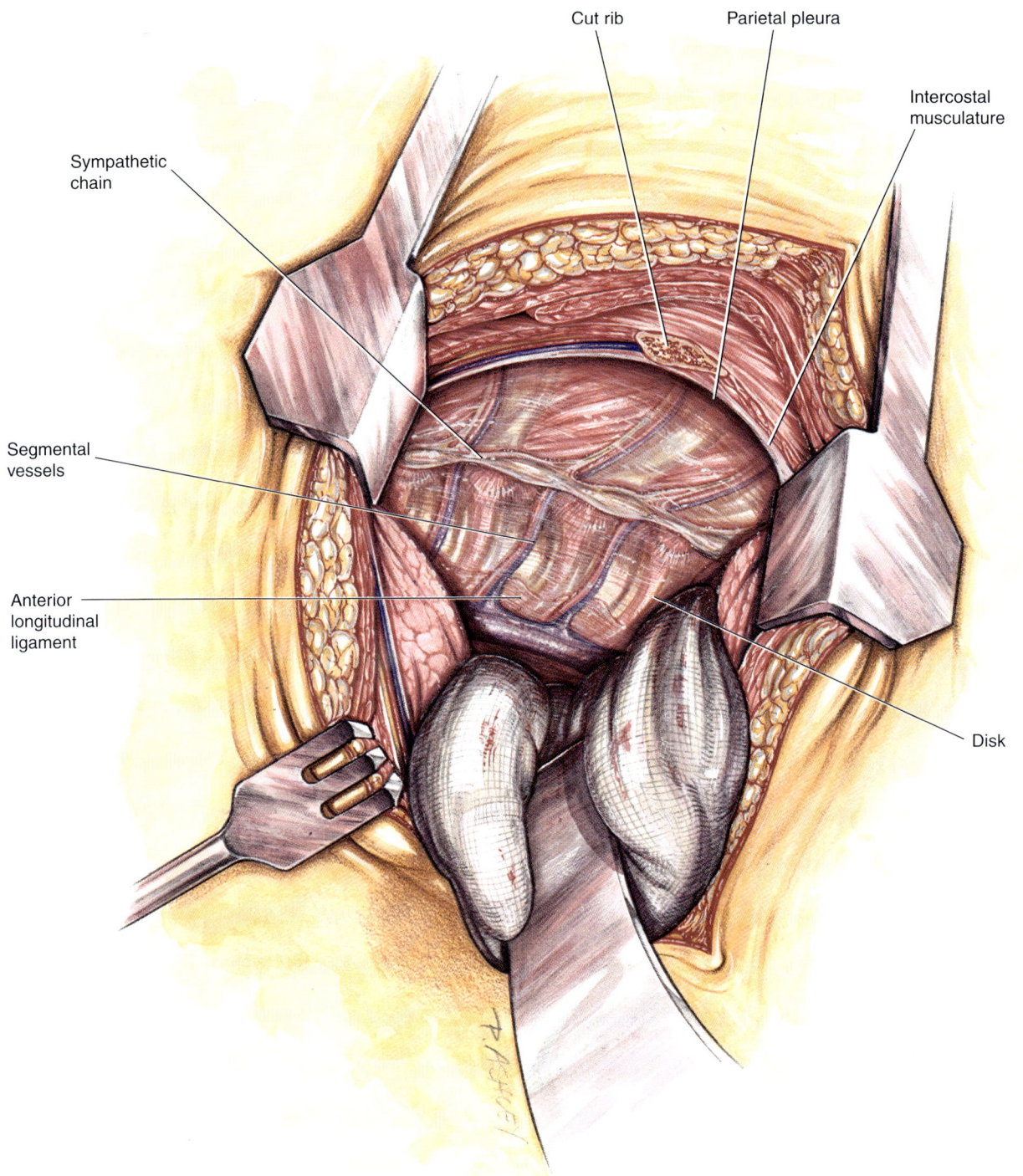

● **Figure 5-11.** Rib resection subperiosteally and lung and rib retraction allow visualization of the spinal column, covered by the parietal pleura.

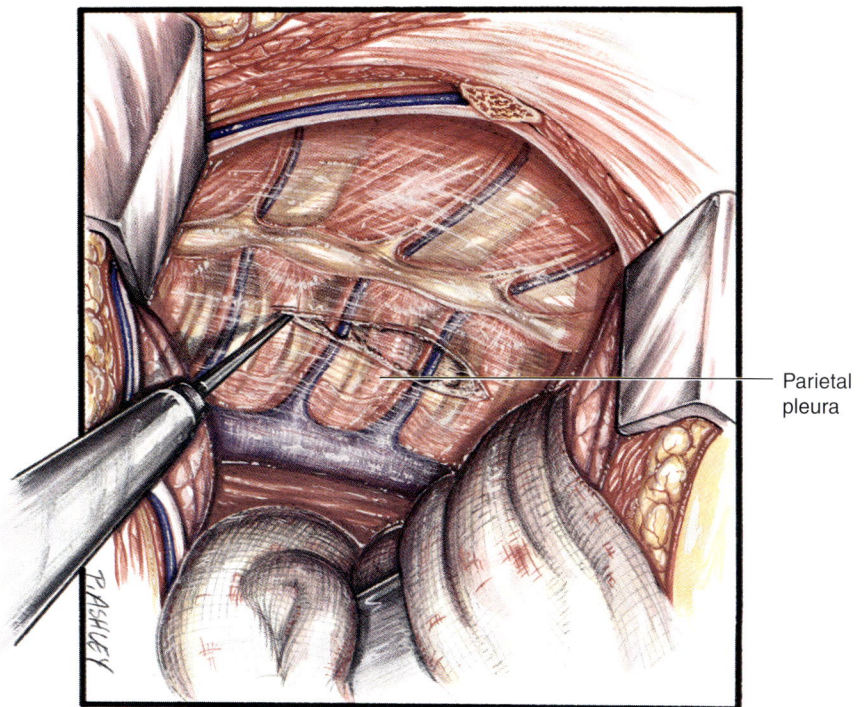

● **Figure 5-12.** Cutting the parietal pleura.

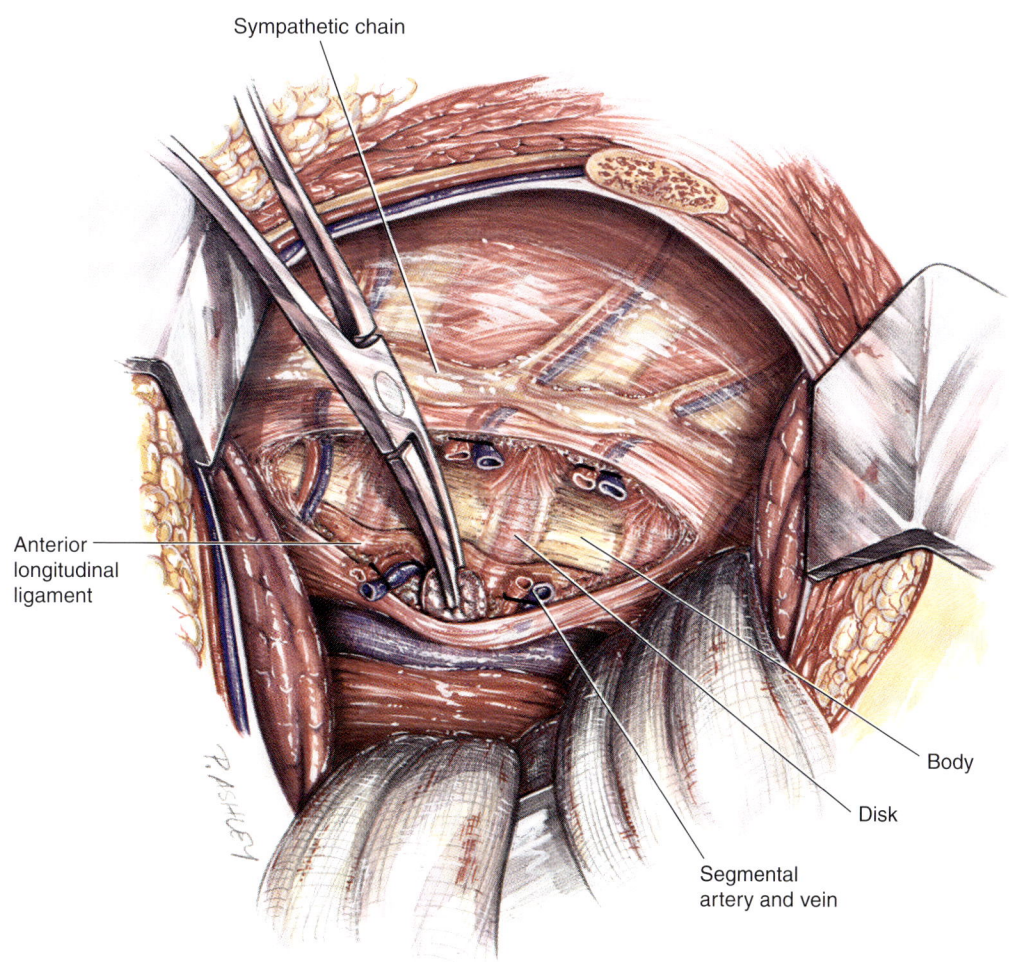

● **Figure 5-13.** After segmental vessels are ligated, blunt dissection is used to clear the parietal pleura.

Sternum-Splitting Approach

Because splitting the sternum alone will not yield any significant exposure of the spine, it must be combined with an anterior cervical incision to obtain any useful exposure.

General endotracheal anesthesia is induced with the patient supine on the operating table. A rolled towel is placed between the scapulae. A vertical incision is made through the skin from the manubrial notch to the tip of the xiphoid process. At its most proximal end, the incision is extended proximally and obliquely to the left. This portion should overlie the anterior border of the left sternocleidomastoid muscle (Figure 5–14). The vertical portion of the incision is carried down through minimal subcutaneous tissue, and the periosteum is incised over the anterior surface of the sternum.

Before the sternum is cut, the retrosternal space must be developed and cleared. The inferior thyroid vein, just proximal to the suprasternal notch, must be avoided. Blunt dissection can be used to reflect the parietal pleura from the posterior surfaces of the costal cartilages and the sternum. The sternum is then cut longitudinally with either an oscillating or a Gigli saw. The anterior neck incision begins through the skin. The platysma muscle is incised the length of the skin incision, and then the anterior sternocleidomastoid fascia is separated from the more medial strap muscles. An interval is found, and then the sternocleidomastoid muscle and carotid sheath are retracted laterally while the strap muscles, esophagus, and trachea are retracted medially. The split sternum is then spread with a self-retaining sternal retractor (Figure 5–15).

After dissection through some retropleural fascia, the retraction allows exposure of the vertebral bodies from C3 to T4: the esophagus, trachea, and right brachiocephalic artery and vein are pulled inferolaterally to the patient's right, and the left carotid sheath, left subcla-

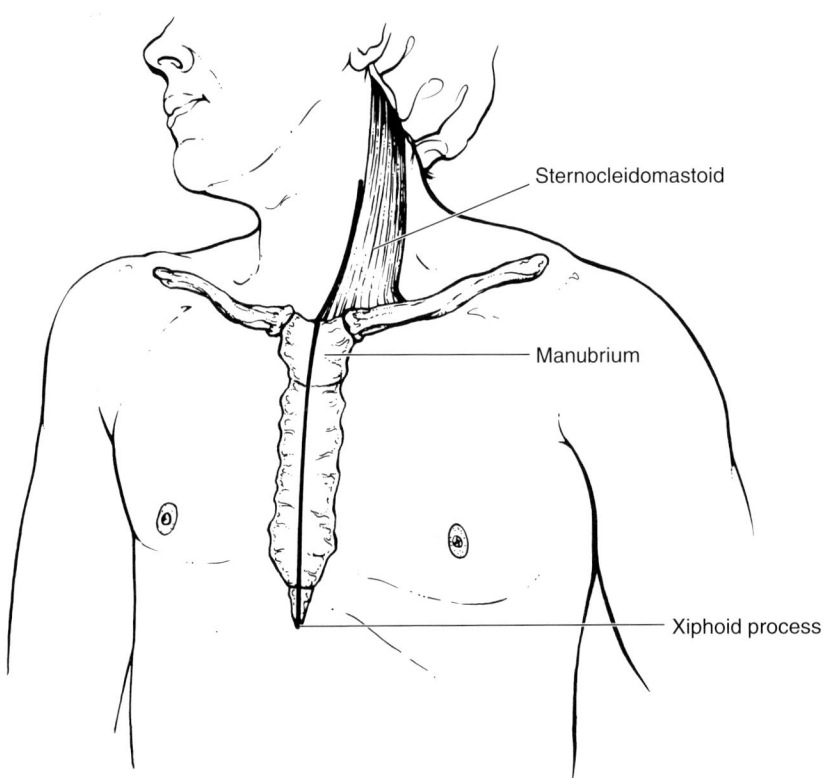

● **Figure 5-14.** Skin incision for sternum splitting approach to cervicothoracic junction.

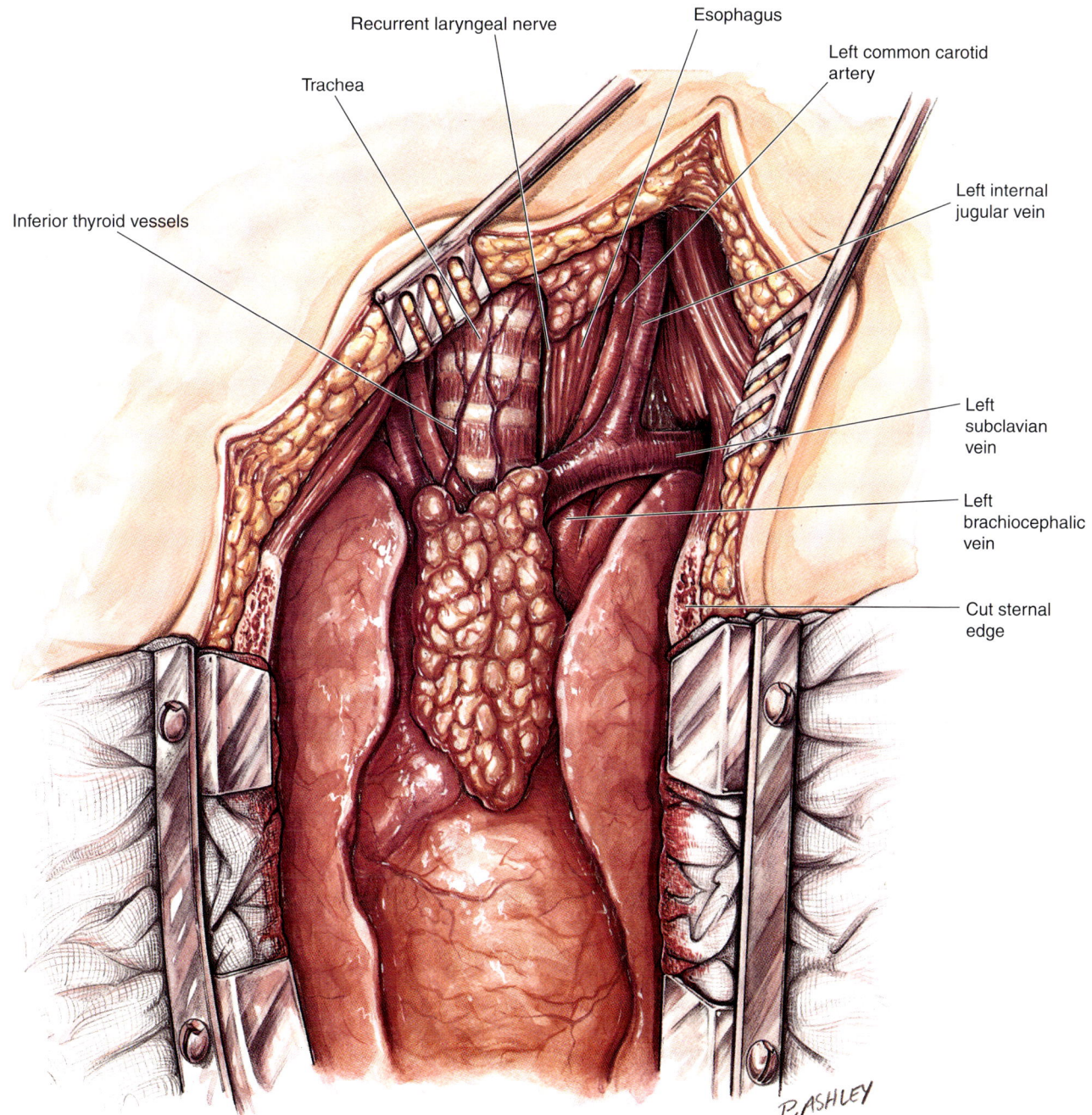

● **Figure 5-15.** After sternal retractor is placed and superficial and middle cervical fasciae are dissected, the cervicothoracic junction is covered only by the outlet vasculature and tracheoesophageal complex.

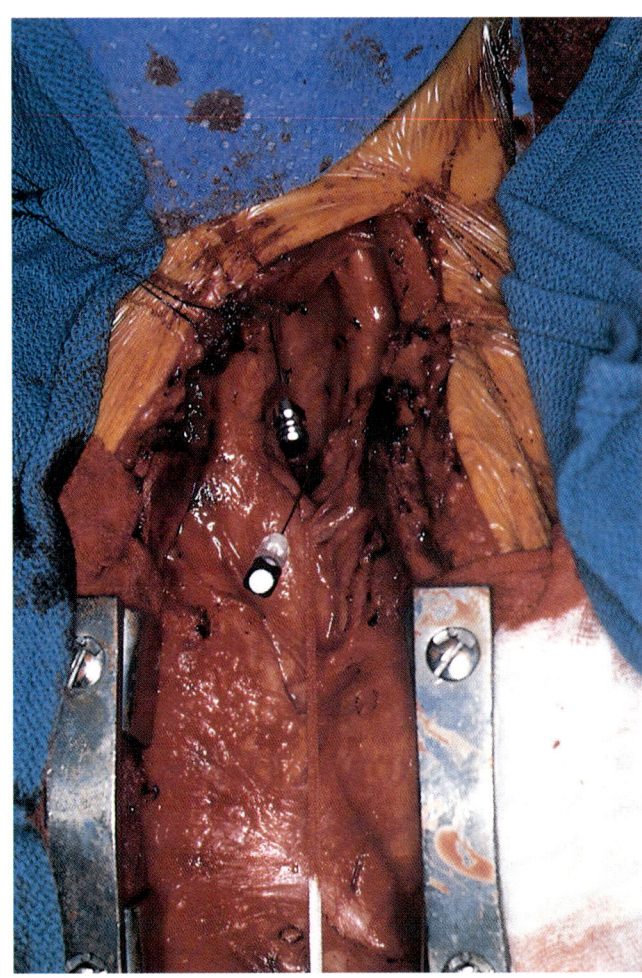

● **Figure 5-16.** Clinical photograph after sternal split with proximal extension showing needles placed into upper thoracic disks.

vian artery, and brachiocephalic vein are retracted inferolaterally to the patient's left. After the prevertebral fascia is dissected free, the vertebral bodies come into view (Figure 5-16).

Complications

Complications of these three approaches are somewhat similar to those seen for the more superior approaches in the neck, with the added morbidity that can be associated with entering the lung or injuring the vessels of the thoracic inlet. Possible injury to the thoracic duct, if the surgeon strays laterally to the carotid or with an aberrant thoracic duct, is a significant complication leading to a lymph leak. Attempts should be made to close the duct if it is injured. Tissues are fragile and very difficult to hold with stitches. Arterial injury in the area of the thoracic inlet can lead to significant blood loss and a need for venous or arterial repair. Recurrent laryngeal nerve injury can lead to voice changes as well as swallowing problems. Unrecognized esophageal injury, as in the upper cervical spine, can be catastrophic, leading to retropharyngeal abscess and mediastinitis. When a sternotomy is attempted, sternal wound infection can be catastrophic and often requires muscular flap reconstruction.

Although we have not seen this in practice, when dissecting the medial clavicle many surgeons worry about shoulder disability from disconnection of the sternoclavicular joint.

BIBLIOGRAPHY

Birch R, Bonney G, Marshall RW: A surgical approach to the cervicothoracic spine. J Bone Joint Surg Br 72:904, 1990.

Charles R, Govender S: Anterior approach to the upper thoracic vertebrae. J Bone Joint Surg Br 71:81, 1989.

Eismont FJ, Bohlman HH, Soni PL: Pyogenic and fungal vertebral osteomyelitis with paralysis. J Bone Joint Surg Am 65:19, 1983.

Felding JW, Stillwell WT: Anterior cervical approach to the upper thoracic spine. Spine 1:158, 1976.

Hodgson AR, Stock FE, Fang HSY, Ong GB: Anterior spinal fusion: The operative approach and pathological findings in 412 patients with Pott's disease of the spine. Br J Surg 48:172, 1960.

Kurz LT, Pursel S, Herkowitz HN: Modified anterior approach to the cervicothoracic junction. Spine 16(Suppl):542, 1991.

Micheli IJ, Hood RW: Anterior exposure of the cervicothoracic spine using a combined cervical and thoracic approach. J Bone Joint Surg Am 65:992, 1983.

Standefer M, Hardy RW, Marks K, Cosgrove CM: Chondromyxoid fibroma of the cervical spine: A case report with a review of the literature and a description of an operative approach to the lower anterior cervical spine. Neurosurgery 11:288, 1982.

Sundaresan N, DiGiacinto GV: Surgical approaches to the cervicothoracic junction. In Sundaresan N, Schmidek HH, Schiller AL, Rosenthal DI (eds): Tumors of the Spine: Diagnosis and Clinical Management p 358. Philadelphia, WB Saunders, 1990.

Sundaresan N, Shah J, Feghall J: The trans-sternal approach to the upper thoracic vertebra. Am J Surg 198:473, 1984.

Sundaresan N, Shah J, Foley KM, Rosen G: An anterior surgical approach to the upper thoracic vertebrae. J Neurosurg 61:686, 1984.

CHAPTER 6

POSTERIOR CERVICAL EXPOSURES

Thomas G. Andreshak, M.D.
Howard S. An, M.D.

The posterior approach to the cervical spine allows a complete exposure of the posterior elements of the cervical spine and is one of the safest and most utilized exposures for the treatment of problems of the entire cervical spine. Indications for the posterior cervical approach include posterior cervical fusions, exploration and excision of tumors, decompression of nerve roots or the spinal cord, and treatment of posterior element fractures and dislocations. The vast majority of posterior procedures involve some element of stabilization and fusion, and these can be performed from the occiput to the thoracic spine without a complexity of anatomic structures to become entangled as in anterior cervical procedures.

The posterior approach may also be indicated for procedures at the atlantoaxial articulation. These procedures include stabilization for traumatic and late instabilities and various fractures of C1 or C2, including type II odontoid fractures. The surgeon must choose the most appropriate form of treatment for these problems, and this depends on the pathologic process present, the surgeon's skill and familiarity with the technique, and the mechanism of injury. The utilitarian posterior approach is discussed along with its relevant anatomic landmarks, specifics on various surgical techniques using the posterior approach, and the potential complications that can be encountered.

Clinical Anatomy

The bony landmarks are the key to determining that the surgery will be at the appropriate levels. The spinous processes are palpable posteriorly, with those of C2, C7, and T1 the most evident. Because of the narrowed interspaces and the inferior sloping of the spinous processes, overdissection of the posterior spine may lead to unnecessary fusion of uninvolved levels.

The posterior cervical spine is covered with thick muscular layers, and a direct approach through the muscular planes is used. The superficial layer of the deep cervical fascia is found investing the trapezius posteriorly and fuses with the intermuscular septum and the spinous processes. The prevertebral fascia continues posteriorly from the intermuscular septum and inserts on the vertebral spinous processes.

The ligamentum nuchae, a fibrous septum with few elastic fibers, inserts on the spinous processes and the cervical paraspinal muscles and in humans provides minimal support.[1] The supraspinous ligaments are essentially in continuity with the ligamentum nuchae and spinous processes and blend with the interspinous ligaments anteriorly. These ligaments are poorly defined in the upper cervical spine and become well developed in the lower. The ligamentum nuchae acts as the primary origin or insertion point for most of the muscles in the posterior neck.

The trapezius lies most superficial just deep to the superficial fascia. The rhomboid minor and serratus attach to the seventh cervical spinous process and course distally. The intermediate muscles deep to the trapezius include the splenius capitis and splenius cervicis. The deep muscle group includes the semispinalis capitis and cervicis, and it is penetrated by the greater occipital nerve. The deepest group of muscles is the iliocostalis and the longissimus cervicis (Figure 6–1). Smaller muscles that assist in extending the head are found at the occipitocervical junction and include the rectus capitis posterior major and minor and the superior and inferior capitis obliques, which all attach to the spinous process or transverse process of the axis (Figure 6–2).

The posterior approach uses an internervous plane in the midline that separates the muscles from the segmental innervation supplied by the right and left posterior rami of the cervical nerves. The remainder of the dissection is in this plane, and denervation is not a problem, owing to the segmental pattern.

The atlantoaxial and occipitocervical regions have the potential for a significant risk of complications and operative morbidity if the anatomy peculiar to each region is not under-

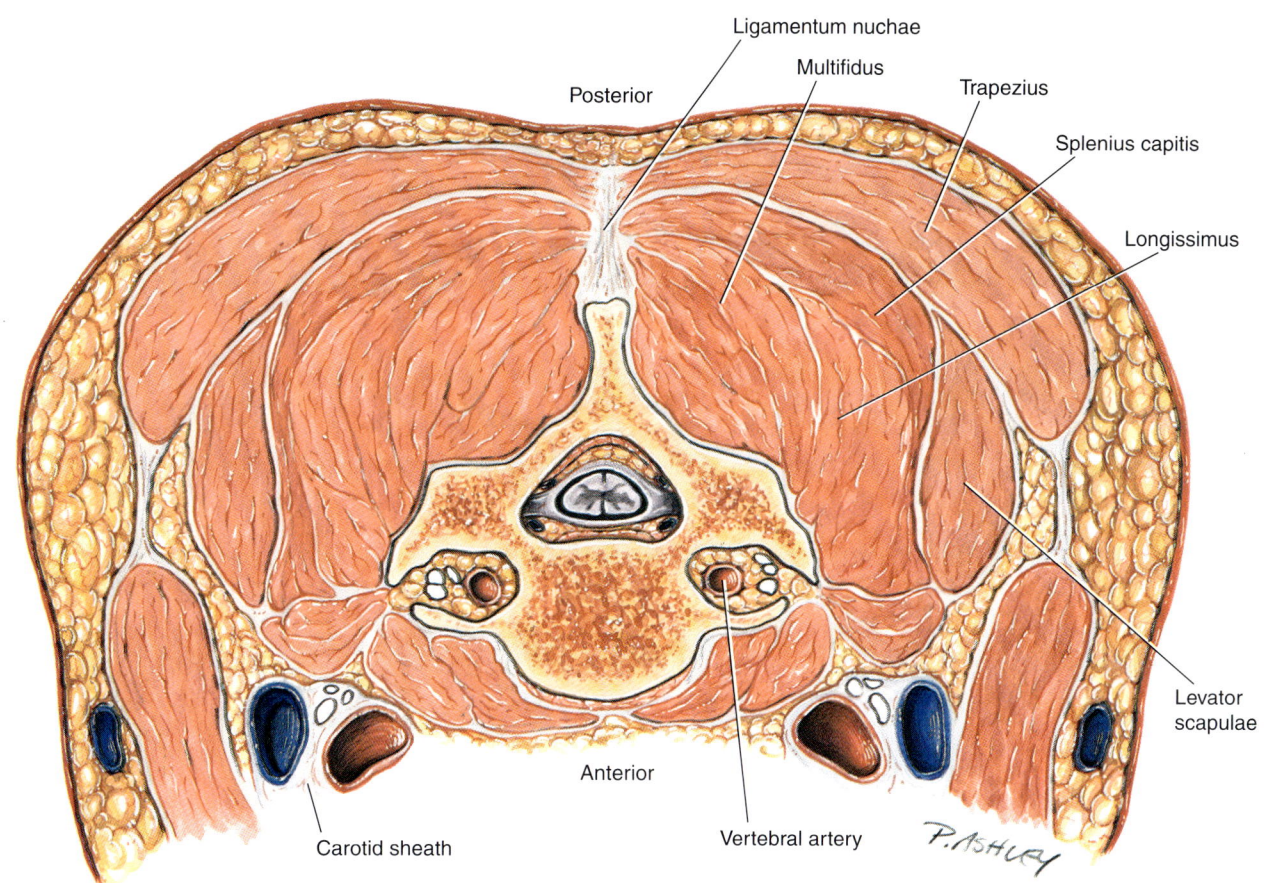

● **Figure 6-1.** A cross section of the neck demonstrates the direct midline approach to the cervical spine and the attachments of the paraspinal muscles to the posterior tubercle and ligamentum nuchae. The individual muscle layers are bound by the cervical fascial layers, which all attach to the ligamentum nuchae. Note the paucity of vital structures that are encountered posteriorly.

stood before undertaking the exposure. The course of the vertebral arteries should be thoroughly understood. The course of the artery along the posterior arch of C1 makes it prone to injury if the dissection on the posterior arch is performed more than 1.5 cm from the midline of the posterior tubercle. This distance is only 1 cm in the child. The posterior ring of C1 is also very fragile and small, and it is therefore prone to fracture if vigorous dissecting of the ligamentum flavum is performed. Slippage of a periosteal elevator into the canal can occur on the narrow posterior arch if caution is not used. A great number of the muscles in the upper cervical spine attach to the spinous process of C2, and these should be preserved if this level is not involved in the fusion to prevent the possibility of instability developing at C2-C3.

Posterior Approach

The posterior approach requires careful positioning to minimize the risk of neurologic injury and maximize exposure of the required level. The use of somatosensory evoked potentials should be routine for myelopathy or with neurologic deficits. The intubation should be controlled and the head stabilized with Mayfield tongs or a holder to permit atraumatic turning to the prone position. A Stryker frame may need to be used in traumatic situations. The elbows and ulnar nerves must be well padded, and an axillary or chest roll will avert

84 • SURGICAL APPROACHES TO THE SPINE

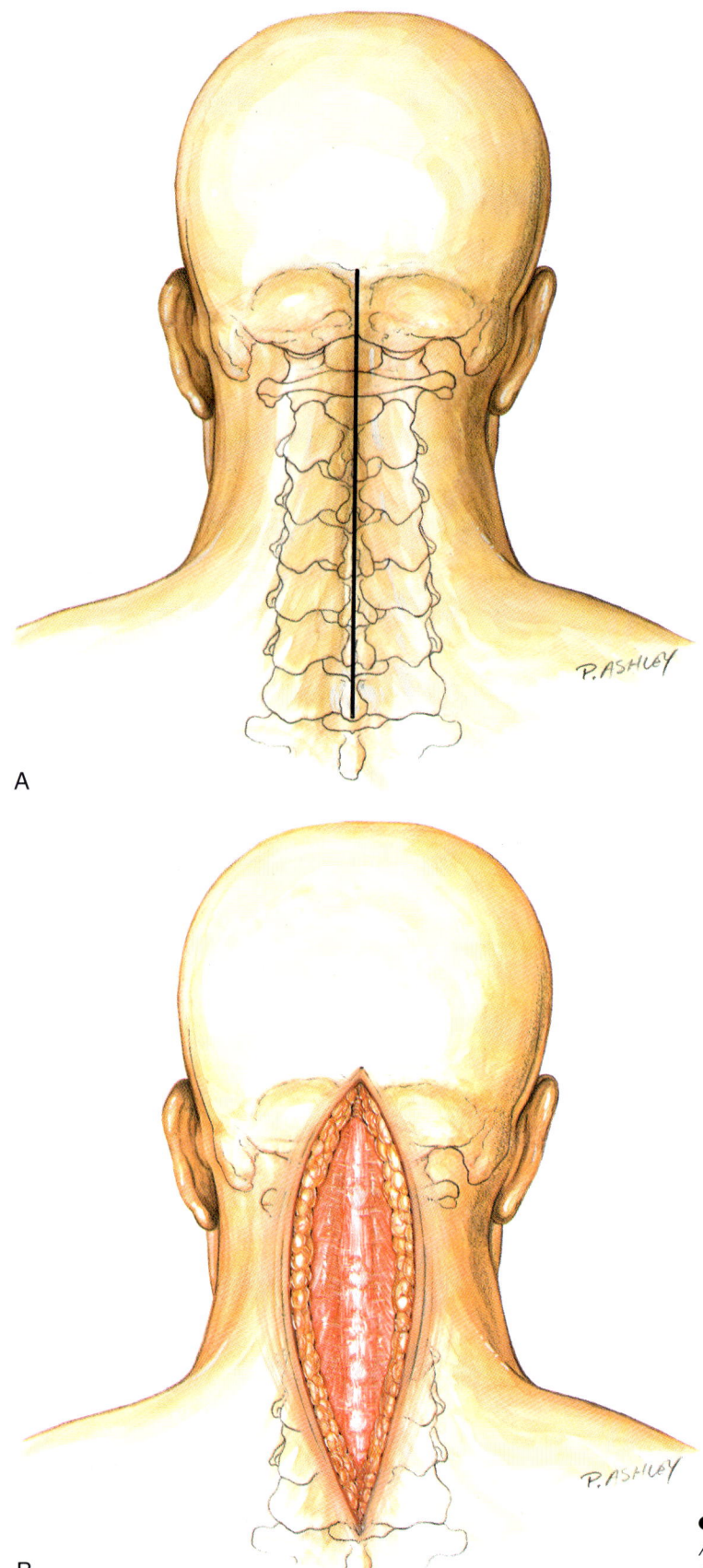

● **Figure 6-2.** *A* through *D*, Posterior approach. *A,* Skin incision over midline. *B,* Extensive posterior exposure from C2 distally is very dry if performed by splitting ligamentum nuchae.

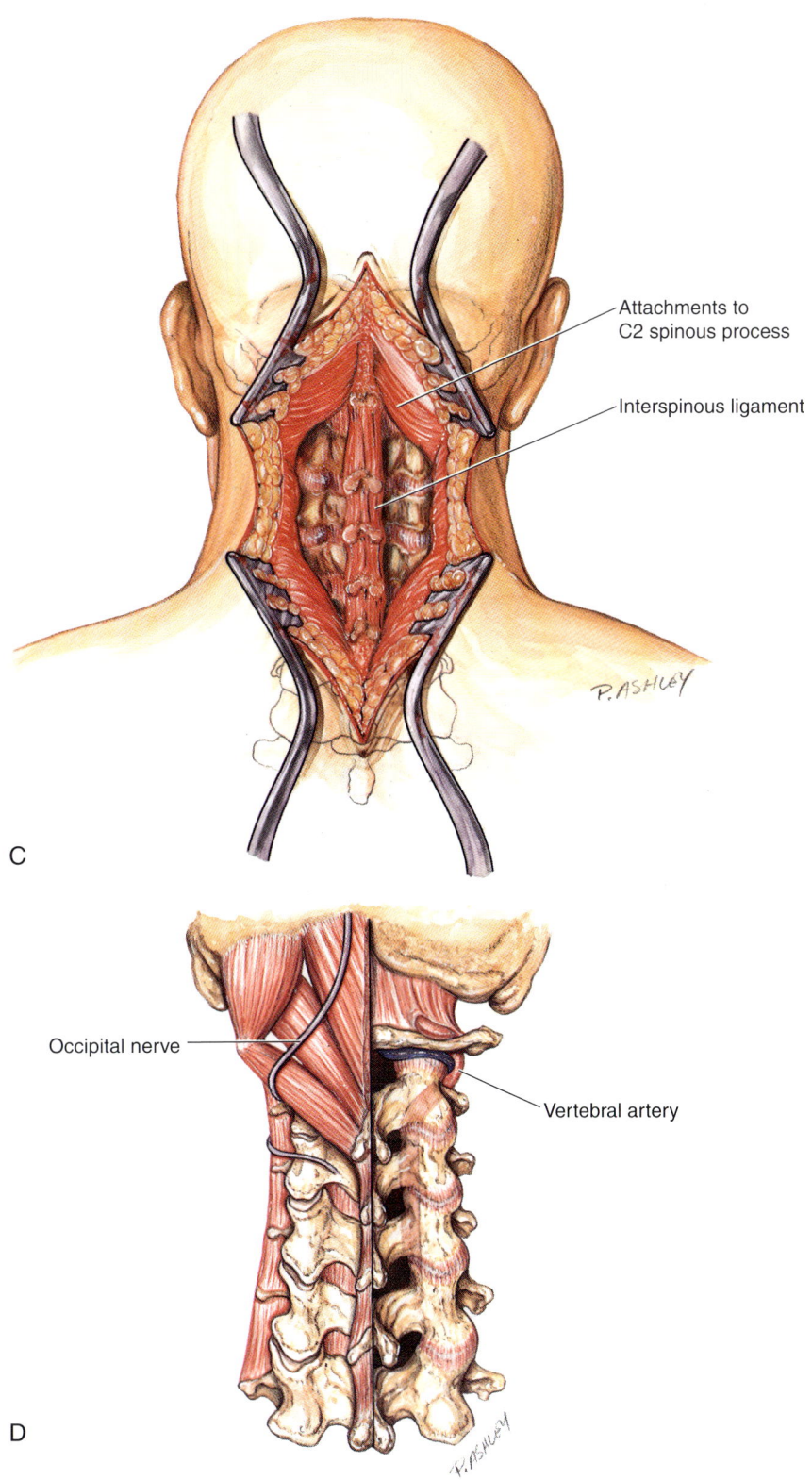

● **Figure 6-2.** *Continued C,* Interspinous ligament is preserved as are attachments to C2. *D,* The posterior approach should be midline to avoid injury to the occipital nerves or the vertebral artery. The posterior muscles of the occipitocervical region form a triangle that provides a landmark to the location of the vertebral artery. These muscles provide stability to the C2 articulations and should not be dissected off the spinous process of C2 to prevent any late instability from occurring.

any undue pressure on the brachial plexus. The head and neck should then be positioned, if appropriate, in the degree of flexion or extension to facilitate the proposed procedure. A reverse Trendelenburg position minimizes venous bleeding and lower cerebrospinal fluid pressure (Figures 6–3 and 6–4). Care must be taken to avoid any pressure on the eyes.

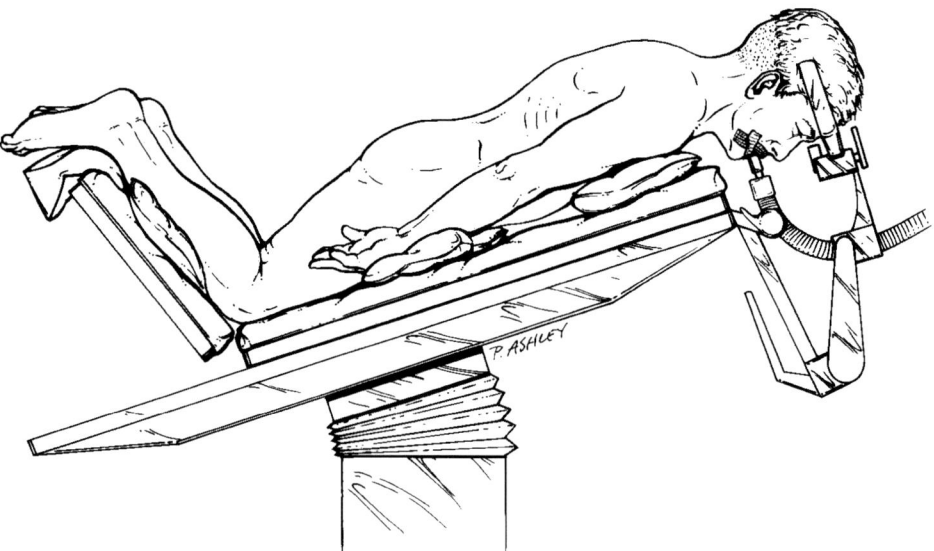

● **Figure 6-3.** The position for most posterior cervical spine surgery is the reverse Trendelenburg position. Note the head tongs or holder to stabilize the head and neck. The chest should be supported by rolls to allow expansion, and the knees should be bent to relax the sciatic nerve and stabilize the patient.

The posterior approach uses a longitudinal midline incision that extends above and below the segments required for the procedure. This extension of the skin and subcutaneous tissues is necessary because the skin of the posterior neck is less mobile and thicker for retraction. The skin is incised sharply, and then electrocautery is used to dissect to the ligamentum nuchae. The ligamentum nuchae is incised in the midline, and dissection is done subperiosteally down the spinous processes. It is prudent to stay subperiosteal because the bifid nature of the spinous processes may result in a bulbous expanse and the dissection may

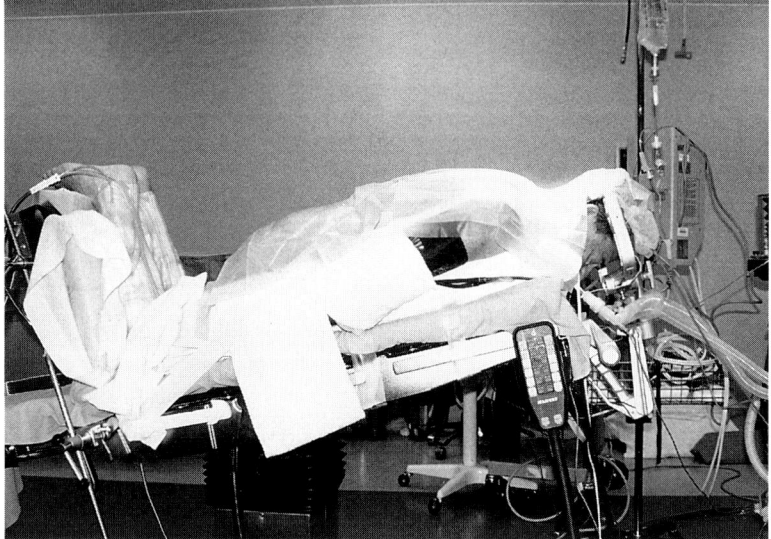

● **Figure 6-4.** Patient in reverse Trendelenburg position for posterior foraminotomy. The position minimizes bleeding during procedures by allowing venous drainage.

err into the paraspinal musculature. A superficial plexus of veins may be encountered and should be cauterized as needed (Figure 6–5). A wide, flat periosteal elevator such as a Cobb elevator should be used to carefully dissect the paraspinal muscles off the spinous processes, using the electrocautery knife for the attachments to the interspinous ligament. The preoperative films should be examined for any evidence of spina bifida or other bony defect to avoid inadvertent entry of an instrument into the canal.

The laminae of the cervical spine are angulated at 45 degrees from medial to lateral and cephalad. In the cervical spine, the laminae do not override each other as much as in the thoracic spine; therefore, the interlaminar space may be inadvertently penetrated if caution is not taken during the exposure of the laminae. A "hill" is encountered that is the lateral mass that includes the facet joint. Care should be taken at the lateral edge of the joint as the nerve root and vertebral artery lie anterior to the spinolamellar membrane of the adjoining transverse processes. Vigorous decortication or stripping may damage the thin bone and, subsequently, the nerve root and vertebral artery. The segmental artery at the lateral edge of the facet joints may be cauterized as it exits between the transverse processes.

Various retractors may be used to facilitate exposure, and a small Taylor retractor may be used at the lateral edge of the articular mass to facilitate a unilateral exposure (Figure 6–6). To safeguard the nerve roots, care must be taken not to insert the tip of the Taylor retractor too anteriorly.

After the appropriate procedure has been performed, the closure includes an initial

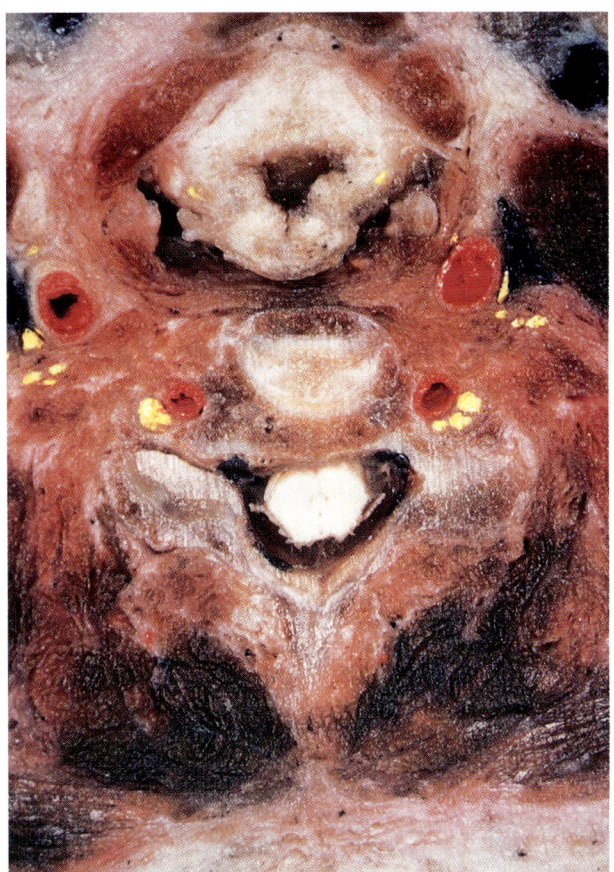

● **Figure 6-5.** Cadaveric cross section at the C4-C5 level. The vertebral artery lies anterior to the facet joints and articular masses. The midline can be seen to be relatively avascular with numerous small venous plexi seen in the muscular layers. Dissection should remain subperiosteal and therefore minimize bleeding. Note the epidural plexus of veins seen in blue directly adherent to the lamina.

irrigation of the wound and then a tight closure in layers, with the muscle and ligamentum nuchae closed separately to avoid dead space. Nonabsorbable sutures may be used to close the ligamentum nuchae. A strong suture should be used on the ligamentum nuchae because the incision tends to spread with time from the strong broad pull of the trapezius. A bloodless field should be accomplished before closure by cautery to minimize the formation of a hematoma, which may compromise any of the neural structures. A drain is placed deep and removed in 48 hours.

Posterior Foraminotomy and Laminectomy

In decompressive procedures, all of the dissection is done under 3.5× loupe magnification and with headlamp illumination. The head is stabilized with Mayfield tongs to protect the spine from extraneous motion during the surgical procedure, and somatosensory-evoked potentials are monitored routinely in myelopathy and decompressive cases. The table is placed at 45 degrees of reverse Trendelenburg to minimize venous bleeding. The sitting position is an option, but air embolism may be a complication. The head is positioned in

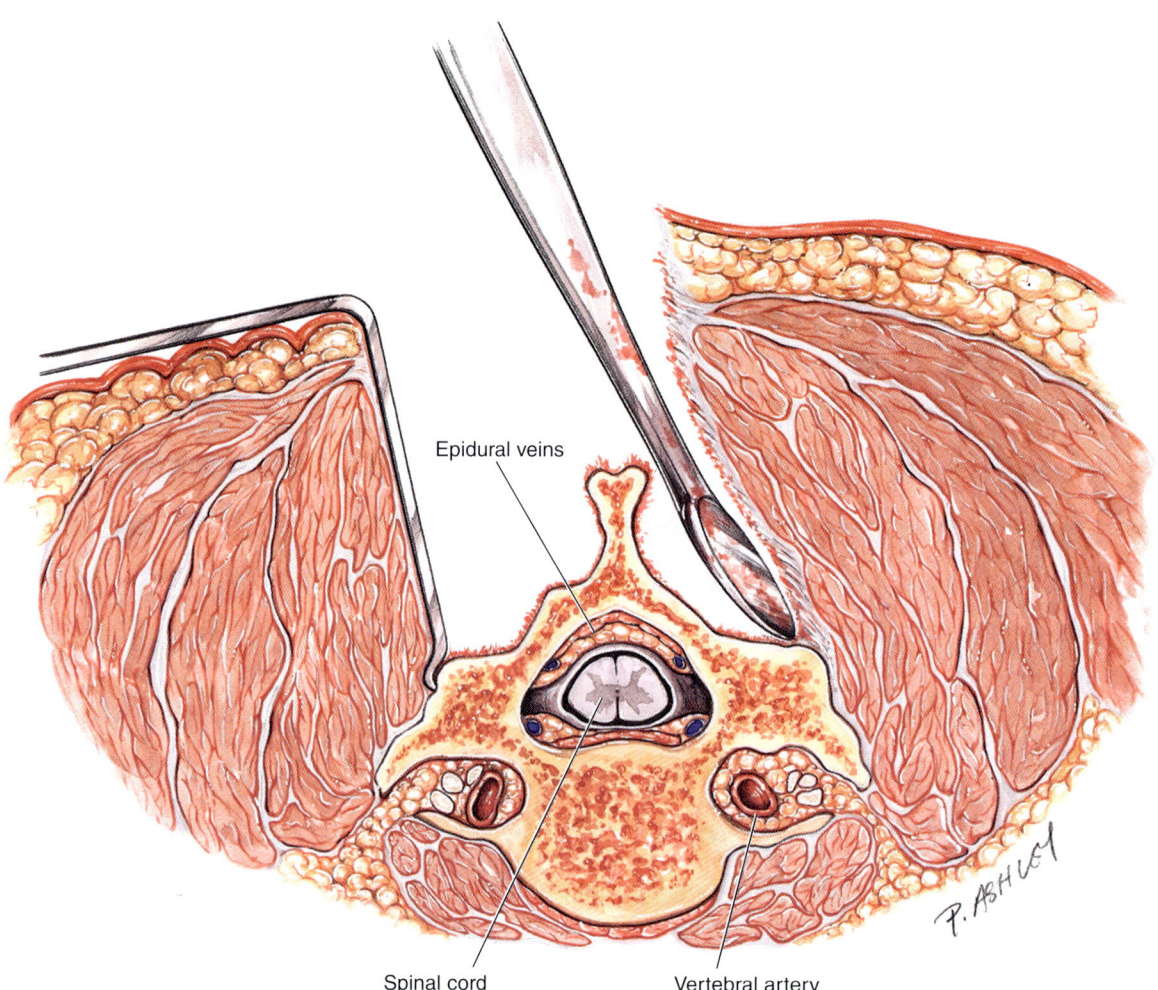

● **Figure 6-6.** The posterior dissection is performed subperiosteally along the lamina out to the lateral margin of the lateral masses. The paraspinal muscles are removed unilaterally or bilaterally as needed. Note the single Taylor retractor on the border of the lateral mass for a unilateral approach.

flexion unless the patient has cervical spondylotic myelopathy, in which case the head is placed in neutral position. This prevents any cord compression from the spondylotic bars.

The approach is midline, and the dissection is subperiosteal out to the lateral edge of the articular masses. A Taylor retractor is placed lateral to the lateral mass; the retractor should not be placed too deep to possibly impinge the nerve root. A Kerrison rongeur may be used to remove a portion of the inferior and superior laminae. Partial facetectomy or foraminotomy is performed by thinning the facets with a power bur. We use an air-powered

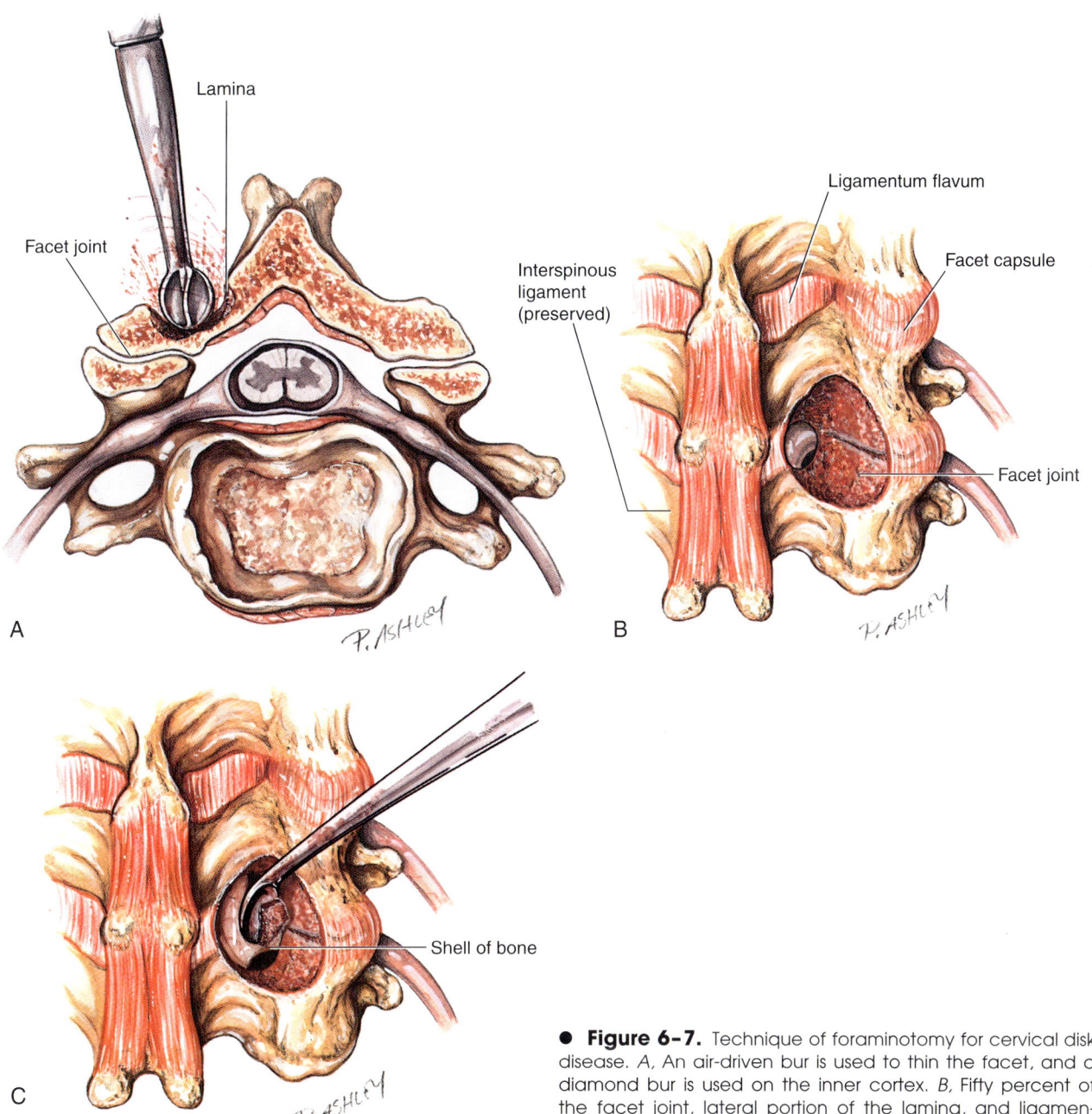

● **Figure 6-7.** Technique of foraminotomy for cervical disk disease. *A,* An air-driven bur is used to thin the facet, and a diamond bur is used on the inner cortex. *B,* Fifty percent of the facet joint, lateral portion of the lamina, and ligamentum flavum are removed. *C,* A small, angled curet is used to remove the remaining shell of bone.

high-speed bur to thin the cortex over the foramen or laminae involved and then finish the thinning with a diamond-tipped bur (Figure 6–7). Caution during the use of power instruments is vital. The surgeon should hold the instrument with both hands and rest the wrists or forearms on the patient carefully to obtain proprioceptive feedback and avert any unexpected deviation of the instrument.

The lamina and thinned bone should then be gently lifted off the cord or nerve with small, angled curets. Placement of a Kerrison rongeur under the lamina may result in injury to the neural elements. Once the bone is removed, the dura and nerve root are exposed and the abundant venous plexus in the cervical canal may need to be cauterized with the bipolar cautery to minimize bleeding. Meticulous hemostasis is essential to avoid complications, owing to lack of exposure or hematoma formation, which may lead to an epidural hematoma and spinal cord compression. The nerve root may be gently retracted if necessary, but manipulation of the nerve root may cause neurologic injuries. The nerve root is usually well decompressed by removal of the overlying facet, and removal of disk material is not routine by the authors unless the herniated disk is acute, soft, and large.

Laminectomy is performed by thinning of the cortices at the laminar and facet junction with a power bur (Figure 6–8). A small Kerrison rongeur may be used to finish the cut, and a small angled curet is then used to lift the lamina. Somatosensory-evoked potentials should be monitored in most cases of laminectomy. The adherent, underlying venous plexus should be cauterized to minimize hematoma formation.

Approach to C1-C2

The posterior approach to the C1-C2 complex is indicated for spinal fusions, decompression, and treatment of tumors. The head should be slightly flexed to open the space between the ring of C1 and the occiput. The external occipital protuberance and the spinous process of C2 can be palpated and the incision made from the inion caudad approximately 8 cm. The dissection is continued through the ligamentum nuchae, and the paraspinal muscles are stripped from the posterior of C3 to the occiput. The posterior tubercle of the atlas is deeper anterior than the occiput and C2 spinous process, and the facet joint of C1-C2 lies about

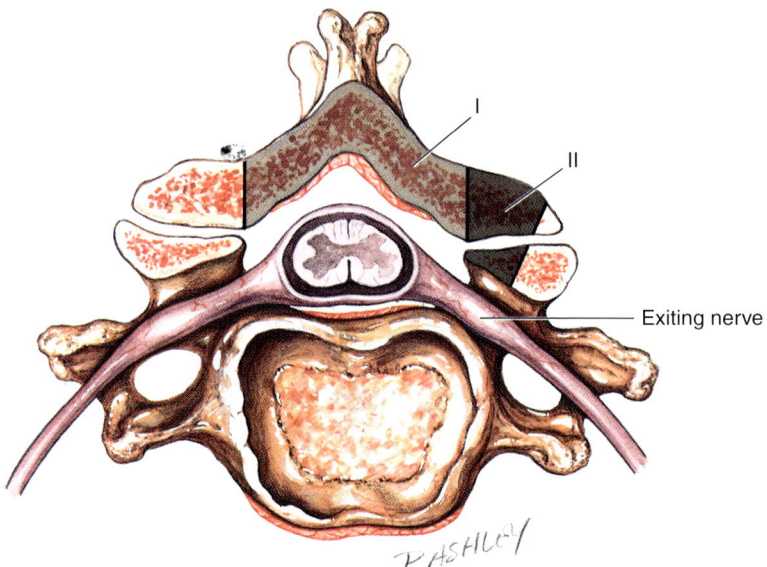

● **Figure 6-8.** This illustration shows the area of bone removal for laminectomy (I) and partial facetectomy (II).

2.5 cm anterior than the C2-C3 joint (Figure 6–9). The use of a large broad elevator to dissect the posterior paracervical muscles from the arches of C1 and C2 will help avert plunging into the spinal canal. A small curet can be helpful to remove the muscular attachments on the bifid spinous process of C2 while stabilizing the arch of C2. Rarely is the removal of the atlantoaxial ligament or atlanto-occipital membrane indicated. Careful separation of the membrane or ligament from the bone is all that is usually needed to pass sublaminar wires. This can be performed with a small angled curet or a small Freer elevator. One should use caution at the inferior edge of the foramen magnum because uncontrollable bleeding may be encountered. An additional technique to strip the arch of C1 or C2 is to cut the periosteum along the arch and then use a small Freer elevator to lift the periosteum. This allows the vertebral artery to be additionally protected at the lateral margins. Dissection should not proceed laterally from the midline more than 1.5 cm in an adult nor 1 cm in a child to avoid injuring the vertebral artery as it courses over the arch of the atlas and pierces the lateral angle of the posterior atlanto-occipital membrane (Figure 6–10). The spinal cord should never be retracted at this level because death from respiratory paralysis can result. The greater occipital nerve (C2) and the third occipital nerve cross the field and course laterally in the paracervical muscles. Subperiosteal dissection and avoidance of a lateral dissection should prevent injury to these nerves.

The spinal canal at C1-C2 is very capacious and allows the extensive motion that is required at that level. Passage of sublaminar wires at the C1-C2 level is not uncommon, but passage at other levels is associated with increased risk of neurologic injury. The Brooks fusion is preferred in extension injuries, whereas the Gallie fusion is good for flexion injuries and avoids the passage of sublaminar wires under the C2 arch by utilizing the spinous process. Greater rotational stability is provided by a Brooks fusion.

We prefer the modified Gallie fusion as described by Simmons[2] and use an H-shaped graft from the iliac crest (Figure 6–11). The wire is doubled and passed from inferior to superior under the arch of C1, and the graft is shaped to fit the space between C1 and C2. The wire is then passed over the graft, securing it, and is looped around the spinous process.

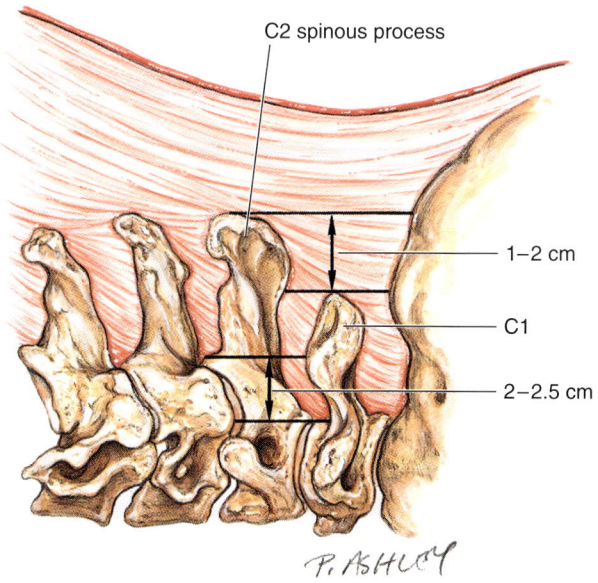

● **Figure 6-9.** The location of the arch of C1 to the spinous process of C2 is crucial during the dissection to the C1-C2 junction. The posterior arch of C1 lies 1 to 2 cm anterior to the spinous process of C2 and the facet joint of C2-C3 lies 2 to 2.5 cm posterior to the facet of C1-C2. Dissection should be performed carefully on the fragile ring of the atlas.

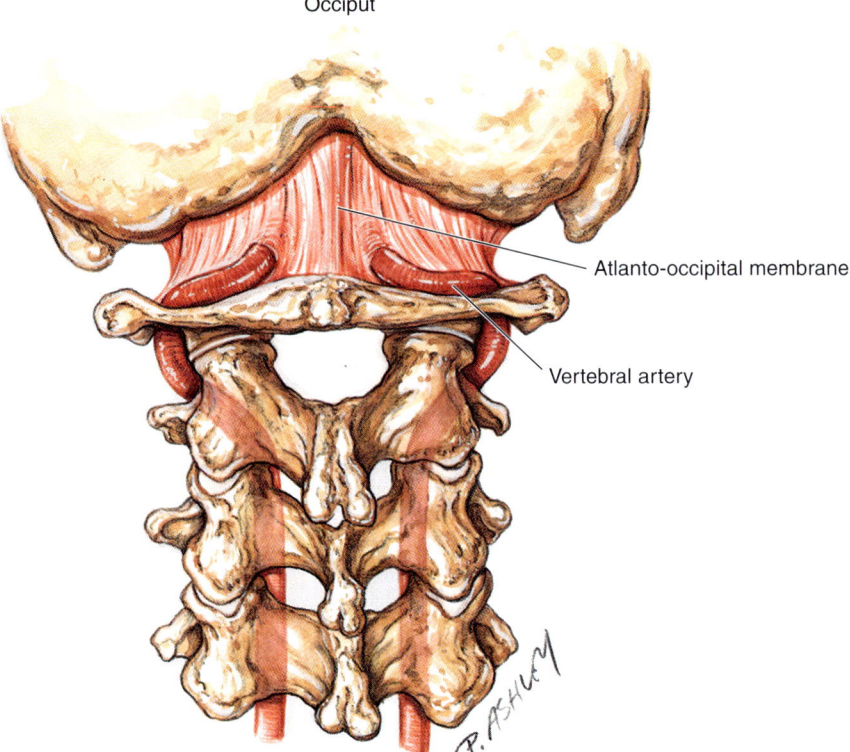

● **Figure 6-10.** The vertebral artery lies along the posterolateral border of the rim of the atlas and is protected by the posterior atlanto-occipital membrane directly midline. It is vulnerable to injury as it exits the foramen transversarium at the C1-C2 facet joint and the lateral margin of C1. Dissection should not be performed laterally more than 1.5 cm from the midline in the adult. Note the wide interspaces between the occiput, C1, and C2.

The ends are then securely tightened over the graft. The graft should have a contoured surface to fit in the groove of C1 and C2, which adds stability to the segment. Additional cancellous graft is placed in the remaining defects to facilitate fusion. Difficulty in wire passage has led to new techniques and wires that facilitate the procedure and minimize the complications (Figures 6–12 and 6–13). A flexible wire such as Sof'wire (Codman, Johnson & Johnson, Randolph, MA) allows contouring and passage under the arch of C1 with control in fixation and tightening that a rigid wire lacks.

The Brooks fusion is more complex requiring the passage of doubled wires of 24-gauge steel under the arch of C1 and C2 (Figures 6–14 and 6–15). This is usually easiest if passed under C1 first then C2. The use of a small right-angled clamp may facilitate the passage of the wires. Two wedge-shaped iliac crest grafts, approximately 1.25 by 3.5 cm, are fashioned and beveled to fit the interval between the arch of C1 and the lamina of C2. A notch is cut in the superior and inferior cortical edges to secure the wires, and the wires are then tightened securely and lock the graft in place, with additional graft added for optimization of fusion. The wires may be passed through the grafts as described by Meyer.[3] A triple wire technique may also be used for the upper cervical spine in addition to its many uses for the lower cervical spine.

A transarticular fixation of the atlantoaxial joint is described by Magerl for use in those patients with a deficient posterior arch or to improve biomechanical strength.[4] This procedure requires meticulous dissection at the level of the facet joints but obtains a rigid fixation. A midline exposure of the upper cervical spine is made, and K-wires are used to retract the soft tissues containing the greater occipital nerve and associated venous plexus. The screws

Text continued on page 98

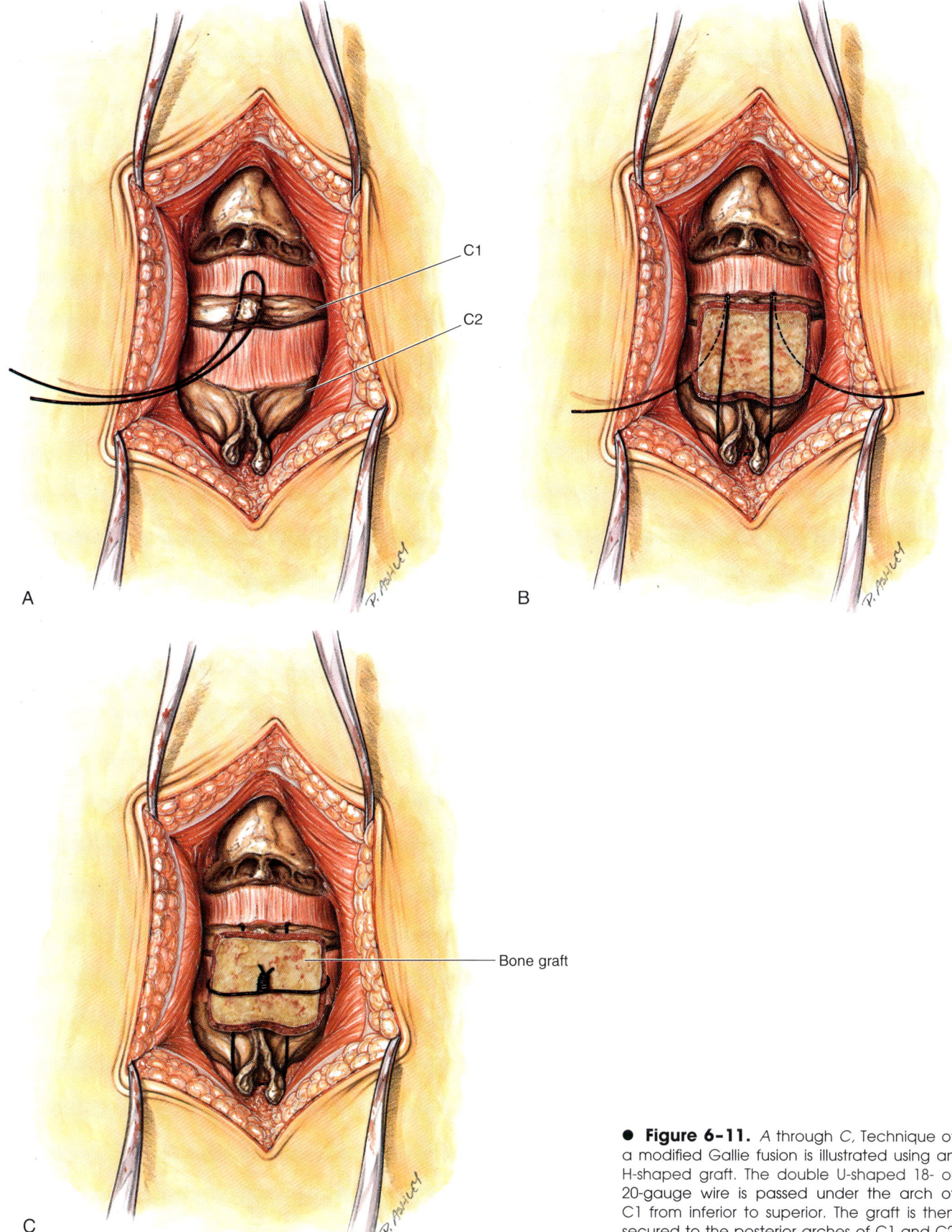

● **Figure 6-11.** A through C, Technique of a modified Gallie fusion is illustrated using an H-shaped graft. The double U-shaped 18- or 20-gauge wire is passed under the arch of C1 from inferior to superior. The graft is then secured to the posterior arches of C1 and C2 with the wire.

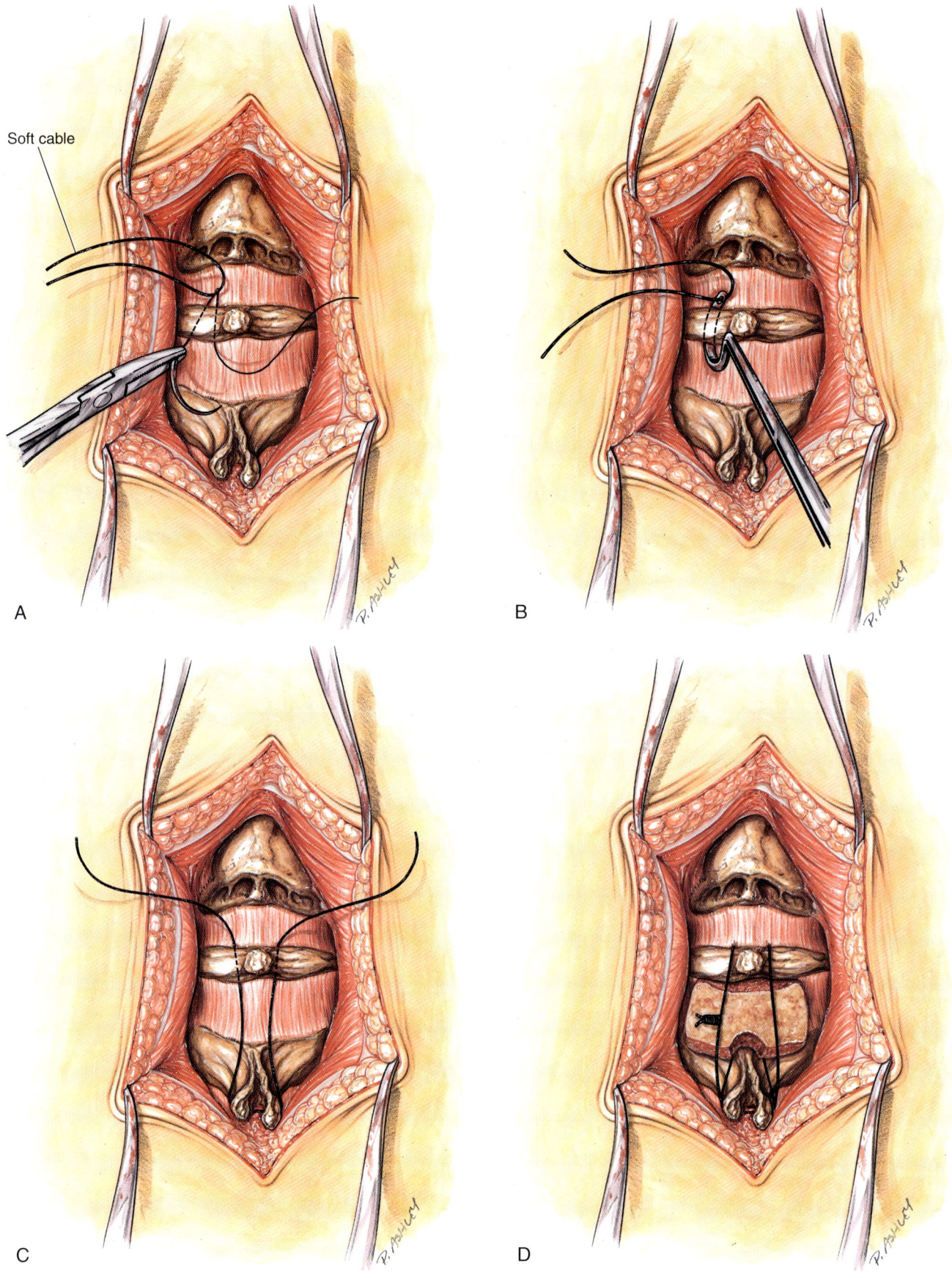

● **Figure 6-12.** Modified Gallie fusion can be performed by using a flexible wire to allow better conformity to bony structures with minimal distortion. *A,* The sublaminar wire passage may be enhanced with a specially designed cable guide. *B,* A suture may be used to pass the flexible wire because its conformity to the bony contours allows minimal trauma to the dura or cord during passage from superior to inferior. *C,* Cable is looped around the spinous process. *D,* Bone graft is contoured and positioned.

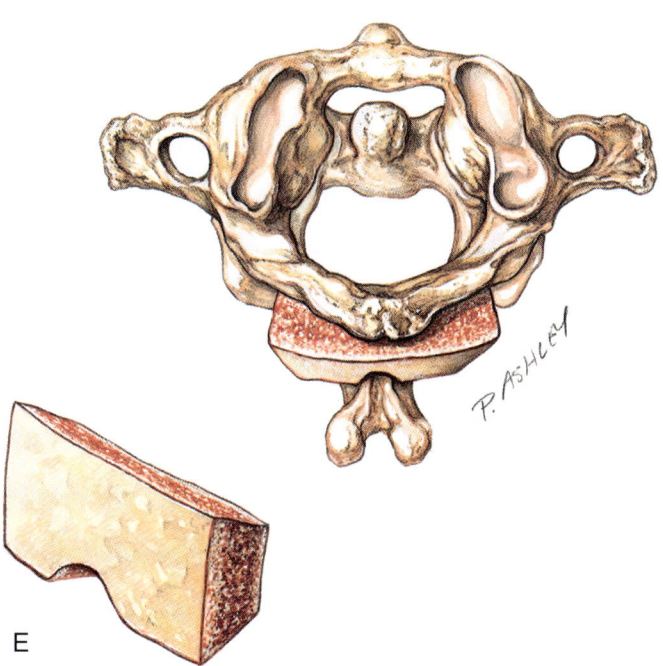

● **Figure 6-12.** *Continued E,* Superior view of graft. The cable is then used to secure the graft.

96 • SURGICAL APPROACHES TO THE SPINE

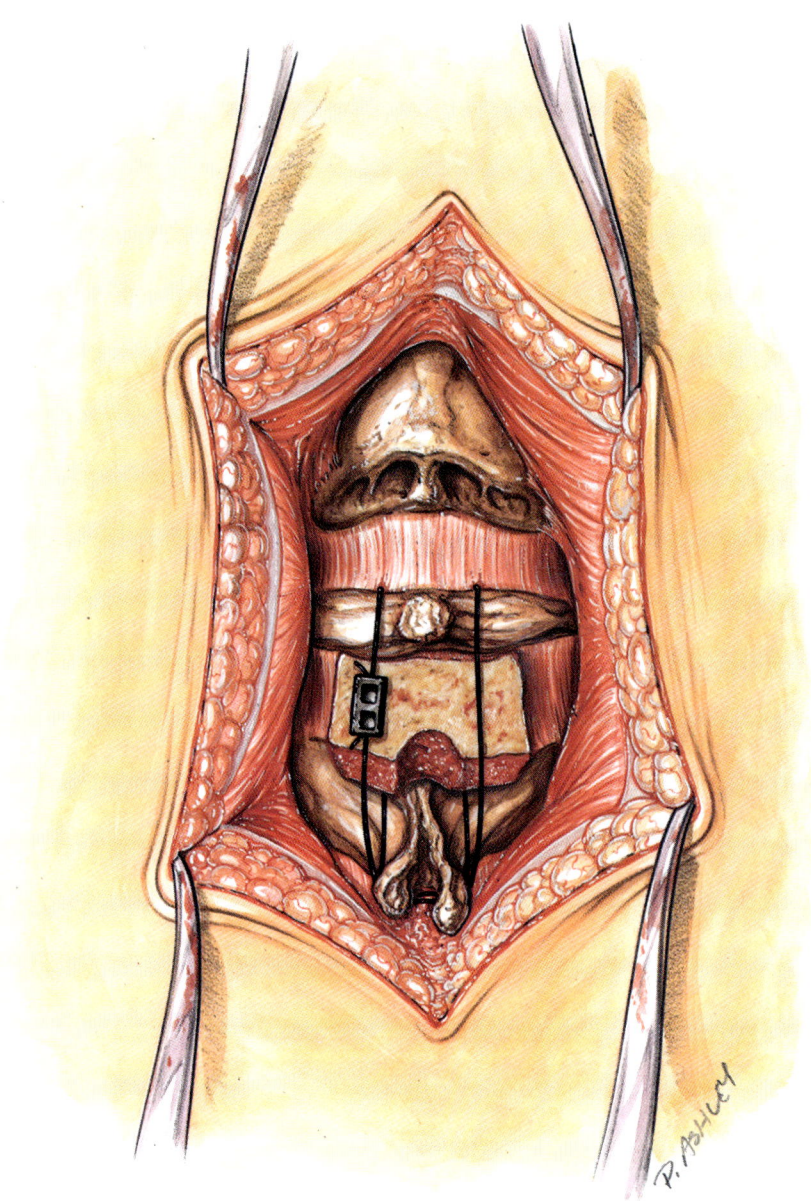

● **Figure 6-13.** Modified Gallie fusion with cable and locking cinch in place. This construct allows controlled tension to be placed on the graft.

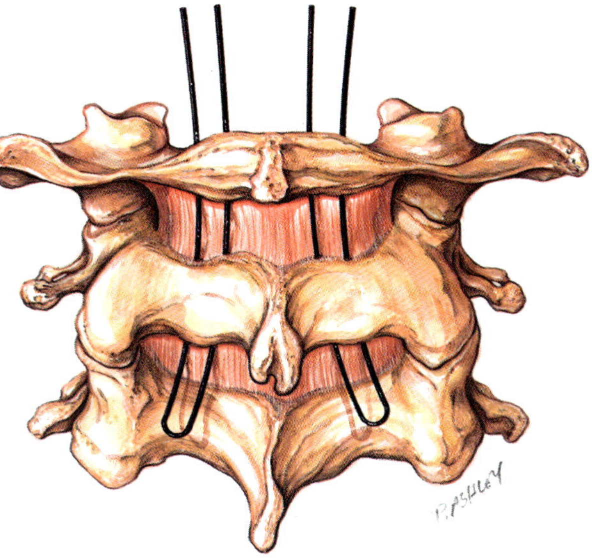

● **Figure 6-14.** *A*, The Brooks-type fusion uses double-twisted 24-gauge wires that are passed sequentially under the arch of C1 and C2 from superior to inferior. *B*, Bone grafts are contoured to the interval between C1 and C2. *C*, Twisted wires hold the grafts securely in place.

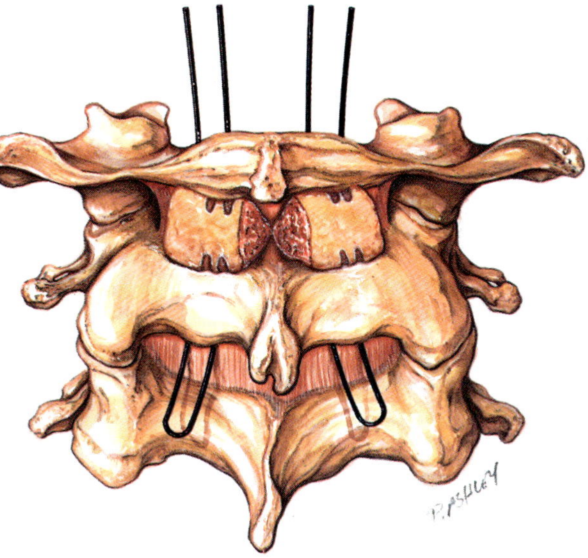

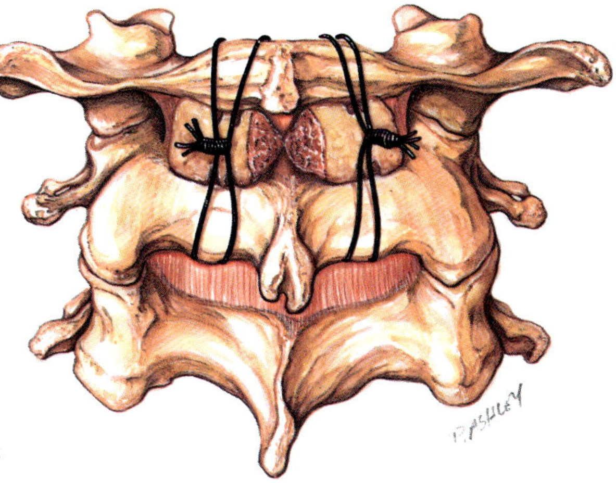

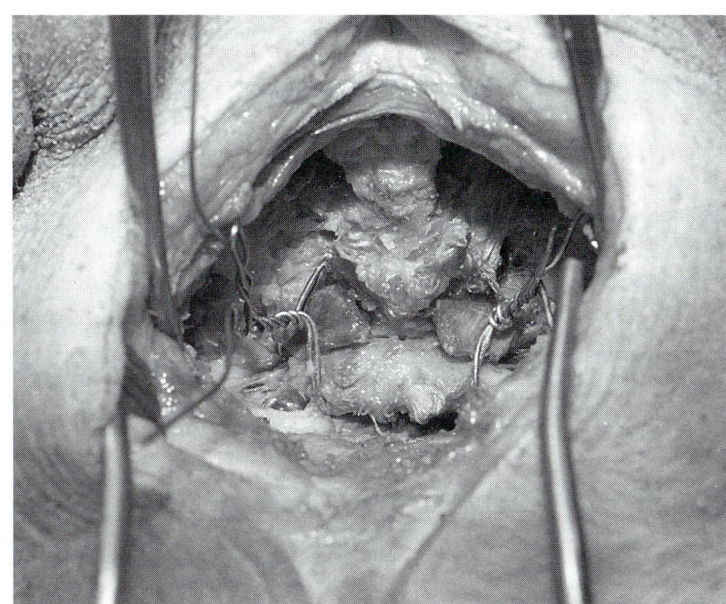

● **Figure 6-15.** Cadaveric model showing a Brooks-type fusion using doubled wires. Extra cancellous graft is then placed for enhancement of fusion. Note extended skin incision for facilitation of exposure.

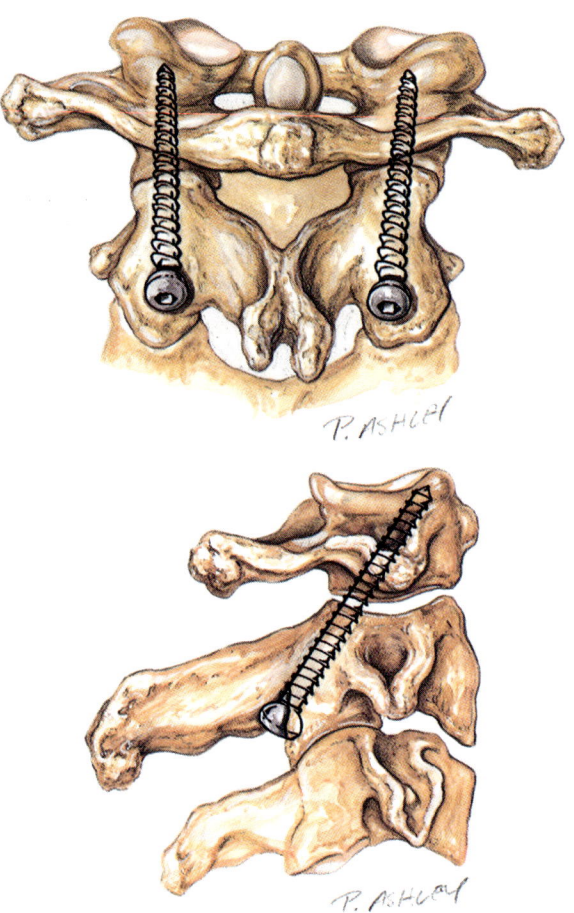

● **Figure 6-16.** Magerl's transarticular screw fixation of the C1-C2 articulation. Note the orientation of the screws through the articular masses and into the lateral masses of C1.

are inserted at the inferior aspect of C2, angle toward the lateral mass, and exit at the posterior aspect of the upper articular process (Figure 6–16). The screws cross the facet joint and enter the lateral mass of C1. This procedure is performed with the aid of radiographic fluoroscopic control.

Approach to Occipitocervical Fusion

The approach to the occipitocervical junction is not commonly used but may be the primary procedure for stabilization of basilar impression, tumor, or fractures of the odontoid with a concurrent fracture of C1. A posteriorly opening halo is usually used to stabilize the head, and a midline incision is made from the inion to the spinous process of C2. Capsular ligaments of the facets should be preserved to maintain stability. Sharp subperiosteal dissection of the external occipital protuberance and lamina is performed, and care is taken to protect the vertebral arteries from injury at the lateral borders of the atlas. The external occipital protuberance is thick and allows the passage of wires without the trouble of going through both tables. We prefer the method of Wertheim and Bohlman.[5] A high-speed bur is used to make a trough on both sides of the protuberance 2 cm above the foramen magnum. A towel clip or tenaculum clamp is used to make a hole in the ridge. A wire loop is then passed through the hole (Figure 6–17). The ring of C1 is cleaned using small angled curets,

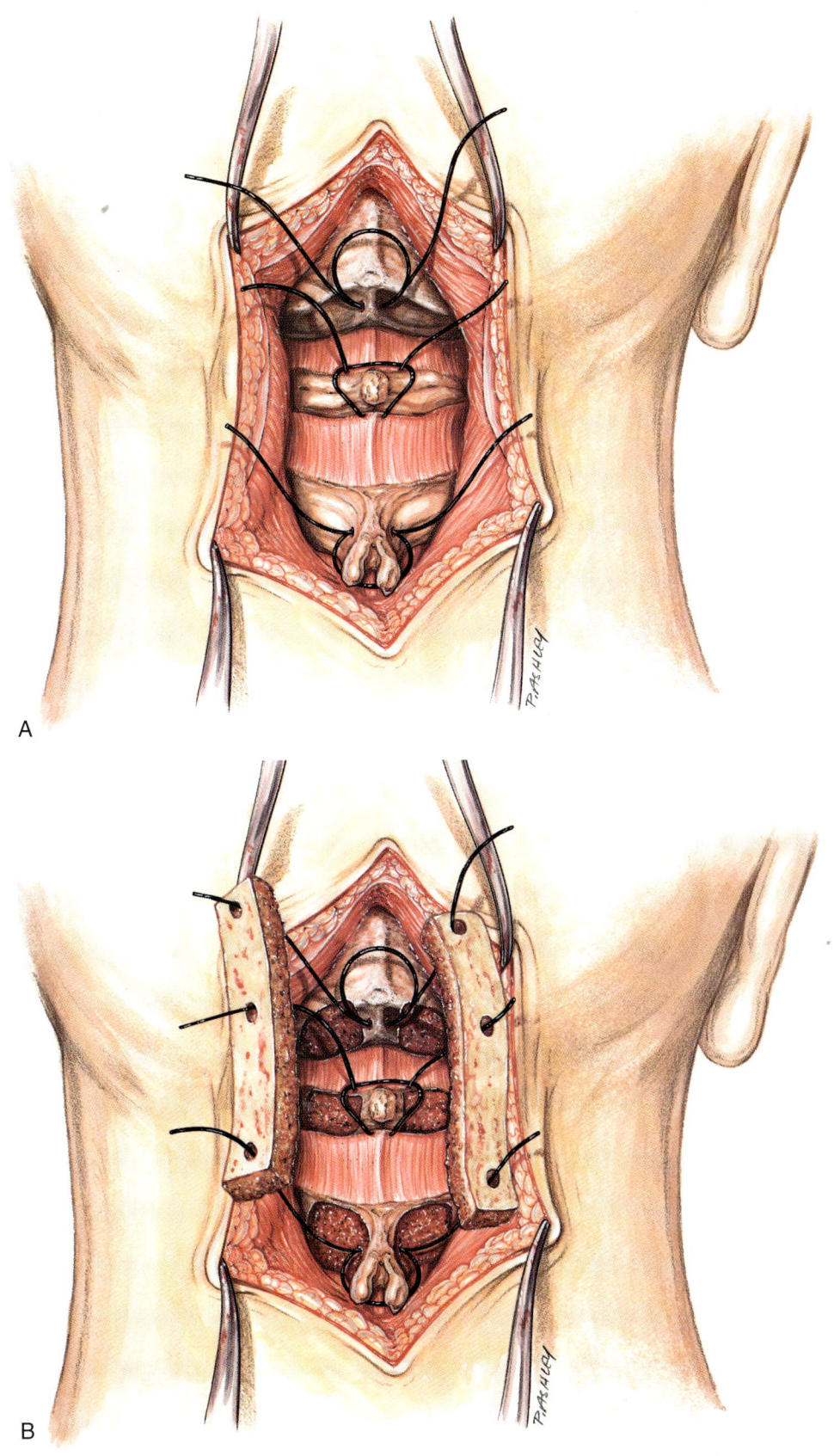

● **Figure 6-17.** Occipitocervical fusion as described by Wertheim and Bohlman uses wires passed through the external occipital protuberance and around the spinous processes of C2 and C3. Graft is wired over cancellous bone, securing the fusion.

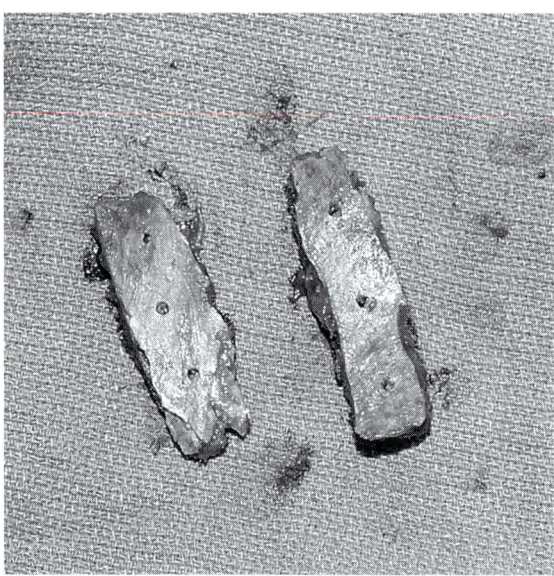

● **Figure 6-18.** Large unicortical autogenous grafts are obtained from the iliac crests, and holes are drilled for the corresponding wires of the occipitocervical fusion. Abundant cancellous bone should be left attached to the cortical rims.

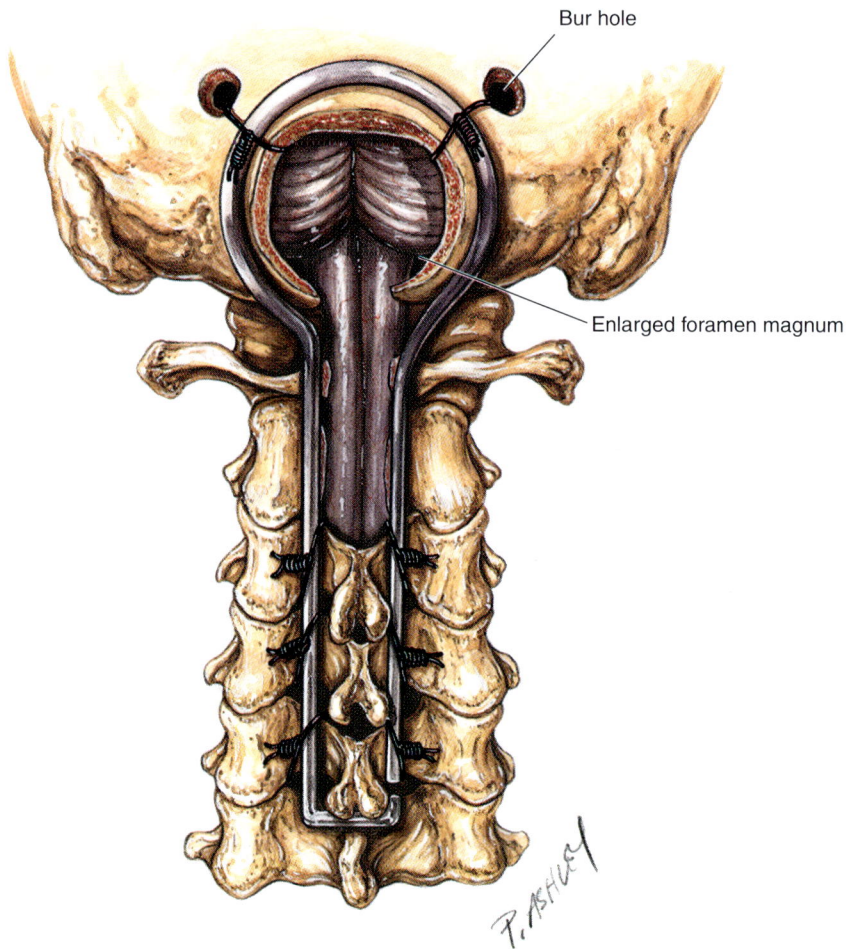

● **Figure 6-19.** Ransford loop for occipitocervical fixation and fusion. (From Ransford AO, Crockard HA, Pozo JL, et al: Craniocervical instability treated by contoured loop fixation. J Bone Joint Surg Br 68:173, 1986.)

and a wire is then passed around and locked on itself. The third wire is then wrapped around the base of the spinous process of C2. Two large, thick, corticocancellous grafts are harvested from the iliac crests and three holes are drilled in these (Figure 6–18); the wires are then passed through these holes and the grafts are securely tightened with additional cancellous graft placed to fill the defects. A halo jacket is placed for 3 months to ensure healing. Various methods of fixation have been devised, utilizing plates, rods, or combinations of hardware and bone, with each requiring meticulous attention to detail. Ransford and associates[6] described a contoured loop with sublaminar wiring for occipitocervical fusions and noted good results (Figure 6–19). Potential complications with sublaminar wires limit their routine use, but they may be advantageous in those patients requiring a multilevel fusion from the occiput to the lower cervical spine. Facet wires may be used instead of sublaminar wires. If the posterior elements are absent or if more rigid fixation is required, we prefer plate fixation by Roy-Camille contoured plates or by malleable pelvic AO reconstruction plates. Bicortical purchase of the screws is recommended for the occiput.

Posterior Interspinous Wiring

Interspinous wiring and fusion as described by Rogers[7] or Bohlman[8] is a safe and effective technique that provides adequate stabilization for the patient with the postoperative external support of a cervicothoracic brace or halo until the fusion matures. Posterior interspinous fusion is a less complex procedure and restricts flexion and anterior translation if the facet joints are intact, but interspinous wiring has little control of extension or rotation.

The patient should be placed in the three-point head rest or skull traction on a Stryker frame, and slight distraction is applied when the patient is turned prone. The skin and subcutaneous tissue are incised deep to the ligamentum nuchae. Dissection of the muscular attachments off the spinous processes is performed, and a radiograph is obtained to confirm the level of the procedure. Subperiosteal dissection is continued through the avascular midline plane to the laminae. The facets and capsular ligaments contribute to the stability of the spine and should be preserved at uninvolved levels. A 3- to 4-mm drill hole is made with a bur at the base of the spinous process. The hole should be at the proximal and distal extent of the cephalad and caudal spinous process, respectively, to avoid fracture or cutting out. The holes are connected with a towel clip using a rotary motion. Care should be taken to be above the spinolaminar line to avoid injuring the dura or cord with the passage of the towel clip or wire. The wires are passed through the holes, and the middle spinous process is incorporated unless it or the lamina is fractured (Figure 6–20). A general rule regarding the extent of the fusion is if a single level is involved, the involved levels should be fused together, incorporating one level below. A larger area of instability generally requires one level above and two levels below the involved segment. This protects the lower level from early failure. Hyperextension should be avoided to protect the foramen or canal from compromise. The lamina and facets are decorticated with a bur, and the appropriate corticocancellous grafts are harvested and holes drilled for the corresponding wires. The wires are passed and the grafts securely tightened with additional cancellous bone placed on the exposed laminae and facets (Figure 6–21).

Fractures through the facets or instability from bilateral facet dislocations result in shear instability and anterior horizontal displacement of the vertebral bodies. Interfacet wiring gives better control of anterior translation and rotatory displacement than the simple interspinous wiring technique.[9] A 2-mm drill hole is made by placing a Penfield dissector into the facet joint and drilling superior to inferior. The 20- or 22-gauge wire is passed through the hole and looped around the inferior spinous process for a one-level fusion. Adjacent facets may be wired for multilevel instability. The wires may be tied to bone grafts or rods for a more rigid construct and increased stability (Figure 6–22). Sublaminar fixation has been

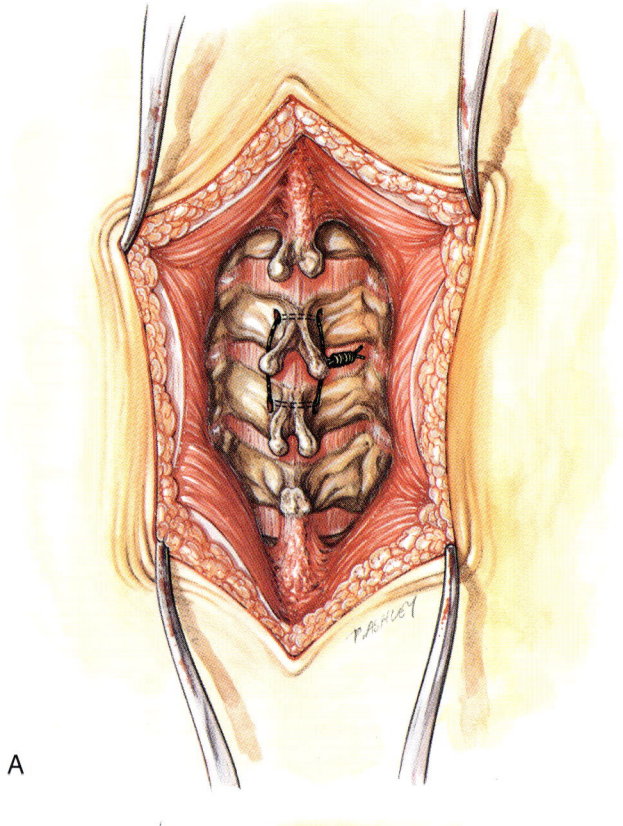

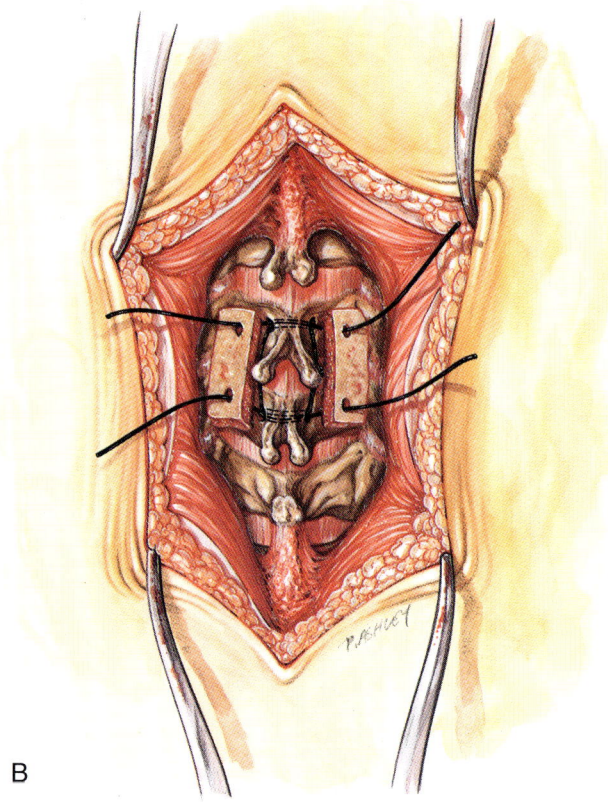

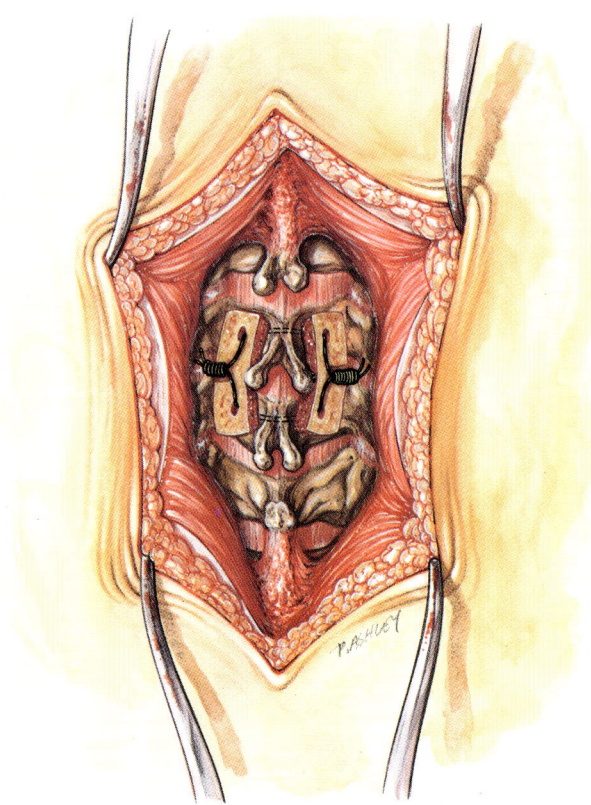

● **Figure 6-20.** Posterior cervical spine stabilization by triple-wire technique. The segment is wired with spinous process wire first (*A*) and then the grafts are secured with additional wires (*B*), compressing the bone to the spinolaminar junction (*C*).

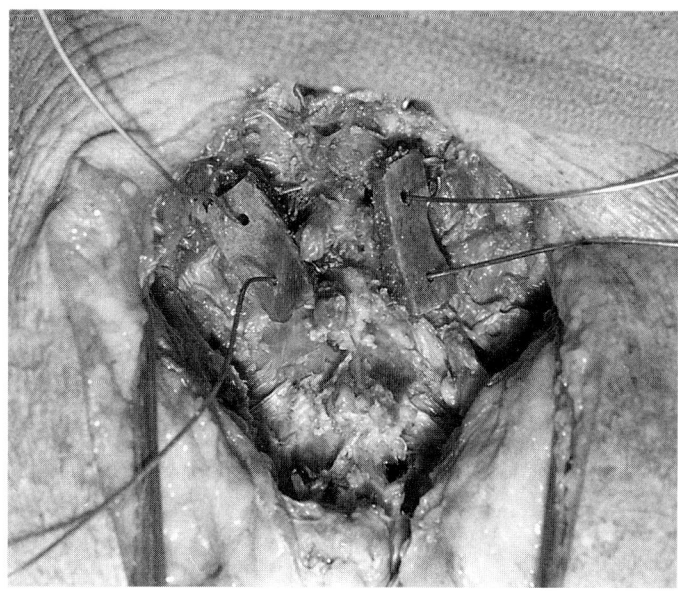

● **Figure 6-21.** Cadaveric model of triple-wire technique with autologous grafts placed on wires and over cancellous graft and ready for tightening.

described, but we do not recommend this procedure in the lower cervical spine because of the increased risk of neurologic injury.

Rigid Internal Fixation

In instances when the posterior elements are deficient or fractured and stabilization is needed, rigid internal fixation methods can be applied from the posterior approach. Multiple levels of stable fixation can be performed easily without increasing the complexity of the procedure as would occur with anterior stabilization. Stable fixation with rods or plates can be performed and is of great benefit in patients with multilevel involvement with a neoplasm or fractures. Early mobilization and minimal external support are benefits of early rigid internal fixation.

Many instrumentation systems have been developed to provide greater stability to the cervical spine. Plating of the posterior cervical spine allows rigid stabilization with a good correction of deformity and maintenance of alignment until fusion. These techniques were pioneered by Roy-Camille in Paris.[10] The technique of posterior plate and screw fixation (Figure 6–23) is exacting and requires attention to detail. Familiarity with the anatomy of the articular pillars and the surgical technique helps prevent potential catastrophic complications. Variation in the placement of the screws may lead to an increased risk of injury to the vertebral artery, nerve root, or spinal cord (Figure 6–24). With most of the modern techniques of screw placement (Figure 6–25), the nerve root and facet joint is at the greatest risk from screw impingement. An anatomic dissection was done to determine the safest direction of screw placement and the safest exit point of the drill.[11] This technique of drilling is described below.

A standard posterior approach is performed, and the dissection is to the lateral limits of the lateral articular masses. The center of the articular pillar is identified, and the cortex is penetrated with a small bur at a point 1 mm medial to the center or the "hill" (Figure 6–

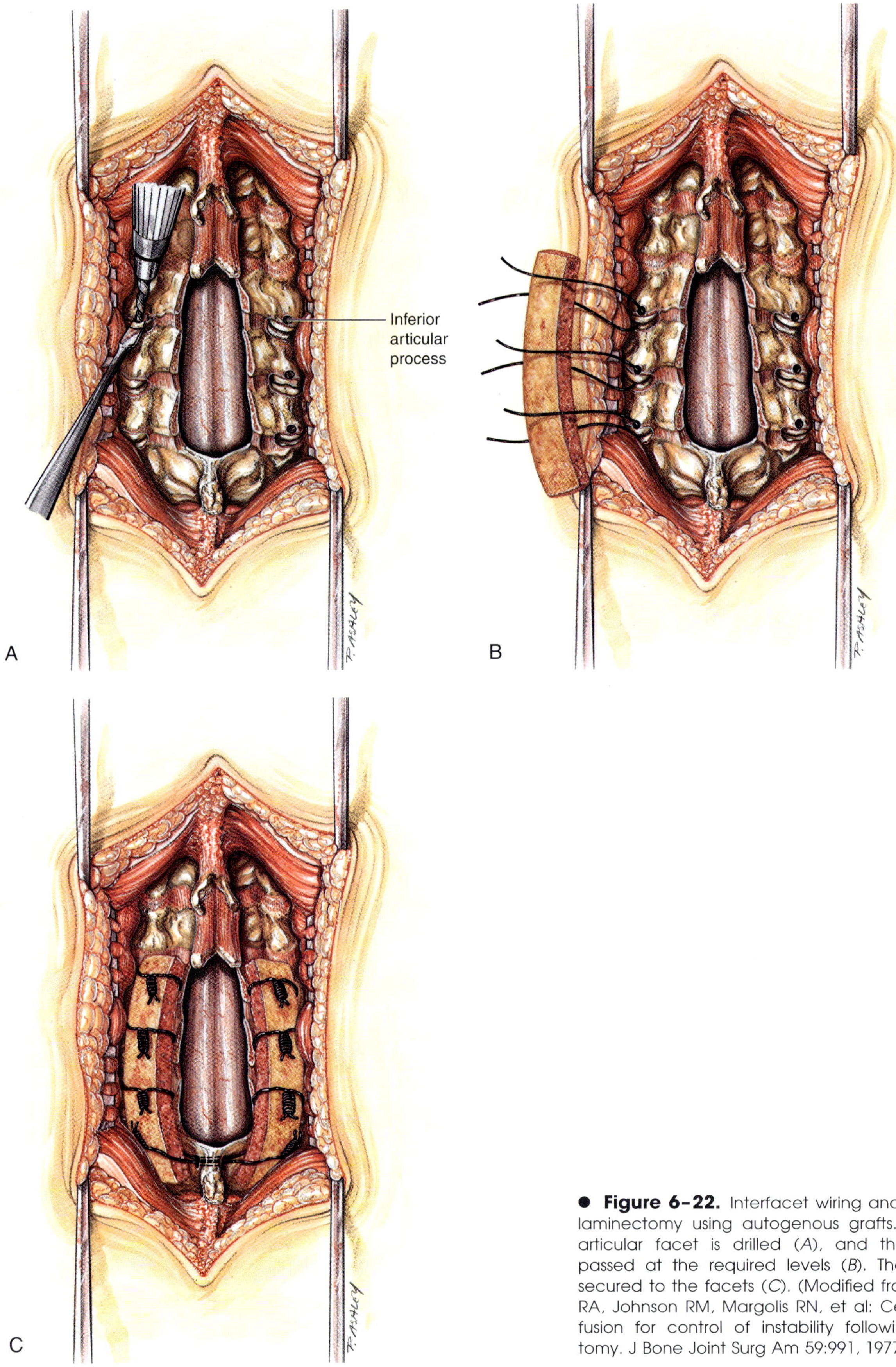

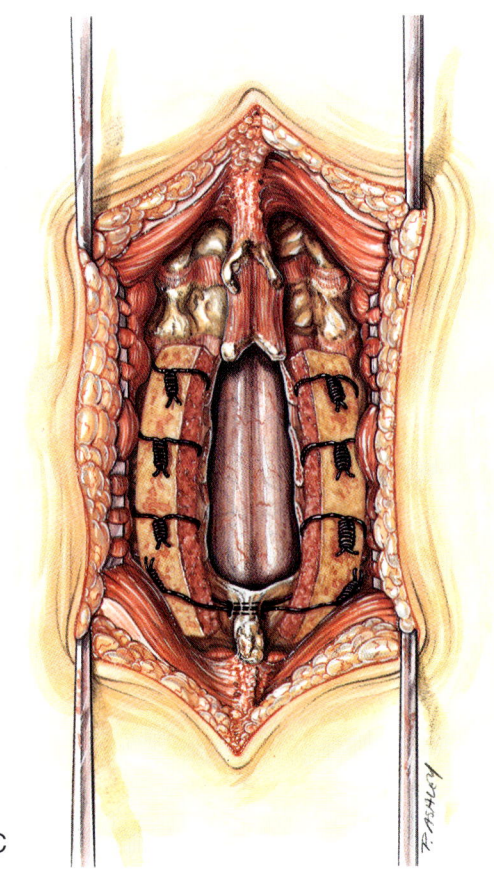

● **Figure 6-22.** Interfacet wiring and fusion after laminectomy using autogenous grafts. The inferior articular facet is drilled (*A*), and the wires are passed at the required levels (*B*). The grafts are secured to the facets (*C*). (Modified from Callahan RA, Johnson RM, Margolis RN, et al: Cervical facet fusion for control of instability following laminectomy. J Bone Joint Surg Am 59:991, 1977.)

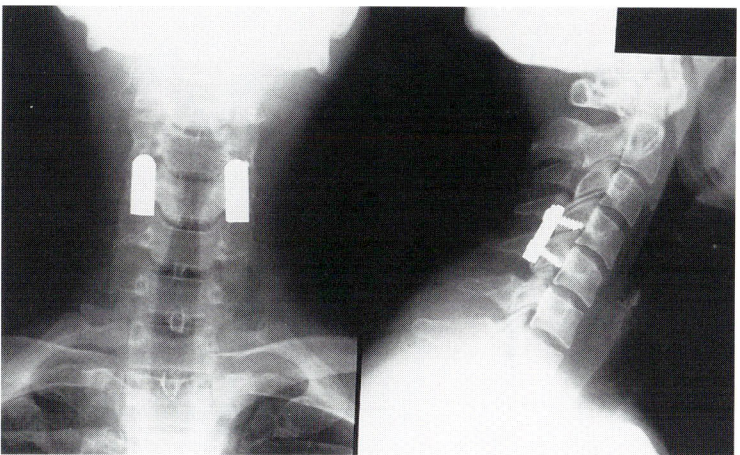

● **Figure 6-23.** Anteroposterior and lateral radiographs of the cervical spine demonstrate rigid Roy-Camille screw-plate fixation of the lateral masses in a patient with C4-C5 instability.

26). With a 2.5-mm drill bit, the pillar is drilled in a direction of 25 to 30 degrees laterally and 15 degrees cephalad for C3 through C6. When drilling at C2, the drill should be angled 10 to 15 degrees medially and 35 degrees superiorly to avoid injuring the vertebral artery, which is exiting the foramen on its course to the C1 arch (Figure 6-27). The direction of the drill is medial and not lateral as in the lower cervical spine and is different from that for transarticular fixation of C1-C2 (Figure 6-28). The opposite cortex should be drilled, except at C2, and a drill stop used to avoid plunging. The hole is tapped with a 3.5-mm tap, and the contoured plate is secured with the correct size 3.5-mm cortical screw. Various plates are available that can be used, with titanium ones becoming widely popular. It is important to then decorticate the surrounding bone, and cancellous graft is added for the fusion.

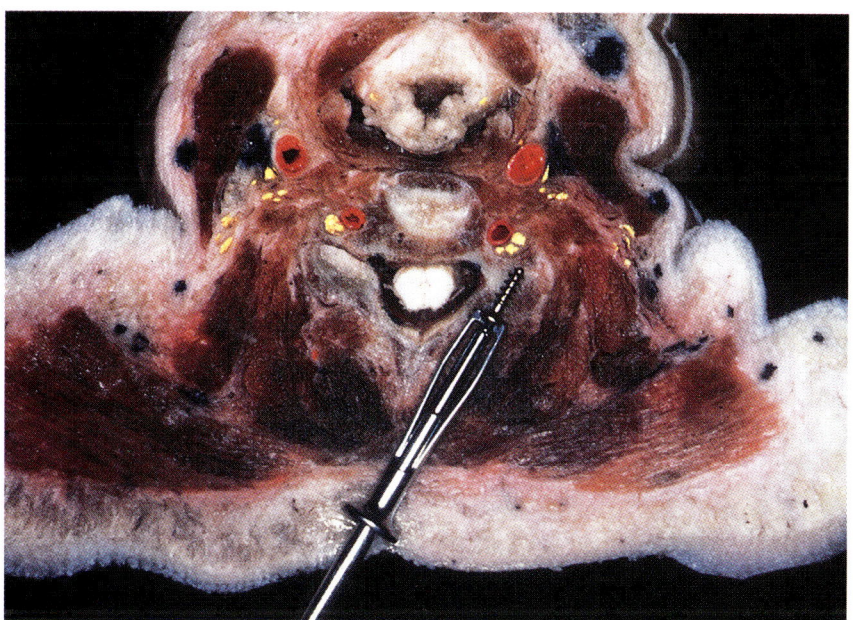

● **Figure 6-24.** Cadaveric cross section at C4-C5 level showing the correct orientation of a lateral mass screw. The consequence of a "straight ahead" approach may injure the vertebral artery, which can be seen directly anterior to the lateral mass.

106 • SURGICAL APPROACHES TO THE SPINE

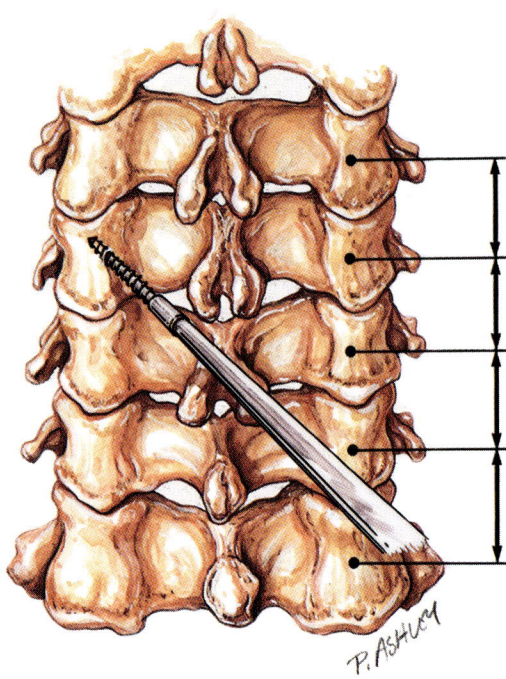

● **Figure 6-25.** The average interfacet distance is 13 mm, but individual variation places the range from 9 to 16 mm.

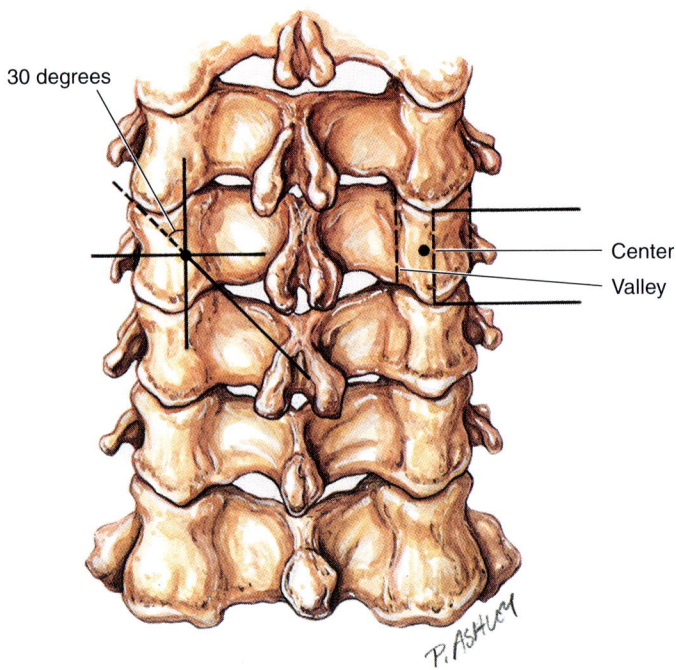

● **Figure 6-26.** The location of the ideal drilling point for starting lateral mass screws is 1 mm medial to the center of the lateral mass on the "hill." The drill should be directed 30 degrees lateral and 15 degrees cephalad to avoid injuring the nerve root as it exits at the anterolateral portion of the superior facet.

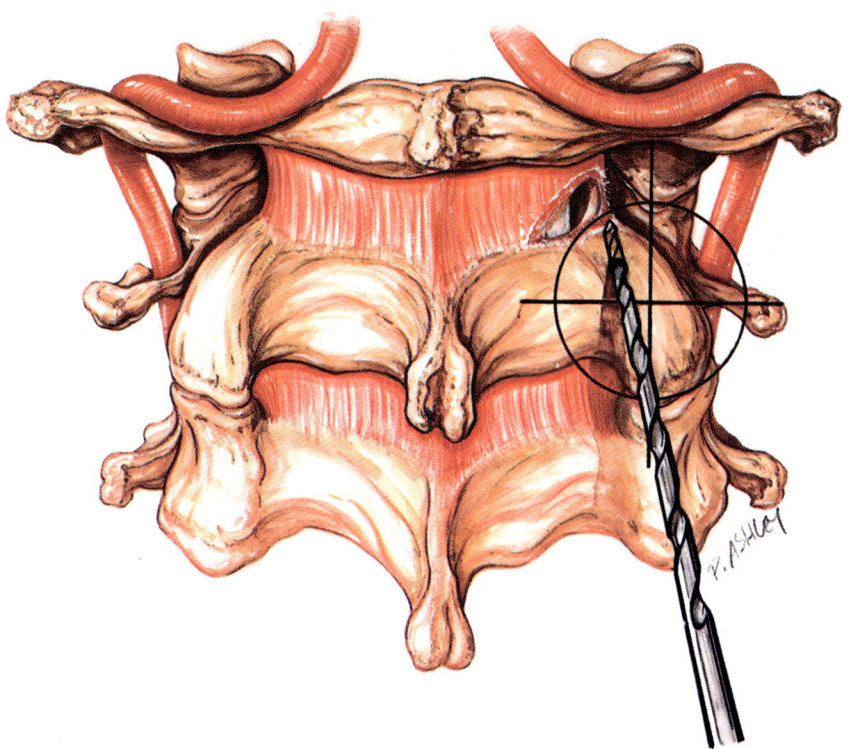

● **Figure 6-27.** The drilling for placement of a screw at C2 is 10 to 15 degrees medially and 35 degrees superiorly to avoid injury to the vertebral artery as it exits the foramen. The opposite cortex is penetrated using a drill with a stop.

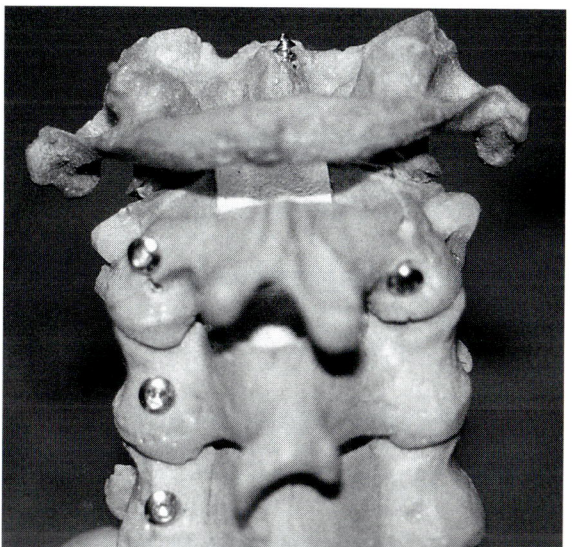

● **Figure 6-28.** Model of the upper cervical spine that demonstrates the different orientation of the screw into the lateral mass of C2 for transarticular arthrodesis of C1-C2 (*right*), and the orientation for fixation of a plate-screw device into the region of the pedicle (*left*). The drill orientation should be 35 degrees cranial and 10 to 15 degrees medial for pedicle fixation.

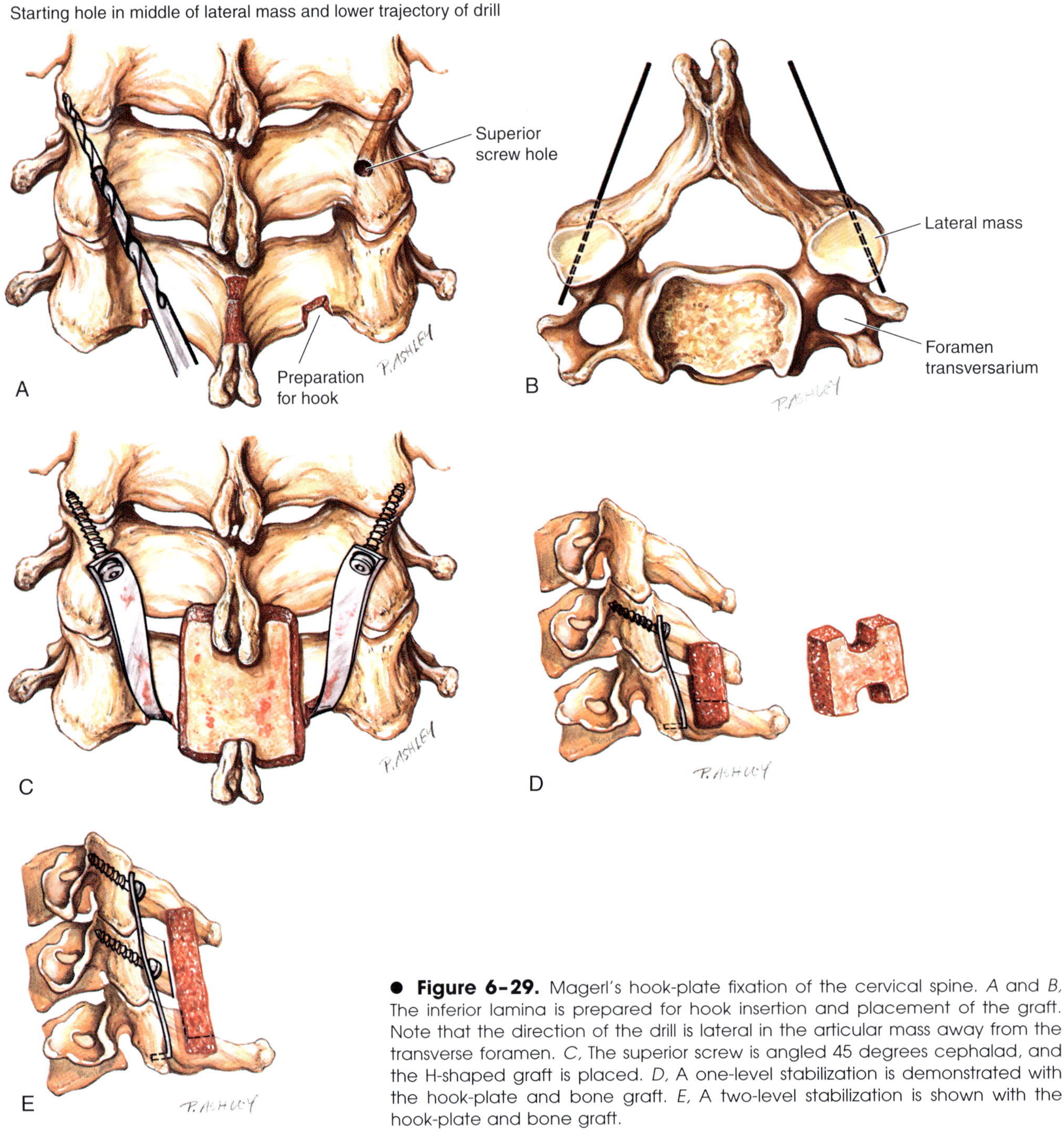

108 ● SURGICAL APPROACHES TO THE SPINE

● **Figure 6-29.** Magerl's hook-plate fixation of the cervical spine. *A* and *B*, The inferior lamina is prepared for hook insertion and placement of the graft. Note that the direction of the drill is lateral in the articular mass away from the transverse foramen. *C*, The superior screw is angled 45 degrees cephalad, and the H-shaped graft is placed. *D*, A one-level stabilization is demonstrated with the hook-plate and bone graft. *E*, A two-level stabilization is shown with the hook-plate and bone graft.

An appropriate closure in layers is performed, and rigid immobilization is unnecessary except in noncompliant patients. Biomechanically, the plate screw systems have been shown to be superior to wiring constructs especially in extension and torsion.[12] The seventh cervical vertebra presents a technical problem in that it is transitional and has a very thin lateral mass. An attempt at a lateral mass screw places the nerve root and facet joint at risk of injury. A hook-plate construct as described by Magerl and associates[13] would be preferred at the C7 region because it provides additional fixation and may obviate the need for an additional screw (Figures 6–29 and 6–30). A pedicle screw-plate system could be used.

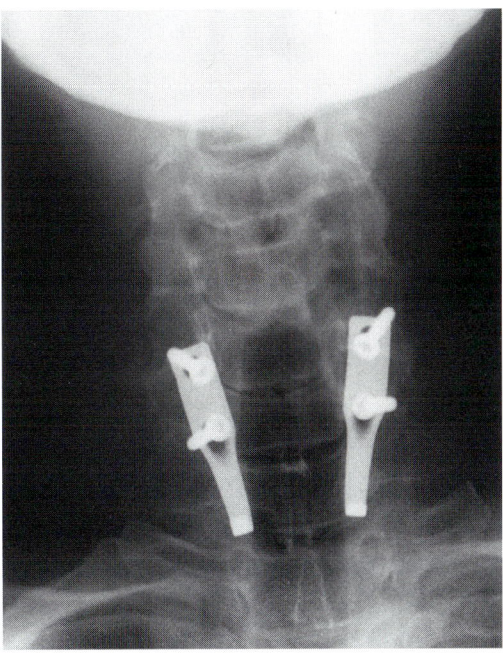

● **Figure 6-30.** Anteroposterior radiograph of a C5-C7 stabilization and fusion with the hook-plate after decompression.

Posterior Techniques at the Cervicothoracic Junction

Lesions at the cervicothoracic junction are generally anterior and require extensive anterior approaches with or without some form of posterior fixation required. Those lesions that may require posterior stabilization include but are not limited to tumors, trauma, postlaminectomy instability, and infection. If the posterior elements are intact, a triple-wiring procedure, rod-

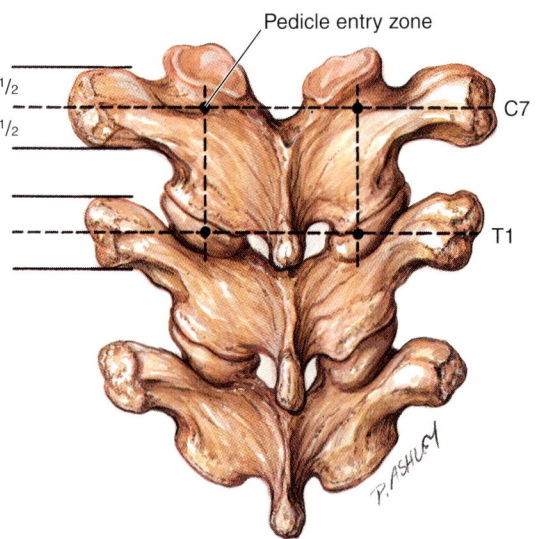

● **Figure 6-31.** Entry point of the pedicle at the cervicothoracic junction. The pedicle is located by crossing a horizontal line at the midportion of the transverse processes and a vertical line at the lamina-transverse process junction or the midportion of the facet. This point is 1 to 2 mm inferior to the facet joint.

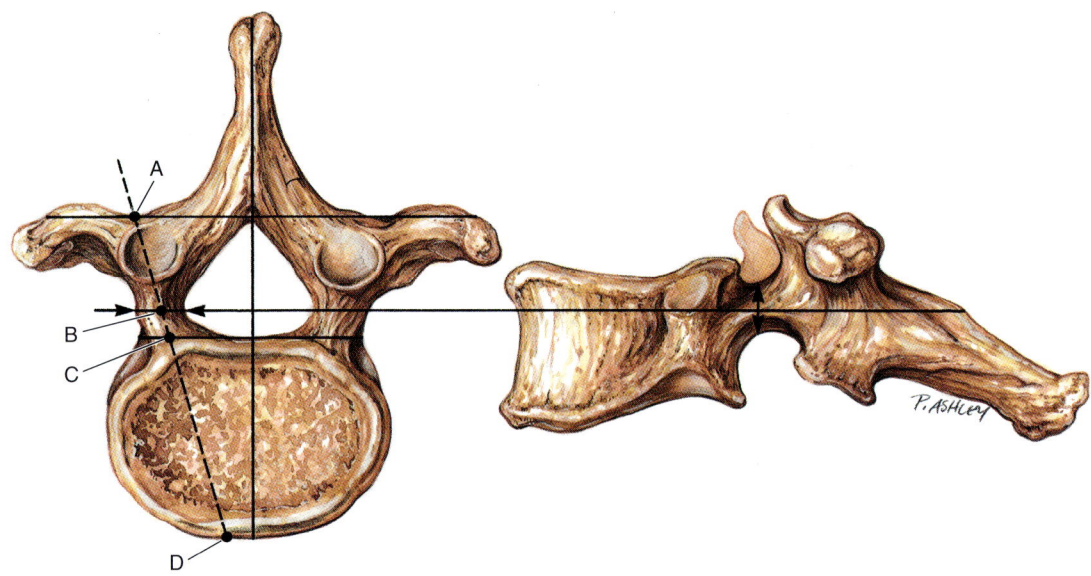

● **Figure 6-32.** Morphometry of the pedicle at the cervicothoracic junction: starting point (A); the middle or narrowest part of the pedicle (B); posterior vertebral line (C); anterior vertebral margin (D). Medial angulation should be 25 to 30 degrees. Superior-inferior diameter is relatively greater than medial-lateral diameter in the thoracic spine as compared with the lumbar spine.

hook system, or Luque segmental fixation may be used. Pedicle screw fixation is an alternative if a decompression including laminectomy has been performed; however, this is an exacting procedure with very little margin for error. Through cadaveric studies, the pedicle landmarks and anatomic characteristics of the cervicothoracic region were found.[11]

A standard posterior approach is used with the dissection performed laterally to the tips of the transverse processes of the thoracic vertebrae. The facet joint is cleaned of its capsule and the articular margins identified. The entry point of the pedicle lies at the intersection of a horizontal line at the midportion of the transverse processes and a vertical line at the lamina–transverse process junction or the midpoint of the facet joint. This intersecting point is 1 to 2 mm inferior to the facet joint (Figure 6–31). The outer cortex is decorticated at this point with a small bur, and a small Penfield elevator or small straight curet is used to probe bluntly and enter the pedicle. Caution should be used to avoid plunging. A 2.5-mm drill may be used to enter the pedicle once it is identified. Medial angulation is required for entry of the pedicle, and it averages 34 degrees at C7, 31.8 degrees at T1, and 26.5 degrees at T2 (Figure 6–32). When compared with the pedicles of the lumbar spine, the superoinferior diameter of the thoracic pedicle is relatively greater than its mediolateral diameter. This leaves little margin for error in the mediolateral plane.

Complications

Complications during surgical procedures on the posterior cervical spine can be related to patient selection, the surgical approach, the technical expertise of the surgeon, the surgical technique, and the pathomechanics of the disease process. Careful patient selection is an important consideration because a procedure with poor rigid fixation in an unreliable and noncooperative patient is doomed to failure and can complicate any future interventions. The experience and expertise of the surgeon in assessing the best procedure and approach to a problem can avert any unnecessary morbidity that may be encountered. A posterior approach to an anterior compressive lesion may increase the instability or neurologic status and not even address the original problem. Poor knowledge of the anatomic region can lead to catastrophic consequences, such as paralysis or even death.

The posterior approach to the cervical spine is relatively safe and universal. The relative internervous plane of muscular dissection prevents any significant denervation if care is taken to stay midline. Once the spinous processes are dissected from the ligamentum flavum, the remainder of the approach is subperiosteal. Meticulous hemostasis is essential because the venous plexus may cause significant bleeding, and it should be cauterized as needed. The development of a hematoma may lead to an epidural hematoma and spinal cord compression and even death. The segmental arteries at the lateral aspect of the facets may be violated and can be coagulated. Although the vertebral artery is uncommonly injured, significant consequences may develop if it is injured. Posterior cervical procedures have the inherent risk of injury to the vertebral artery in the foramen transversarium if dissection is performed lateral to the facets, but there is a greater susceptibility for injury during approaches for C1-C2 fusions.

Reports of posterior vertebral artery injury are rare. Electrocautery was the causative source in three cases reported by Rizzoli,[14] and Stambough and Simeone[15] noted two cases that resulted from vigorous subperiosteal dissection during exposure of C1. The bleeding was controlled by packing, and no neurologic sequelae developed in either case. Strict attention to limiting the dissection to within 1.5 cm lateral to the posterior tubercle of C1 in adults and 1 cm in children and using lateral dissection from the dorsal ramus of C2 between the C1-C2 foramina help avert any complications. Prolonged or excessive retraction of the vertebral artery may lead to occipital cortex ischemia if the collateral circulation is compromised and hence may result in a bilateral homonymous hemianopia or cortical blindness. An injury to the central retinal artery of the eye secondary to pressure from a poorly positioned head rest in the prone position may result in thrombosis and subsequent blindness.[16]

Neurologic complications have a higher overall incidence with posterior procedures than with anterior procedures, according to a survey by the Cervical Spine Research Society.[17] There was an average incidence of 2.18% versus 0.64%, with the potential for injury greater during complete laminectomy in myelopathic patients than during foraminotomy. Extra caution should be used during positioning and intubation, and we recommend an air-driven drill be used to thin the lamina at its junction with the lateral mass and a small angled curet be used to lift off the lamina rather than insertion of a Kerrison rongeur under the lamina.

The possibility of injury is significant during the passage of sublaminar wires, and the use of a needle or instrument to facilitate passage without blind maneuvers minimizes the risk of direct injury. Root injury is fairly uncommon, and although a sensory deficit is rarely of great significance, a motor deficit (particularly of root C5 or C8) can be very serious and of great morbidity to a patient. Decompression without removal of disk or osteophyte decreases the incidence of direct injury; most of the injuries are secondary to traction forces so avoidance of overzealous retraction or manipulation of the root minimizes deficits postoperatively. Most of these are reversible injuries.

Dural tears are a definite risk during posterior procedures and are greater with a complete laminectomy than with a unilateral foraminotomy. Factors that lead to a dural injury may be previous surgery, inexperience of the operating surgeon, or failure to adhere to the principles of spinal surgery. The use of a diamond-tip bur and careful removal of the lamina with small angled curets help avert a dural rent. Meticulous surgical technique minimizes any direct dural injury, and any dural rent should be closed in a watertight fashion with a small atraumatic needle. A blood or fibrin patch may be used.[18] Postoperative cerebrospinal fluid leaks may be managed by lumbar catheter drainage to allow the wound to heal.[19]

The posterior approach is usually done in the prone position with some degree of reverse Trendelenburg, but an alternative is the sitting position. The sitting position for posterior cervical surgery allows the reduction of venous bleeding, but it has the inherent possible complication of air embolism. It may be one of the most serious complications that can occur when an incision is placed above the level of the heart. The risk correlates proportionately with the greater gravitational gradient.[20] All air emboli are not clinically significant, and the incidence of serious complications is fortunately very low. As little air as 0.1 mL of air can be detected by Doppler monitoring as it enters the heart.[20]

Nonunion of the lower cervical spine is rare in posterior cervical fusions and is almost nonexistent in children. Extension of spontaneous fusion is common, and it is therefore prudent to localize the involved level to avoid unnecessary fused segments. Pseudarthrosis of the posterior cervical spine is multifactorial and is related to the approach, surgical technique, age of the patient, use of allograft, and method of fixation. For lower cervical spine fusions, the triple wire technique of spine stabilization as shown by Bohlman in his review had no nonunions in 72 patients.[8] The nonunions from attempts at fusion of the upper cervical spine are more common and include the occipitocervical and atlantoaxial regions.[21]

Conclusion

The posterior approach to the cervical spine is a very simple and safe exposure and allows versatility for the surgeon in addressing a complexity of problems. The dissection is initially midline and subperiosteal, and the greatest danger is in the approaches to the upper cervical spine when dissection is performed laterally. Utmost care with meticulous surgical technique and careful evaluation of preoperative radiographs avert any complications from inadvertent neural injury as a result of bone deficiencies that are not recognized. Good knowledge of the anatomy and landmarks is essential to avoid risks, and a localization radiograph should be obtained to confirm the level. The various definitive techniques of fusion and decompression have the associated increase in risk of possible complications. It cannot be overemphasized that the cause of the lesion, zones of injury, and any subsequent postoperative demands of the patient be addressed carefully before any surgical undertaking. Attention to careful positioning and intubation with stabilization of the unstable cervical spine is mandatory when the posterior approach is used. A tight and thorough closure minimizes any postoperative wound complications or dehiscence.

REFERENCES

1. Fielding JW, Burstein AH, Frankel VH: The nuchal ligament. Spine 1:3, 1976.
2. Simmons EH: Surgery of the spine in rheumatoid arthritis and ankylosing spondylitis. In Evarts CM (ed): Surgery of the Musculoskeletal System, vol 2, pp 85–151. New York, Churchill Livingstone, 1983.
3. Meyer PR Jr: Surgical stabilization of the cervical spine. In Meyer PR (ed): Surgery of Spine Trauma, pp 397–524. New York, Churchill Livingstone, 1989.
4. Magerl F, Seeman P: Stable posterior fusion of the atlas and axis by transarticular screw fixation. In Kehr P, Weidner A (eds): Cervical Spine, vol I, p 322. New York, Springer-Verlag, 1987.
5. Wertheim SB, Bohlman HH: Occipitocervical fusion. J Bone Joint Surg Am 69:833, 1987.
6. Ransford AO, Crockard HA, Pozo JL, et al: Craniocervical instability treated by contoured loop fixation. J Bone Joint Surg Br 68:173, 1986.
7. Rogers WA: Fractures and dislocations of the cervical spine: An end-result study. J Bone Joint Surg Am 39:341, 1957.
8. Bohlman HH: Acute fractures and dislocations of the cervical spine: An analysis of three hundred hospitalized patients and review of the literature. J Bone Joint Surg Am 61:1119, 1979.
9. Callahan RA, Johnson RM, Margolis RN, et al: Cervical facet fusion for control of instability following laminectomy. J Bone Joint Surg Am 59:991, 1977.
10. Roy-Camille R, Saillant G, Mazel C: Internal fixation of the unstable cervical spine by a posterior osteosynthesis with plates and screws. In Sherk HH (ed): The Cervical Spine, 2nd ed, pp 390–403. Philadelphia, JB Lippincott, 1989.
11. An HS, Gordin R, Renner K: Anatomic considerations for plate-screw fixation of the cervical spine. Spine 16(10S):S548, 1991.

12. Cooper PR: Posterior stabilization of the cervical spine using Roy-Camille plates: A North American experience. Trans Orthop 12:43, 1988.
13. Magerl F, Grob D, Seeman P: Stable dorsal fusion of the cervical spine (C2-T1) using hook plates. In Kehr P, Weidner A (eds): Cervical Spine, vol I, p 322. New York, Springer-Verlag, 1987.
14. Rizzoli H: Personal communication, 1985.
15. Stambough JL, Simeone FA: Vascular complications in spine surgery. In Rothman RH, Simeone FA (eds): The Spine, 3rd ed. vol 2, p 1878. Philadelphia, WB Saunders, 1992.
16. Stambough JL, Cheeks ML: Central retinal artery occlusion: A complication of the knee-chest position. J Spinal Disord 5:363, 1992.
17. Graham JJ: Complications of cervical spine surgery. In The Cervical Spine Research Society Editorial Committee (eds): The Cervical Spine, 2nd ed, pp 831–837. Philadelphia, JB Lippincott, 1989.
18. Tew JM Jr, Mayfield FH: Surgery of the anterior cervical spine: Prevention of complications. In Dunsker SB (ed): Cervical Spondylosis, pp 191–208. New York, Raven Press, 1981.
19. Kitchel SH, Eismont FJ, Green BA: Closed subarachnoid drainage for management of cerebrospinal fluid leakage after an operation on the spine. J Bone Joint Surg Am 71:984, 1989.
20. Albin MS, Carroll RG, Maroun JC: Clinical considerations concerning detection of venous air embolism. Neurosurgery 3:380, 1978.
21. Edmunds JO, Goldner JL, et al: Arthrodesis of the unstable upper cervical spine for instability with and without myelopathy. J Bone Joint Surg Am 57:1025, 1975.

CHAPTER 7

THORACOTOMY

Bernard A. Rawlins, M.D.
Todd J. Albert, M.D.
Richard A. Balderston, M.D.

Thoracic surgery can be traced to the 19th century, when sporadic contributions were made in the attempt to treat pulmonary tuberculosis.[1] Tuffier, in 1891, was credited with the first successful lung resection[2]; however, it was Hodgson and colleagues who popularized this approach in the treatment of spinal disorders initially for the treatment of tuberculosis.[3-5] Since these reports, the anterior approach to the spine has become invaluable in the treatment of spinal disorders.[6-12] This trend is related not only to the improved visualization and safety that an anterior approach offers for anterior pathologic processes but also to the growing acceptance of the anterior column of the spine as an important entity for attaining solid fusion and in the correction of deformity or instability.

Indications

The indications for an anterior approach generally fall under three main categories. The first is an anterior lesion—or such as a vertebral body neoplasm, a thoracic disk, or other vertebral lesion causing anterior spinal cord compression—for which a posterior approach would be technically difficult if not impossible. The second category is a rigid deformity that cannot be addressed by a posterior fusion only, thus requiring an anterior release and fusion. Third is the anterior fusion performed to increase fusion rates, as in the treatment of pseudarthrosis. Instruments used for a thoracotomy are shown in Figure 7–1.

Technique

A thoracotomy may technically give you exposure to the 2nd thoracic vertebra craniad and the 12th thoracic vertebra caudad. Access to the second thoracic vertebra is obtained through a third rib incision. This requires division of the dorsal scapular muscles and elevation of the scapula through an incision that parallels its medial border (Figure 7–2). Access to the second thoracic vertebra, however, is relatively hindered, owing to the converging rib cage,

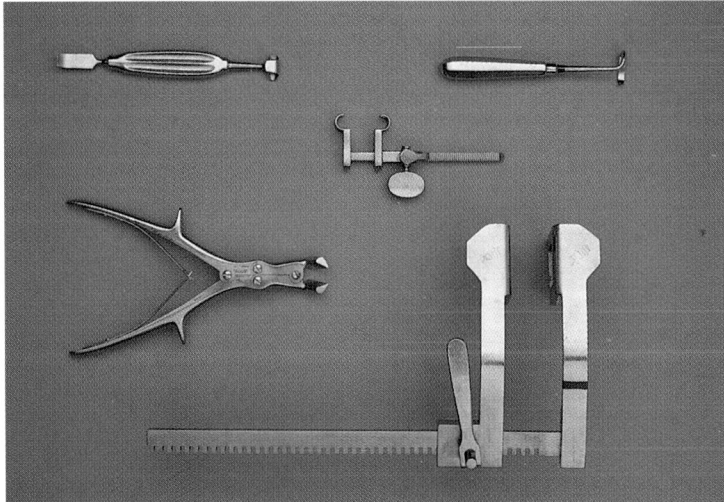

● **Figure 7-1.** Instruments used for a thoracotomy: Finochietto rib retractor *(bottom right)*; Alexander elevator *(top left)*; Doyen rib dissector *(top right)*; rib shear *(bottom left)*; rib approximator *(center)*.

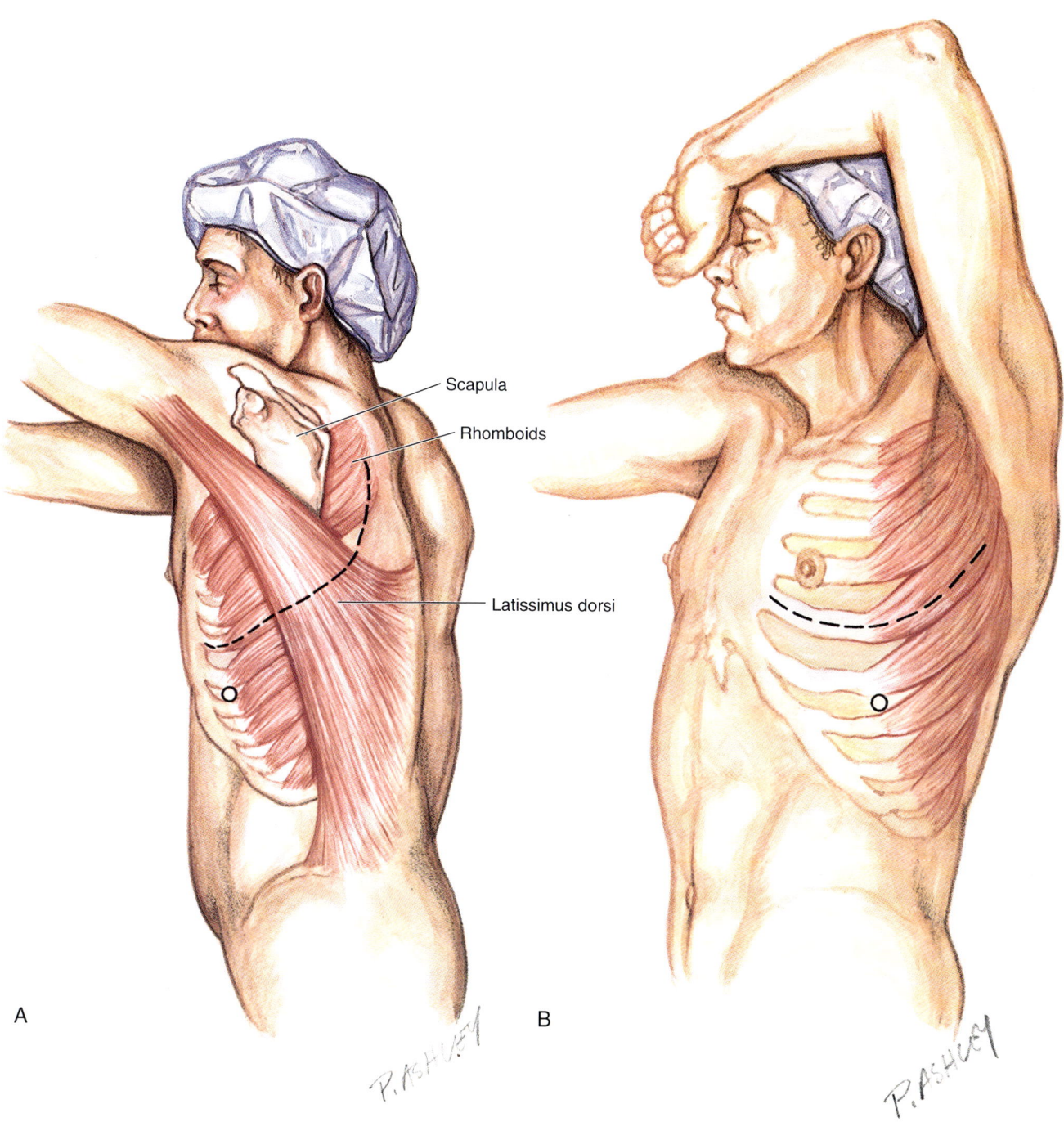

● **Figure 7-2.** Sketch demonstrating the upper thoracic incision (*A*) and the lower thoracic incision (*B*).

thoracic inlet, and difficulty with the presence of the scapula. Alternate approaches to the cervicothoracic junction are more useful when addressing this specific area and are described in a previous section of this book. A thoracotomy can give access to the 12th thoracic vertebra, although division of the medial diaphragmatic insertion may be required for the 12th and sometimes the 11th thoracic vertebrae.

The transthoracic approach may be performed without rib resection. However, rib resection provides improved visualization and autologous rib graft for an anterior fusion either as a free graft or with a vascularized pedicle. Selection of the rib to be resected is crucial to the exposure, and dictates incision placement. Generally the rib at the uppermost level of the anticipated spine dissection should be selected. For example, a lesion at T5 or a deformity from T5 to T9 should be approached through the fifth rib, remembering that approaches above T3 are often not practical. Difficulties will occur in patients with horizontally oriented ribs that tend to limit the caudal extent of the approach. In addition, sloping ribs can limit the cephalic extent of the dissection such that a fifth rib resection may allow only T6 as the most cephalic extent of the spine exposure. This problem may be corrected intraoperatively by dividing the caudal or cranial rib at the angle of the rib and anteriorly to create a focal flat segment. The rib segment is not removed and is incorporated in the final column. Before cutting the rib it is important to ligate the neurovascular bundle beneath the rib at either side of the level of the anticipated rib cut. This maneuver affords additional exposure. A preoperative chest radiograph can be helpful in selecting the rib to be resected. On the radiograph, a perpendicular line is drawn from the vertebra at the apex of the deformity or the level of the lesion to the side of the anticipated thoracotomy. This line forms a perpendicular to the tangent of the rib at the lateral border of the thoracic cage. Selection of this rib provides good exposure to the indicated area, taking into account rib orientation.

The thoracotomy can be performed through the left or right side, depending on the surgeon's preference. When dealing with a coronal deformity, it is easier to approach the convexity of the curve. When there is no deformity, we prefer a left side approach because of the ease in mobilization of the aorta compared with the venous system.

General endotracheal anesthesia should be considered with a double-lumen tube to allow selective collapse of the lung when extensive surgery is planned. Occasional expansion of the lung during the procedure may help to reduce postoperative atelectasis.

The patient is placed in the lateral decubitus position with the right flank directly over an elevated kidney rest that is fitted with abdominal and back supports (Figure 7–3). The lower extremities are carefully padded with the dependent knee flexed and the upper knee extended. A pillow between the legs is helpful. An axillary roll is placed beneath the dependent axilla to protect the brachial plexus. The table is then extended ("broken") and angled in reverse Trendelenburg position to allow the thoracic area to be horizontal to the floor. A pillow is placed between the arms to pad them, and adhesive tape is used over the shoulder, ilium, and legs. A "beanbag" mattress may be used to support the patient; however, this method described without a "beanbag" allows adequate stability while allowing improved access for a thoracoabdominal or retropertoneal approach, which can sometimes be hindered anteriorly if the "beanbag" is placed poorly.

The incision is made directly over the rib to be removed from the tip of the costal cartilage to the angle of the rib. The incision is taken down to the rib through the subcutaneous tissue, latissimus dorsi, and the serratus anterior with an electrocautery unit (Figure 7–4).

With a proximal thoracic approach, the incision anteriorly follows a rib outline and then is gently curved around the scapular tip in the cephalad direction midway between the medial border of the scapular and the spinous process. The incision is carried through the latissimus dorsi. Proximal dissection requires sectioning the trapezius superficially and the

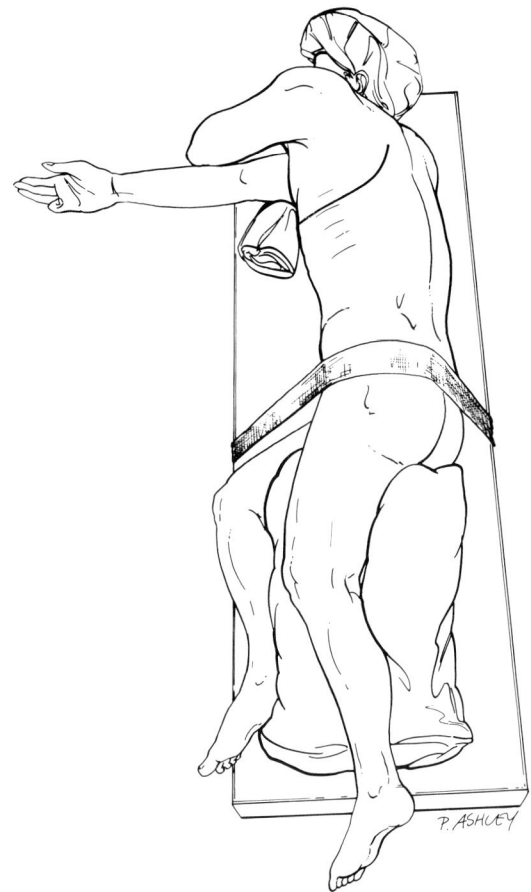

● **Figure 7-3.** Patient in the lateral decubitus position to allow adequate access to the thorax. The same setup may be used for a thoracotomy or the thoracoabdominal approach.

rhomboids deep over the medial scapula to allow proximal retraction of the scapula. The serratus anterior is released close to its muscle attachment to avoid transecting its innervation by the long thoracic nerve. Palpating the space beneath the scapula allows correct identification of the rib to be resected by counting the ribs from cephalic to caudal position. The first palpable rib is usually the second rib.

The rib resection (Figure 7–5) is initiated with an incision into the periosteum on its lateral border, either with a knife or an electrocautery unit, the full length of the incision. Subperiosteal dissection is continued with the periosteal elevator portion of the Alexander elevator to completely remove the periosteum off the lateral aspect of the rib (see Figure 7–5A). The opposite side of the Alexander elevator is used to clean the superior and inferior edges of the rib. Placing the edge of the elevator on the superior edge of the rib posteriorly and running it anteriorly along the entire length of the rib will perform this function. Similarly, the other edge of the Alexander elevator is placed on the inferior portion of the rib anteriorly and is run posteriorly. The dissection or stripping can be recalled with the mnemonic AA-BB (above anteriorly, below backward). A Doyen rib dissector is subperiosteally placed around the rib at one end and, maintaining close contact to the rib, is run the entire length of the incision (see Figure 7–5B). The rib is then cut at each end with the rib shear. Jagged rib edges are excised with a rongeur (see Figure 7–5C).

120 • SURGICAL APPROACHES TO THE SPINE

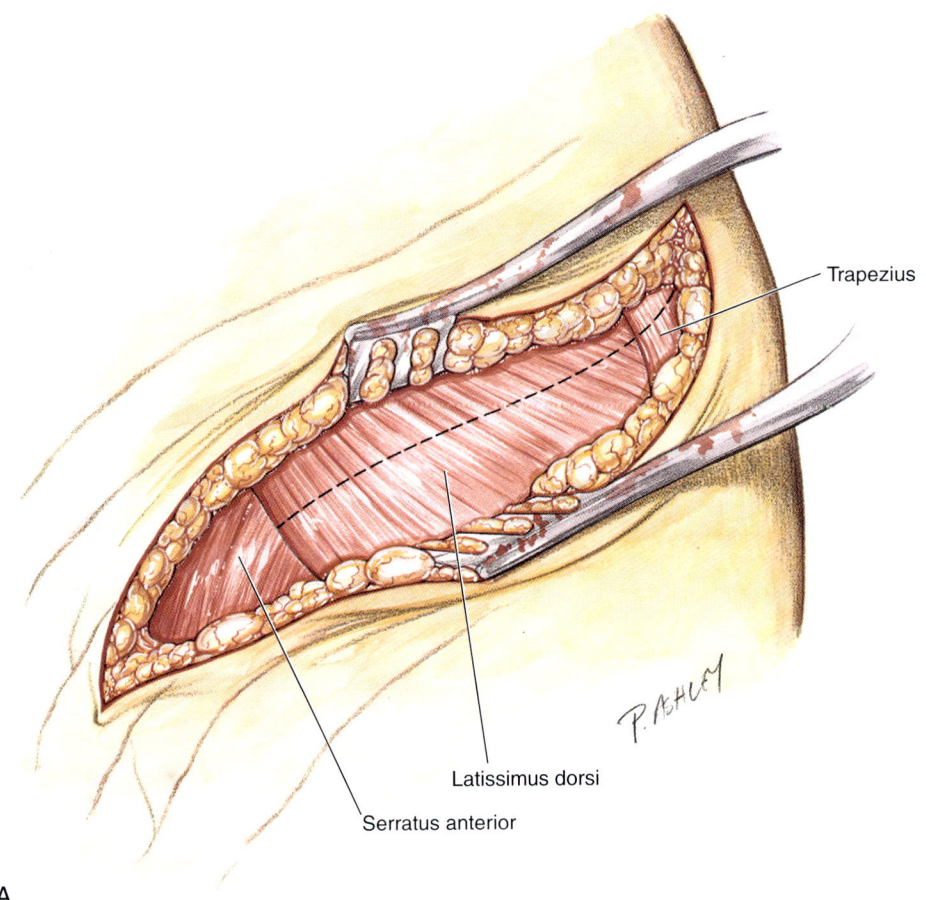

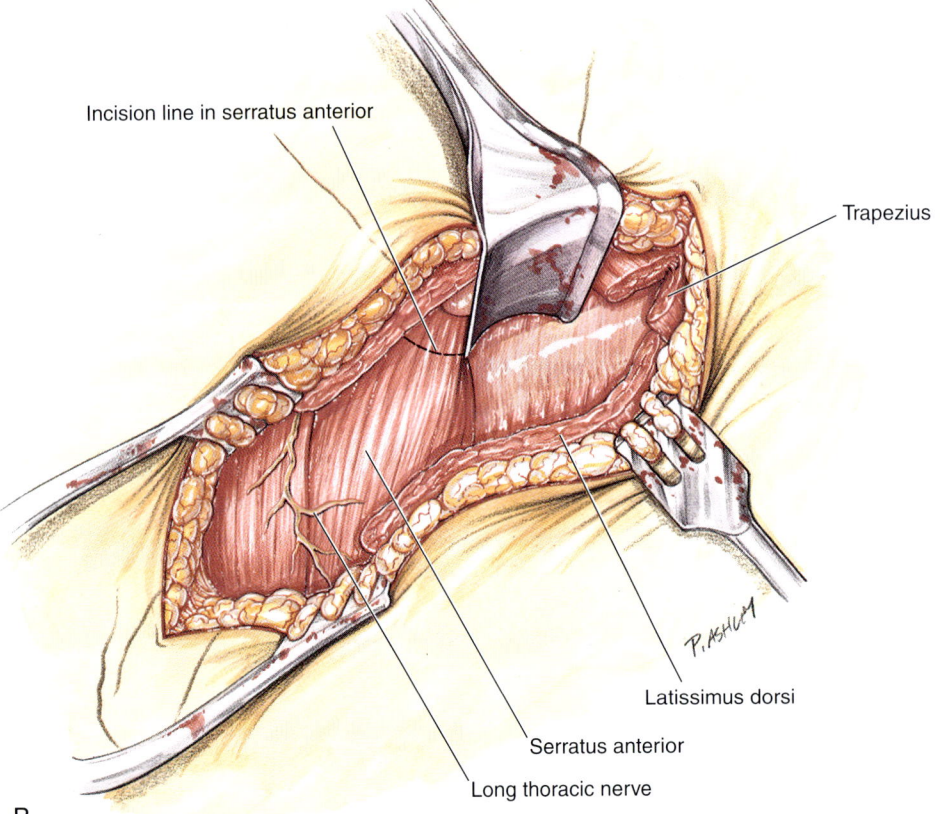

● **Figure 7-4.** *A,* Initial muscle division line to be sectioned with electrocautery. *B,* Latissimus dorsi and trapezius are cut, leaving serratus anterior to be sectioned close to its origin to protect the long thoracic nerve.

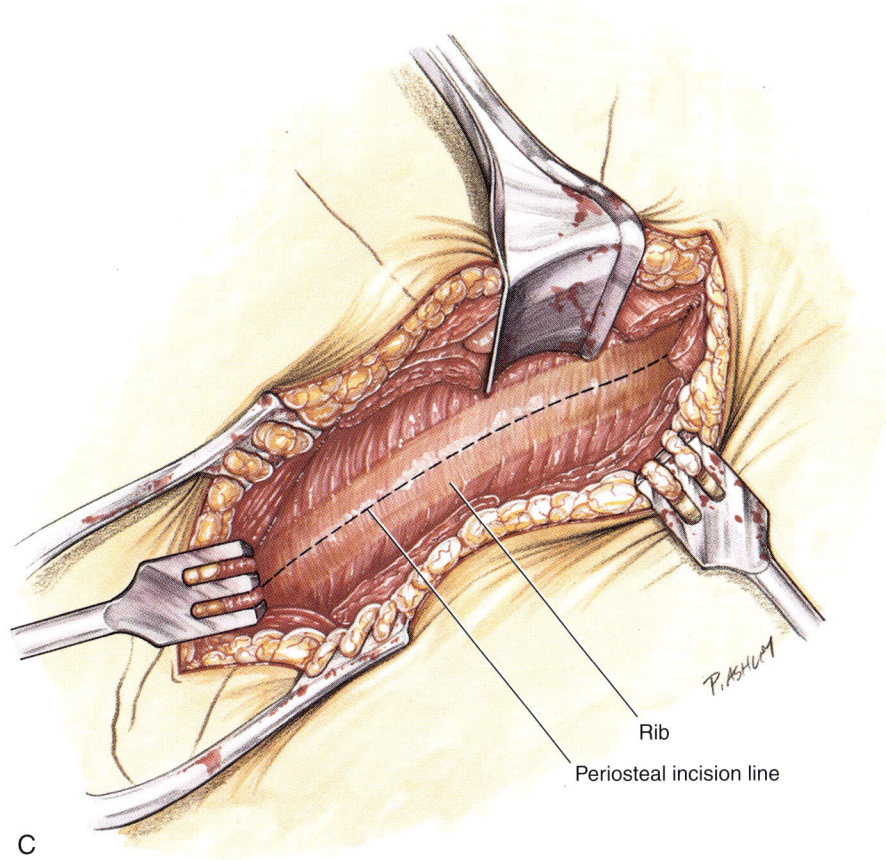

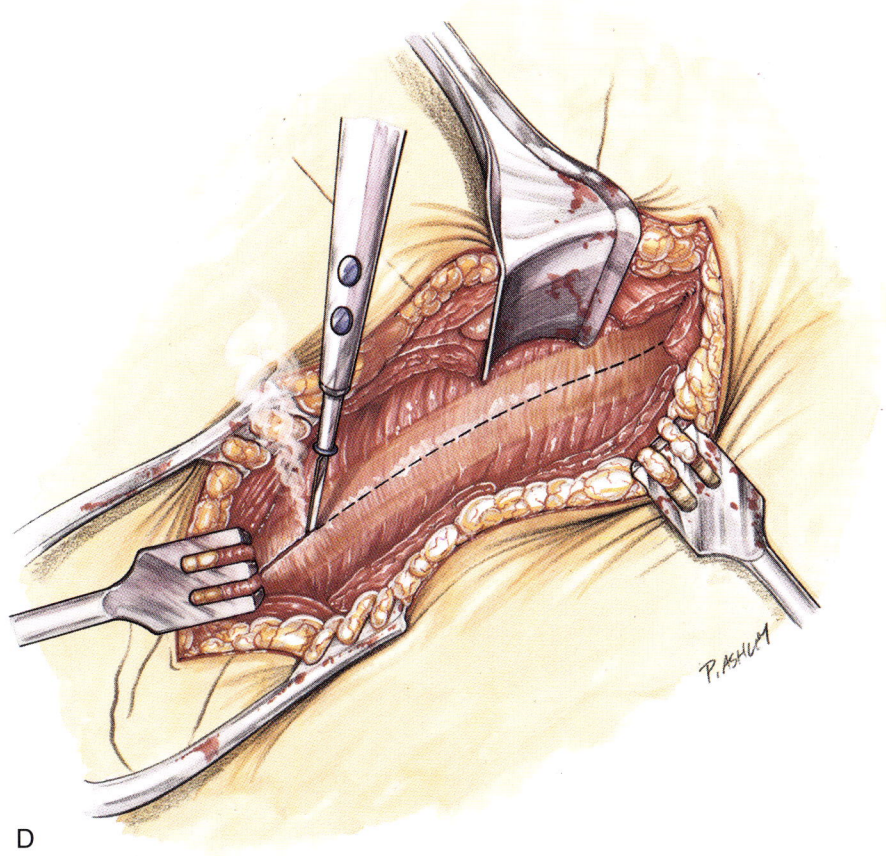

● **Figure 7-4.** *Continued C,* Rib is exposed with periosteal incision line. *D,* Cautery is used to incise the rib periosteum.

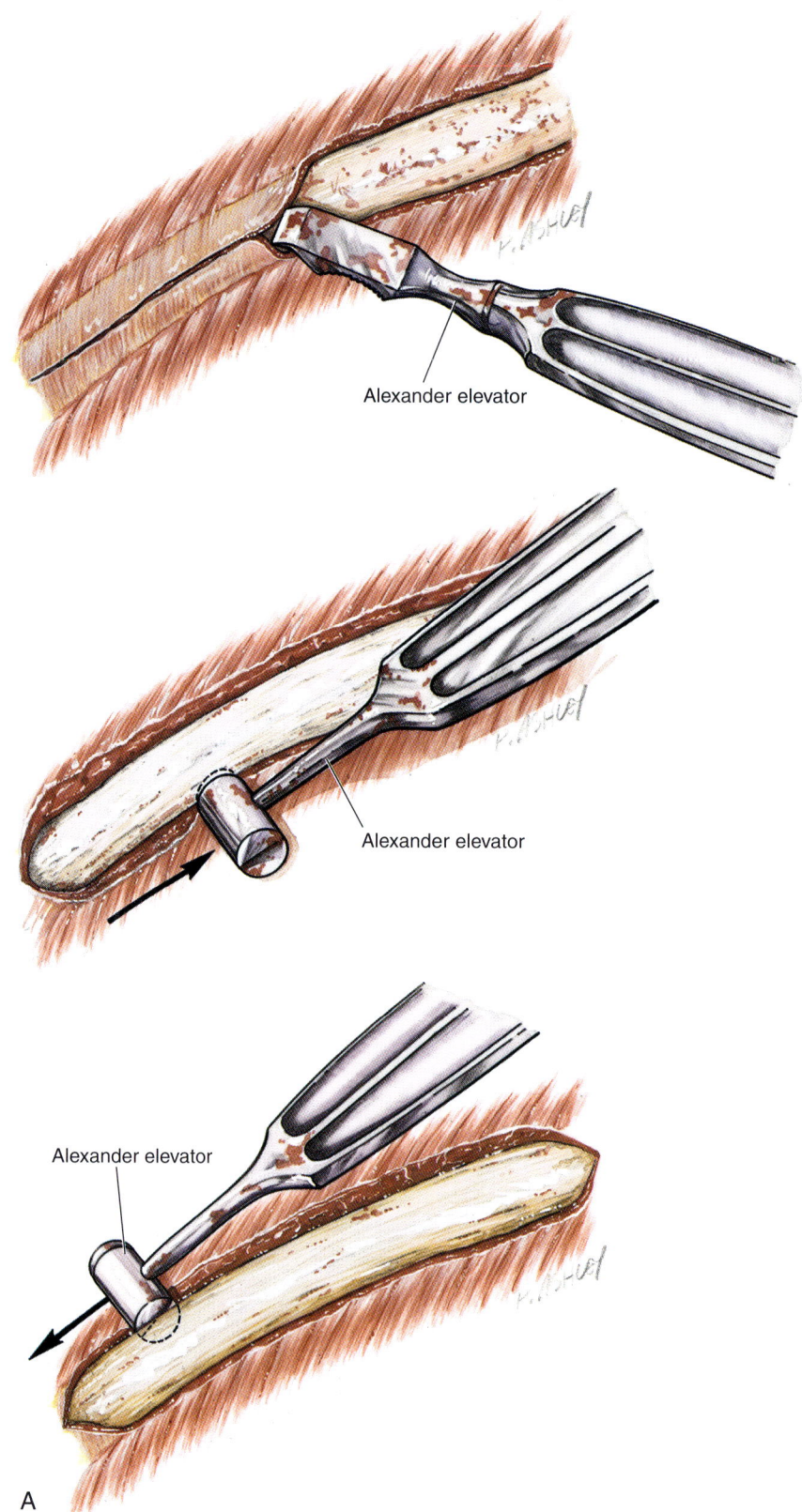

● **Figure 7-5.** *A*, Alexander elevator is used to dissect the lateral rib and the inferior and superior edges.

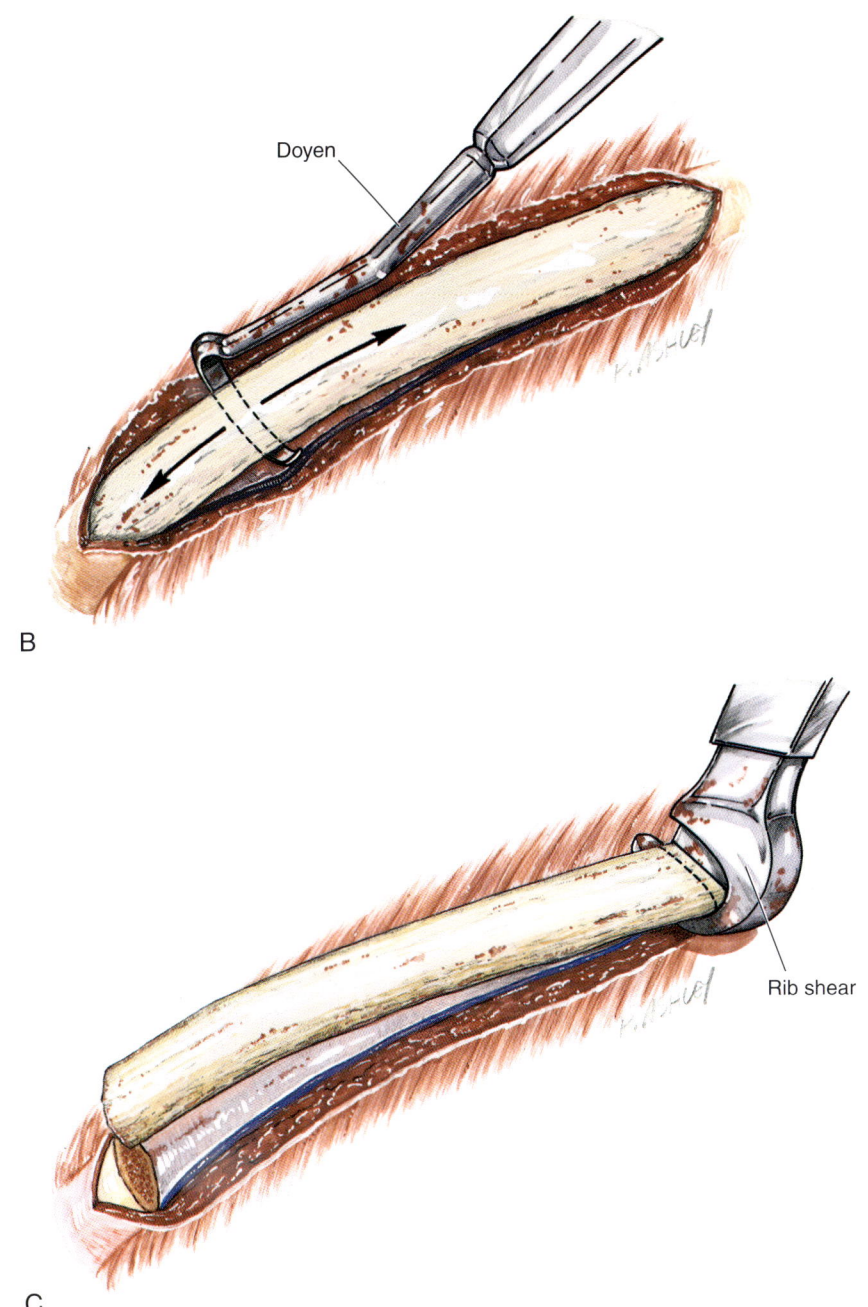

● **Figure 7-5.** *Continued B,* Doyen rib dissector is placed circumferentially about the rib, illustrating the dissection of the medial portion of the rib. *C,* Rib shear is used to cut the rib.

The parietal pleura is then held with two forceps and incised (see Figure 7–5D). The pleural incision is carried the full length of the exposure by placing a finger in the cavity and cutting along the glove with an electrocautery unit to protect the lung (see Figure 7–5E). Moist sponges are placed on the edges of the wound, a Finochietto rib retractor is placed, and the caudal and cephalad ribs are spread (Figure 7–6).

The parietal pleura is then incised over the length of the spine to be exposed. Generally, the vertebral bodies are located in the depressions and the disks over the prominences. The segmental vessels are identified in the depressions by blunt dissection with a Kittner

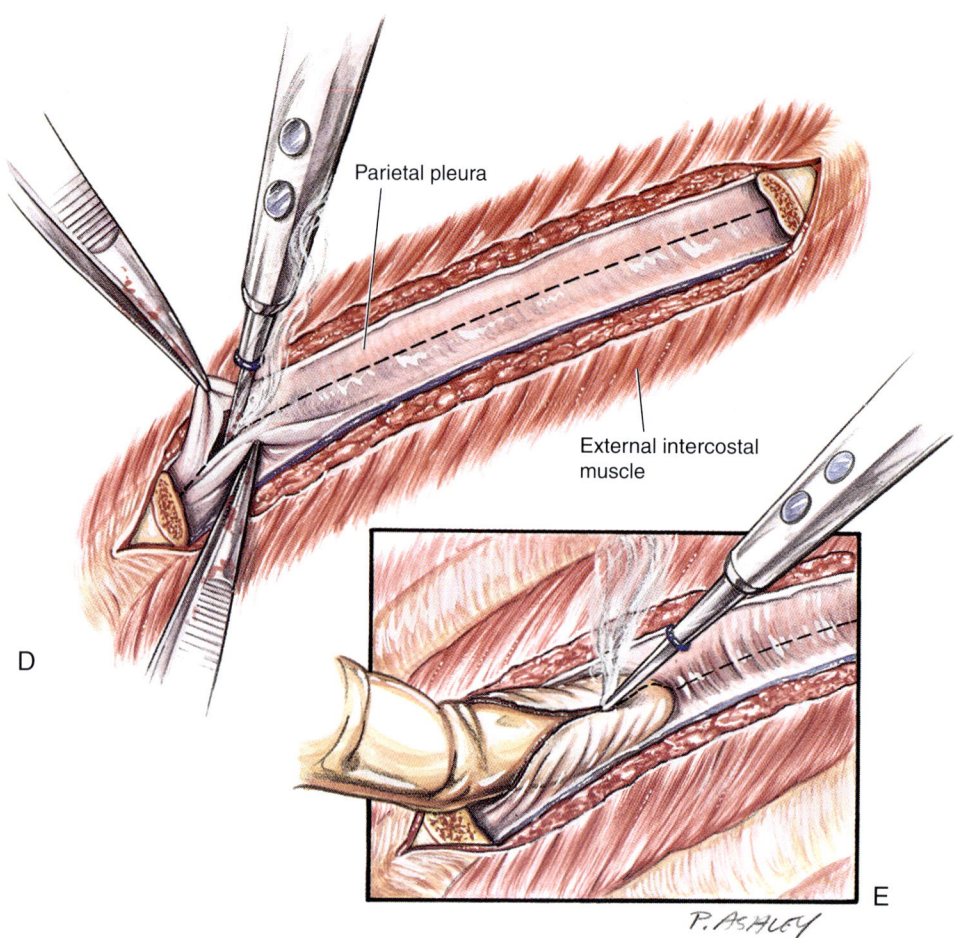

● **Figure 7-5.** *Continued D* and *E,* The pleural cavity is entered with an electrocautery unit.

dissector and a right-angled clamp. The vessels are ligated with sutures or metal clips at the anterior lateral aspect of the vertebral body (Figure 7-7). Ligation that is too close to the foramina can potentially damage the segmental feeder vessels to the spinal cord.[13]

After the definitive spine procedure an attempt is made to reapproximate the parietal pleura with a running chromic suture. This is not always possible but is helpful for hemostasis.

Before closure of the chest cavity, a chest tube should be placed several interspaces from the incision in the midaxillary or anterior axillary region. Chest tubes placed too posteriorly invariably become kinked when the patient is supine, hindering drainage. Patients are generally more uncomfortable when the chest tube is placed too posteriorly.

The skin incision for the chest tube is made slightly smaller than the chest tube selected and is placed at the level of the rib or interspace below the anticipated entrance point into the chest cavity. Tunneling the chest tube in this manner reduces the formation of a pleurocutaneous fistula should the tube remain in for an extended period of time, either because of excessive output or a persistent air leak. A small skin incision and the oblique tunnel will avoid the need for a purse string suture around the chest tube, which would need to be secured when the chest tube is removed. A curved hemostat is inserted subcutaneously

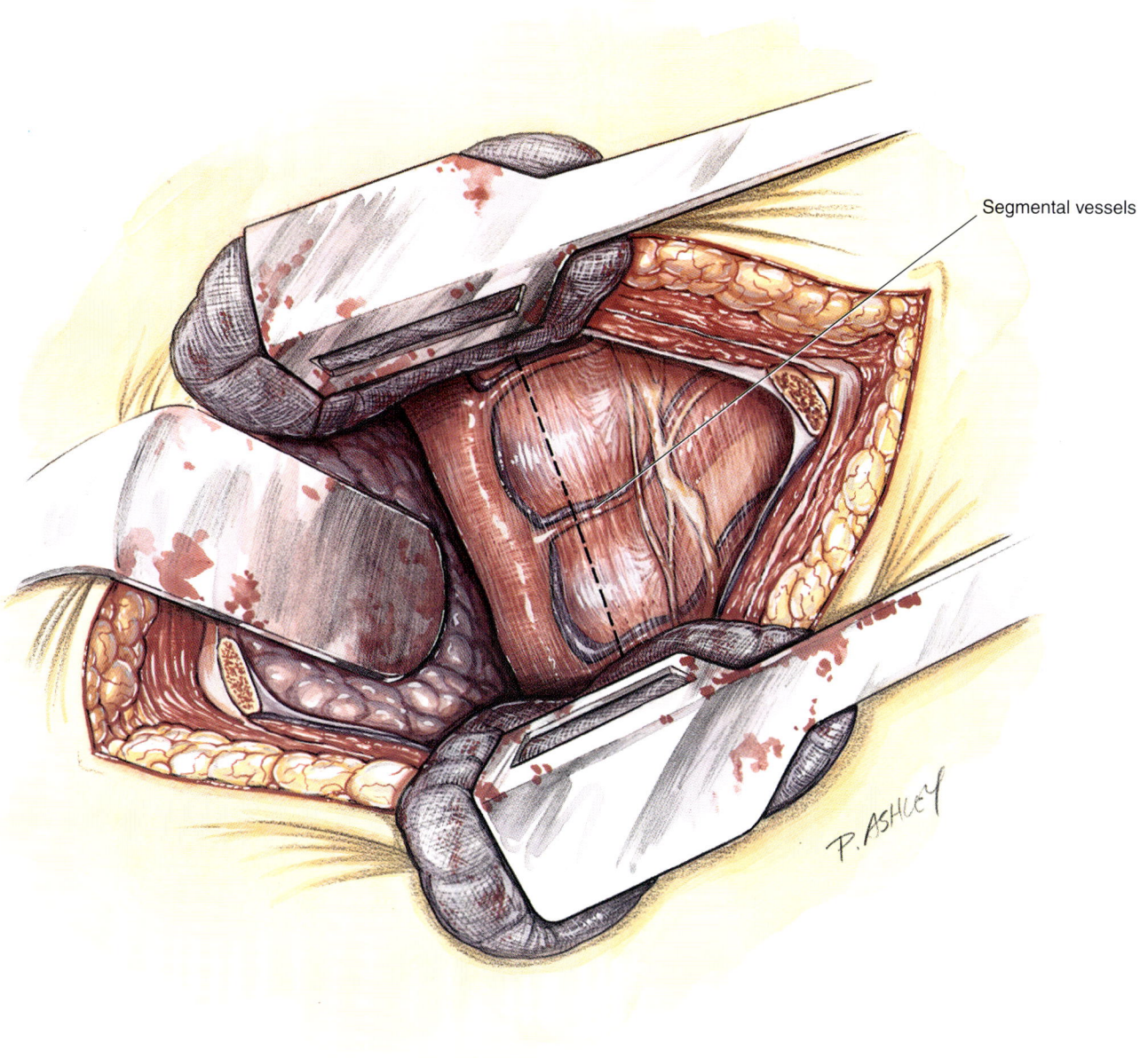

● **Figure 7-6.** Finochietto rib retractor in place. Note segmental vein and artery, and sympathetic trunk over spine.

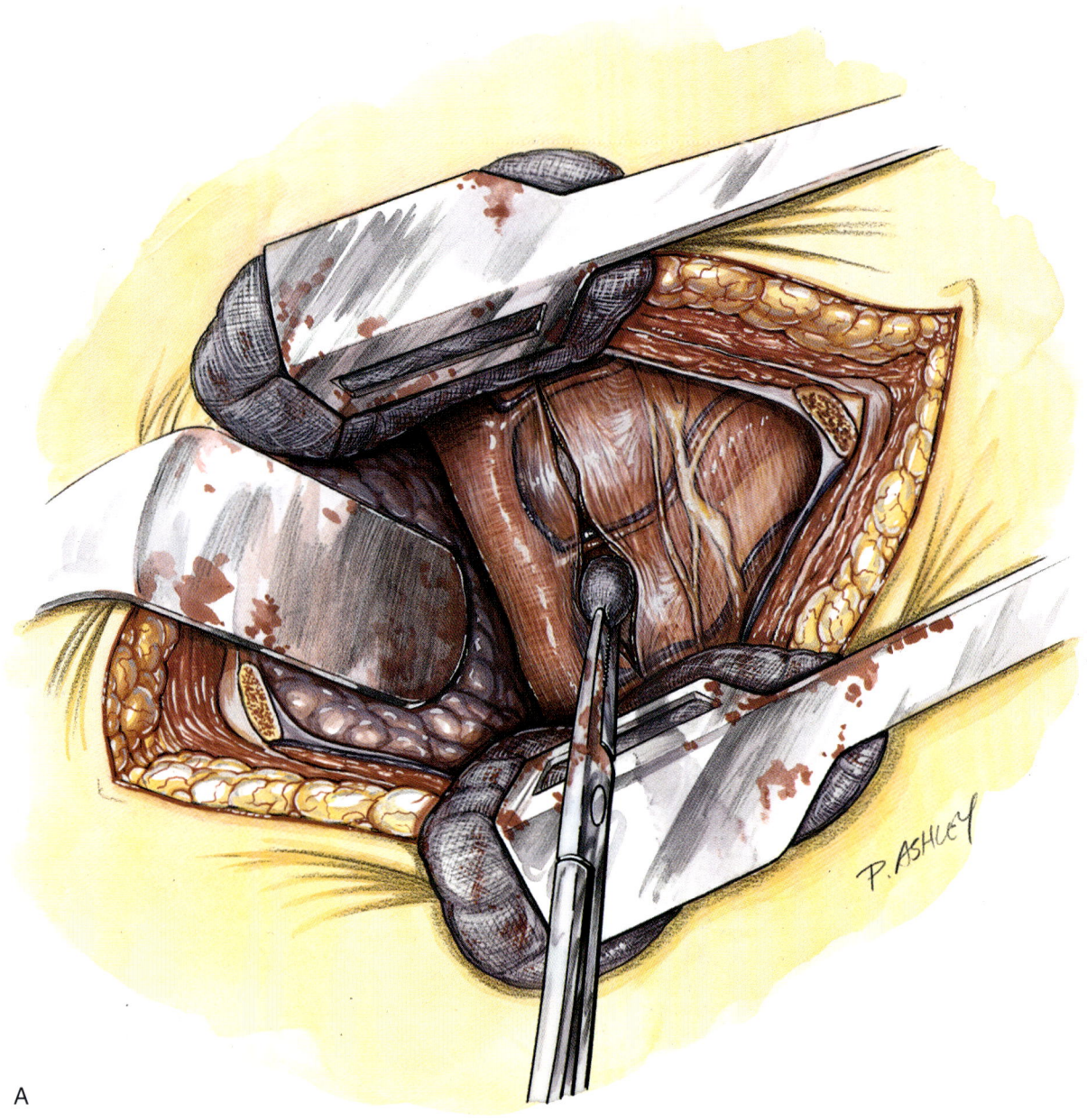

● **Figure 7-7.** *A,* Division of pleura. A peanut dissector is helpful to expose the segmental vessels.

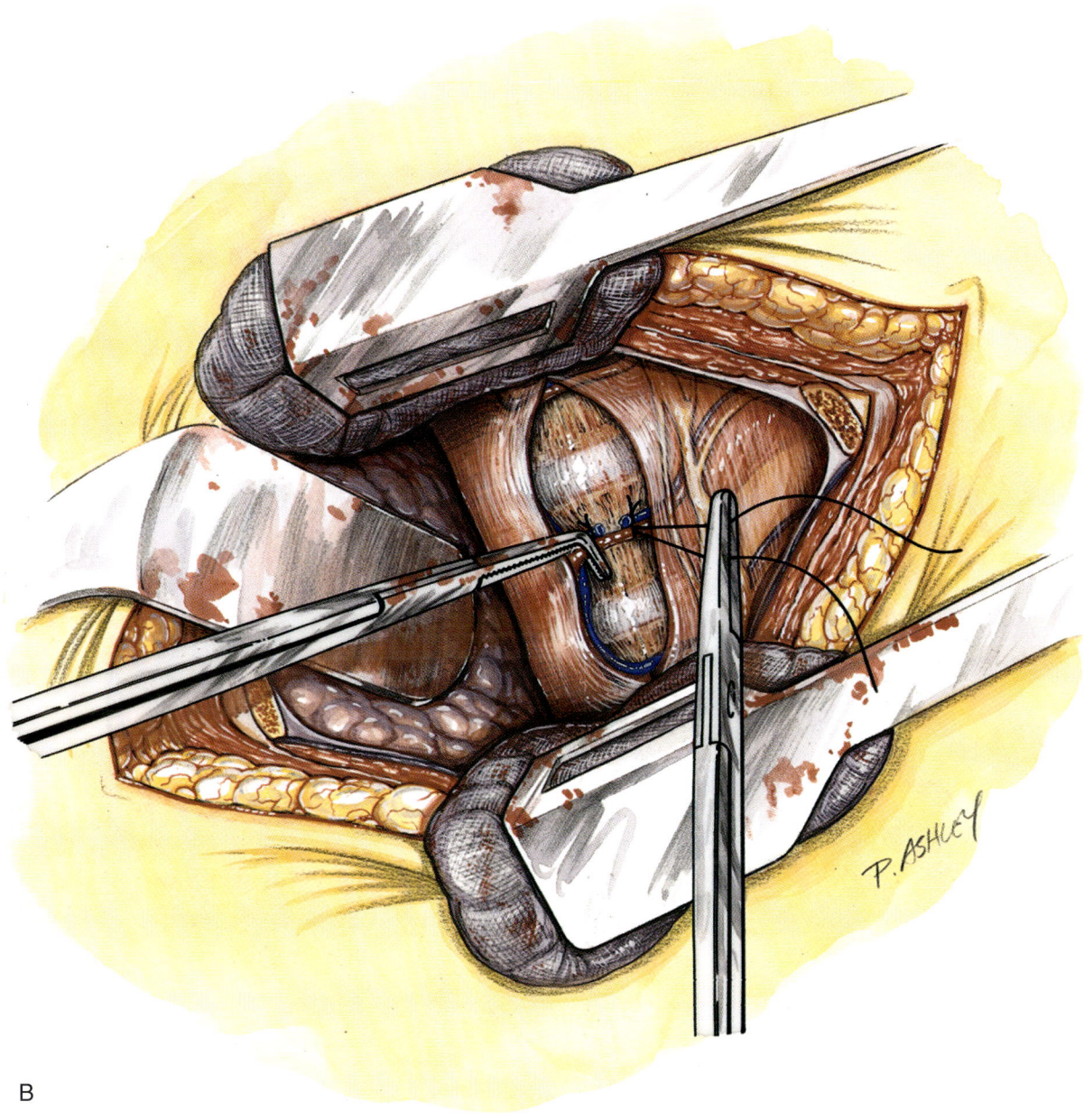

● **Figure 7-7.** *Continued B,* Division of segmental vessels.

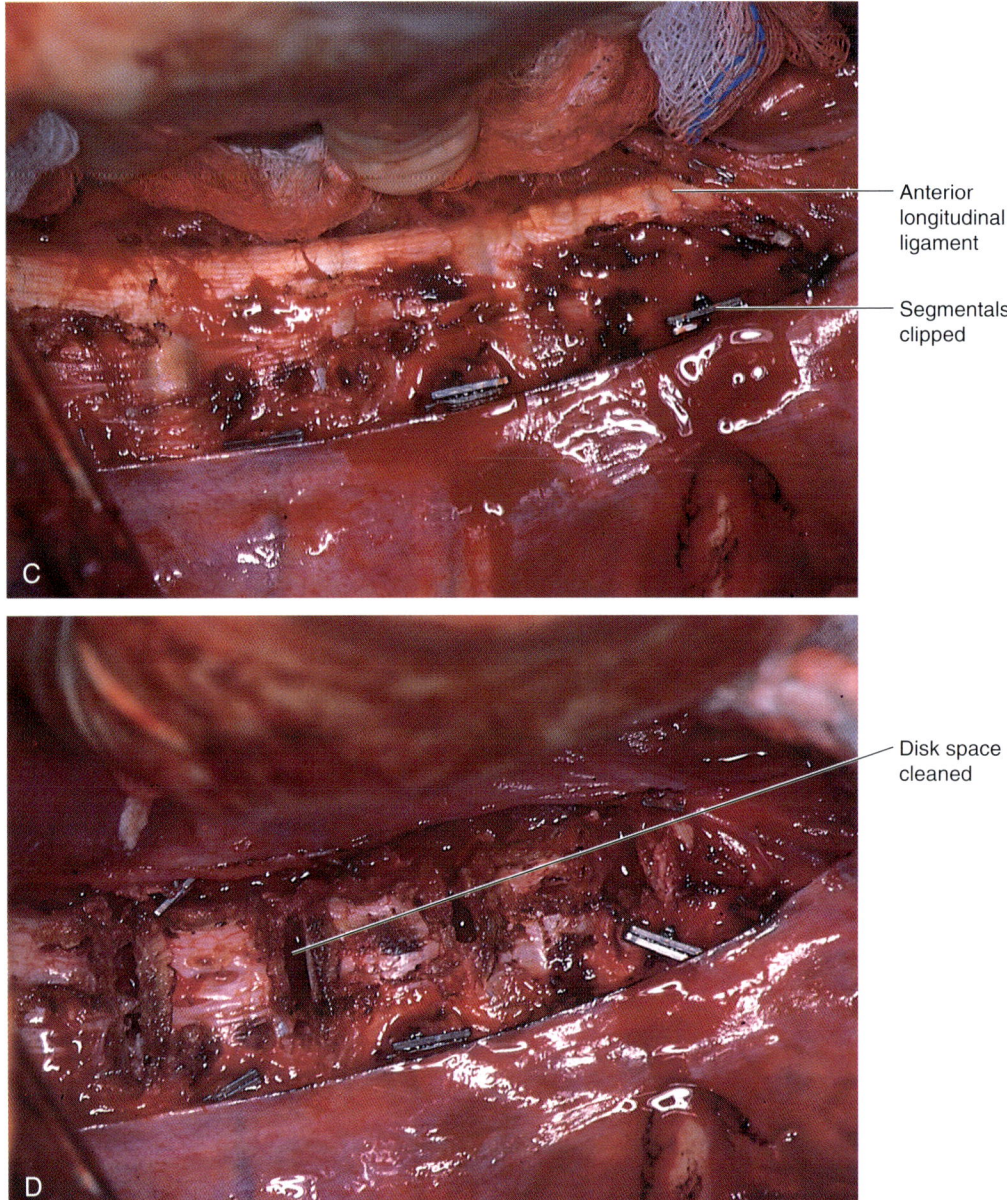

● **Figure 7-7.** *Continued C,* Patient with kyphotic spine showing exposure of anterior thoracic spine (anterior longitudinal ligament) after division of pleura and segmental vessels. *D,* Same patient after multilevel diskectomies and division of anterior longitudinal ligament.

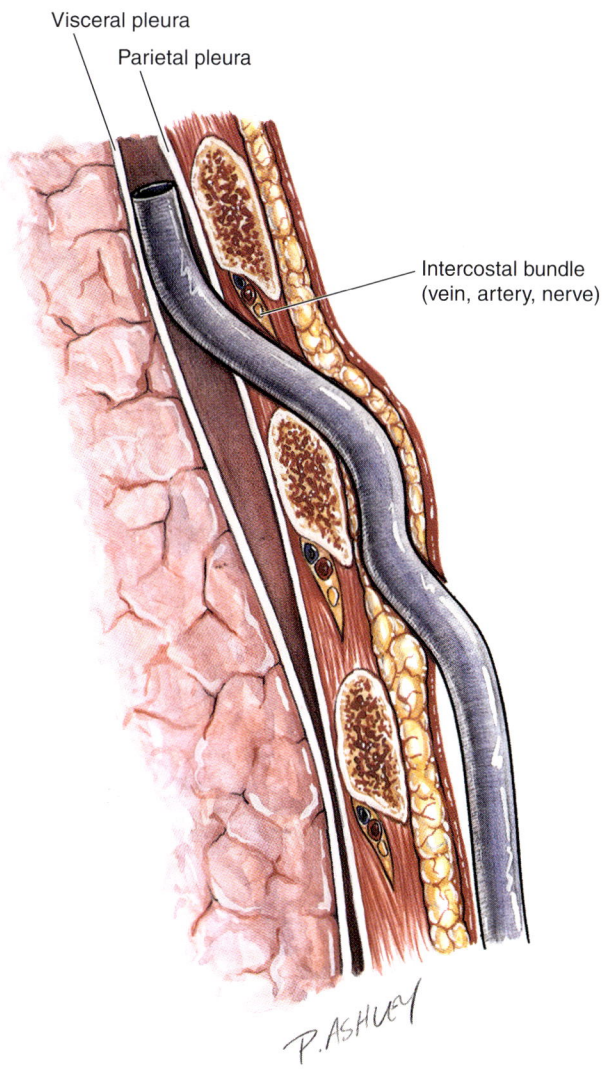

● **Figure 7-8.** Diagram illustrating the oblique path of the chest tube and a method of securing the chest tube.

to the superior edge of the rib where the chest cavity is entered bluntly. This creates an oblique path rather than a right-angled path (Figure 7-8). Separation of the intercostal tissue at the superior edge of the rib by opening the hemostat will assist in the passage of the tube. The curved hemostat is clamped to the chest tube within the chest cavity and fed through the wall from inside out. The chest tube should be secured carefully with a nonabsorbable suture. The suture is placed in the skin adjacent to the chest tube and a knot tied that places no pressure on the skin. A second knot is tied proximal to the first, then each free end of the suture is looped around the chest tube as demonstrated in Figure 7-9. The suture is cinched down tightly to the tube before placement of the final set of knots that will anchor the tube. The lung should then be inspected fully expanded before proceeding to closure of the chest cavity.

Approximately five heavy absorbable pericostal sutures are placed evenly separated along the superior and inferior rib (Figure 7-10). The rib approximator is then placed to

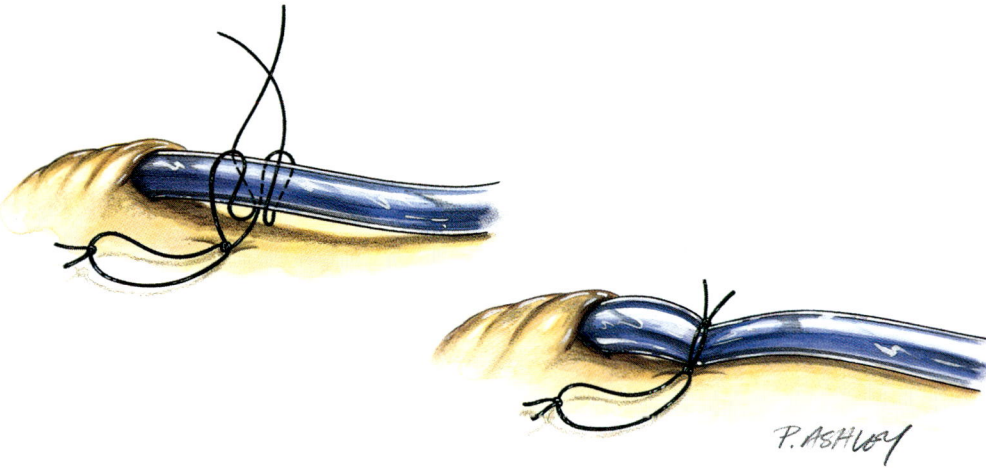

● **Figure 7-9.** Chest tube is secured with a nonabsorbable suture that is looped around tube.

gently bring the ribs together without closing the intercostal space. The periosteal rib bed is then approximated with a running absorbable suture. The pericostal sutures are then secured, and the rib approximator is removed.

The latissimus dorsi, serratus anterior, and rhomboids are approximated accurately. The subcutaneous layer is closed with a running absorbable suture. The skin is approximated with a running suture. Steri-Strips are used for the final closure.

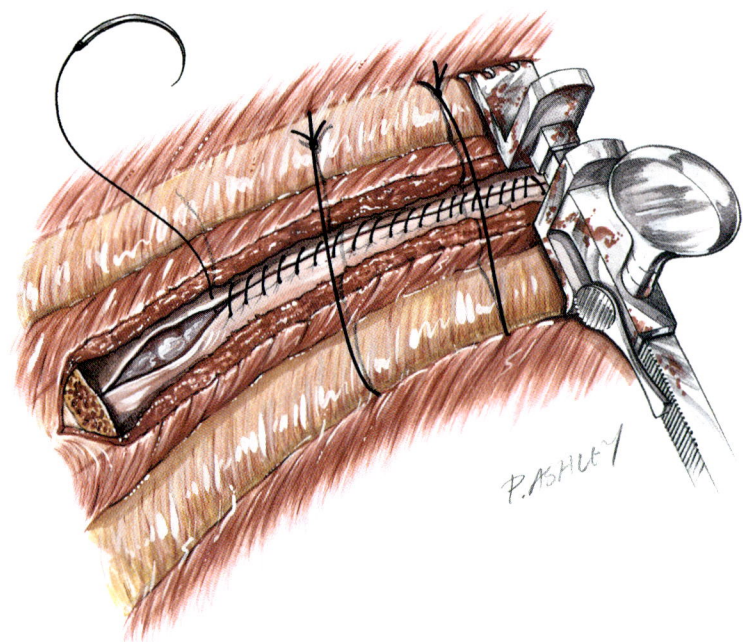

● **Figure 7-10.** Chest closure with rib approximator in place, periocostals positioned, and parietal pleura approximated with a running suture.

REFERENCES

1. Naef AP: The Story of Thoracic Surgery. Kirkland, WA, Hogrefe & Huber Publishers, 1990.
2. Tuffier T: De la résection du sommet du poumon. Semin Med Paris 2:202, 1891.
3. Hodgson AR: Connection of fixed spinal curves: A preliminary communication. J Bone Joint Surg 47:1221, 1965.
4. Hodgson AR, Stock FE: Anterior spinal fusion, a preliminary communication on radical treatment of Pott's disease and Pott's paraplegia. Br J Surg 44:266, 1956.
5. Hodgson AR, Stock FE, Feng HSP, Ong GB: Anterior spinal fusion: The operative approach and pathologic findings in 412 patients with Pott's disease of the spine. Br J Surg 44:266, 1956.
6. Bradford DS, Winter RB, Lonstein JE, Moe JH: Techniques of anterior spine surgery for the management of kyphosis. Clin Orthop 128:129, 1977.
7. Burrington JD, Brown C, Wayne ER, Odom J: Anterior approach to the thoracolumbar spine: Technical considerations. Arch Surg 111:456, 1976.
8. Cook WA: Transthoracic vertebral surgery. Ann Thorac Surg 12:54, 1971.
9. Hall JE: Anterior approach to spinal deformities. Orthop Clin North Am 3:81, 1972.
10. Johnson JTH, Robinson RA: Anterior strut grafts for severe kyphosis. Clin Orthop 56:25, 1968.
11. Riseborough EJ: The anterior approach to the spine for the correction of deformities of the axial skeleton. Clin Orthop 93:207, 1973.
12. Winter RB, Moe JH, Wang JF: Congenital kyphosis, its natural history and treatment as observed in a study of 130 patients. J Bone Joint Surg Am 55:223, 1973.
13. Dommissi EG: The blood supply to the spinal cord. J Bone Joint Surg Br 56:225, 1974.

Chapter 8

Costotransversectomy

Alexander R. Vaccaro, M.D.

The posterolateral approach to the thoracic spine, first described in 1894 by Menard, was initially used for safe and effective decompression and drainage of spinal tuberculous abscesses. Today, in addition to its efficacy in decompressing spinal infections, the costotransversectomy approach allows adequate access to the anterior and lateral aspect of the thoracic vertebrae and is especially important in the upper thoracic spine where anterior transthoracic approaches can be technically difficult. Through this approach, one may perform vertebral body or disk biopsies, thoracic diskectomies, limited anterolateral thoracic vertebral and spinal cord decompression, as well as limited anterior spinal fusions. Some surgeons have found this approach superior with less morbidity than formal anterior thoracoabdominal approaches when performing thoracic diskectomies at the T10 to T12 level. These procedures may be undertaken all while avoiding entry into the thoracic pleural cavity, once a disaster before the emergence of widespread antibiotic use.

Relevant Clinical Anatomy

Muscles

The posterior musculature of the thoracic spine, which may be transversed during this procedure, depending on the level of the lesion, is divided into three layers: (1) the superficial layer consisting of the trapezius, latissimus dorsi, and rhomboid major and minor; (2) the intermediate layer consisting of the serratus posterior superior and inferior, and (3) a deep layer, which includes the erectae spinae muscles (spinalis, longissimus, and iliocostalis) and transversospinalis muscle group (semispinalis, multifidus, and rotatores). The trapezius, thoracolumbar fascia, and rhomboids are divided in lesions of the upper thoracic spine, whereas the trapezius and latissimus dorsi with its associated thoracolumbar fascia, are divided in lower thoracic approaches. Beneath the superficial and intermediate muscular groups lies a deep muscular layer, which can be divided bluntly between the iliocostalis laterally and longissimus muscle medially or, if necessary, transversely for better surgical exposure (Figure 8–1).

Costotransverse Ligaments

To separate the rib from its articulation with the vertebral body and transverse process, four important costotransverse ligaments must be divided: (1) the superior costotransverse ligament, which consists of a strong anterior and smaller posterior division extending between the inferior aspect of the transverse process and the superior border of the adjacent inferior rib; (2) the medial or capsular ligament, which attaches the posterior neck of the rib to the anterior border of the transverse process; (3) the lateral costotransverse ligament, which extends from the posterior tubercle of the rib to the tip of the transverse process, and (4) the anterior costotransverse or radiate ligament, which secures the head of the rib to its respective vertebral body (Figure 8–2).

Neurovascular Structures

The thoracic nerve root exits the neural foramen beneath its respective thoracic pedicle and divides, sending a dorsal ramus posteriorly into the erectae spinae muscle group coursing medial to the superior costotransverse ligament. This is accompanied by the dorsal branches of the posterior intercostal vessels, which may be identified and ligated to prevent excessive bleeding. The thoracic segmental vessels are located at the waist of the thoracic vertebral body and divide laterally into a dorsal and ventral division (posterior intercostal vessels) prior to the level of the neural foramen. The ventral ramus of the thoracic nerve root or the intercostal nerve joins the posterior intercostal vessels and travels laterally to meet with the undersurface of the rib at its posteriormost apex (Figure 8–3). The sympathetic trunk should be identified and protected, along with the parietal pleura as one bluntly dissects between the anterolateral vertebral body medially and the pleura laterally.

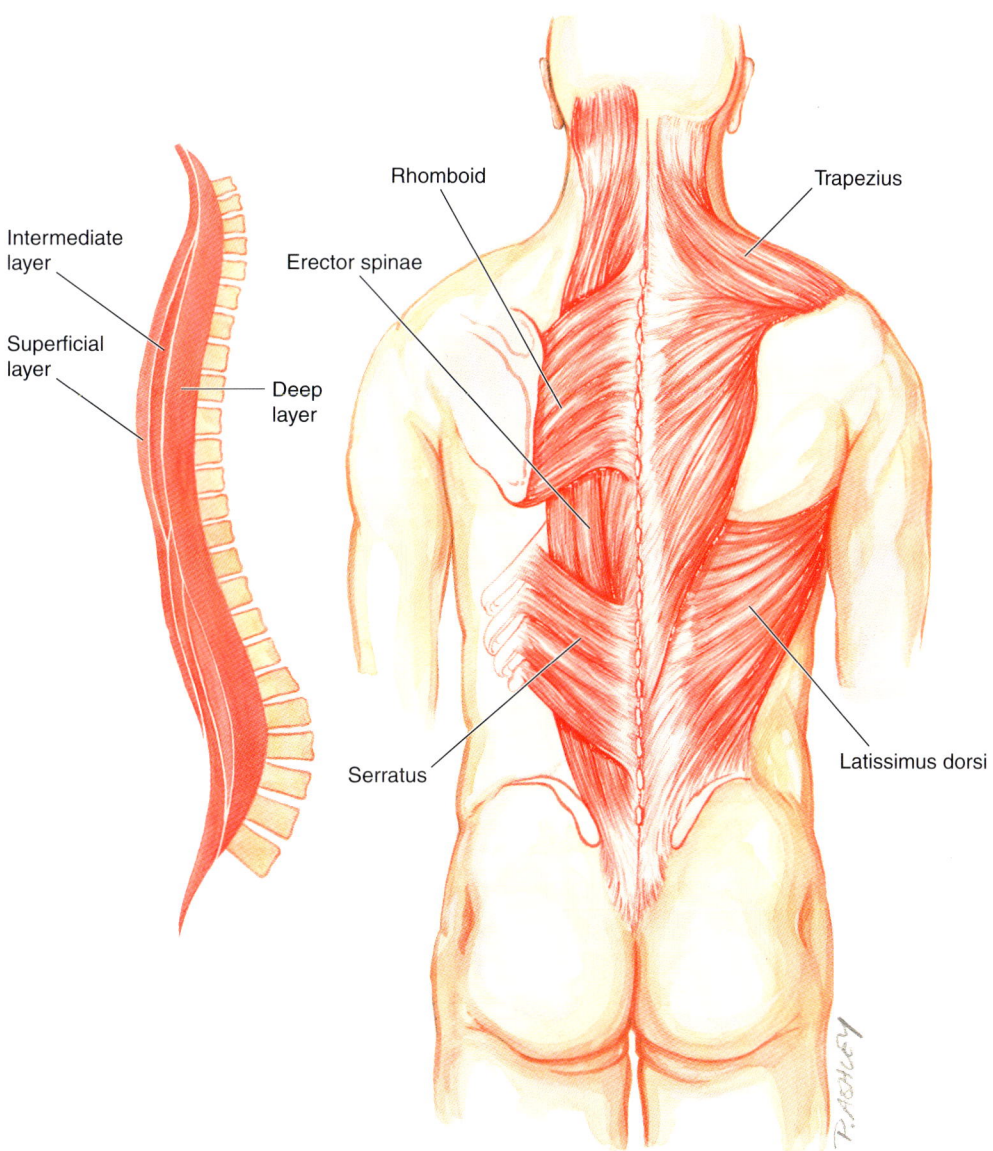

● **Figure 8-1.** The three layers of the posterior thoracic and lumbar spine musculature. The superficial layer consists of the trapezius, latissimus dorsi, and rhomboid major and minor. The intermediate layer is composed of the serratus posterior-superior and posterior-inferior, and the deep layer includes the erectae spinae and transversospinalis musculature groups.

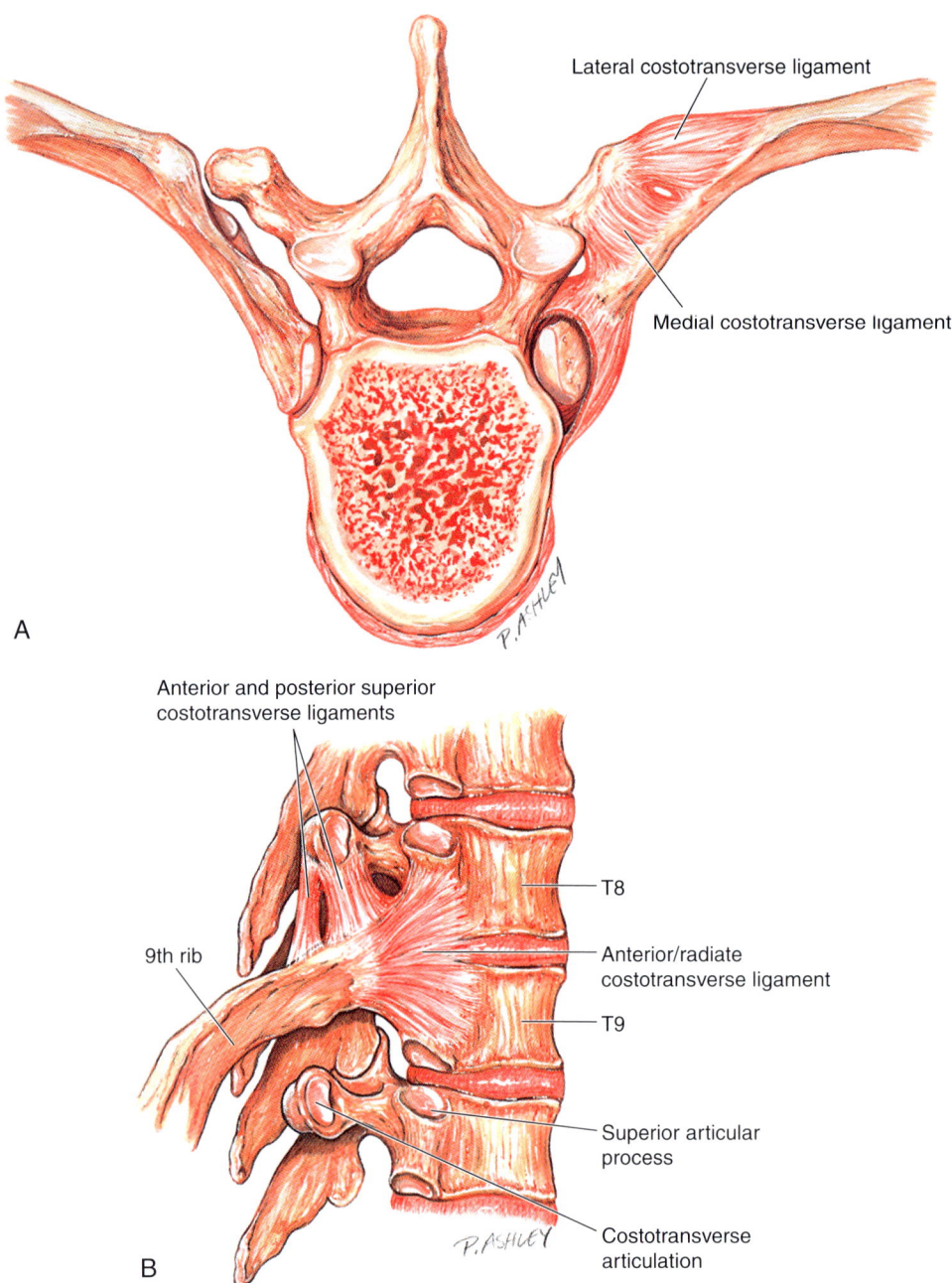

● **Figure 8-2.** The costotransverse ligaments consist of four different ligaments. *A,* The lateral costotransverse ligament extends from the posterior tubercle of the rib to the tip of the transverse process. The medial or capsular costotransverse ligament attaches the posterior neck of the rib to the anterior border of the transverse process. *B,* The anterior and posterior superior costotransverse ligaments extend from the inferior border of the transverse process to the superior border of the adjacent inferior rib, and the anterior or radiate costotransverse ligament secures the head of the rib to the lateral vertebral body. As shown, the articulation of the rib with the vertebral column is over the intervertebral disk of the level of the rib, as well as the vertebral body cephalad to it. Following the base of the rib to its bony pedicle is a safe means of localizing the inferiorly located neural foramen and nerve root.

Bone

The posterior medial border of the head and neck of the rib articulates with the intervertebral disk of its respective vertebral body and the vertebral body cephalad to it. Following the course of the rib to its articulation with the vertebral column allows the surgeon to identify the bony pedicle located at the rib's base as well as the inferiorly located neural foramen (see Figure 8–2).

Surgical Approach

After completion of general endotracheal anesthesia, the patient may be positioned in either the lateral decubitus position with an axillary pad to avoid neurovascular compression, a 15-degree semiprone position with a chest roll placed beneath the elevated chest wall, or, as I prefer, the prone position with two chest rolls or bolsters placed longitudinally, lateral enough to allow adequate chest wall expansion. Draping is performed widely to expose all thoracic ribs that may be approached during this procedure. The posterior iliac crest on either side is also prepped and draped in case one chooses to add a fusion at the completion of the proposed surgical procedure.

A spinal needle may now be placed at the desired level of decompression, and an intraoperative lateral radiograph is taken to confirm the appropriate level. Various incisions

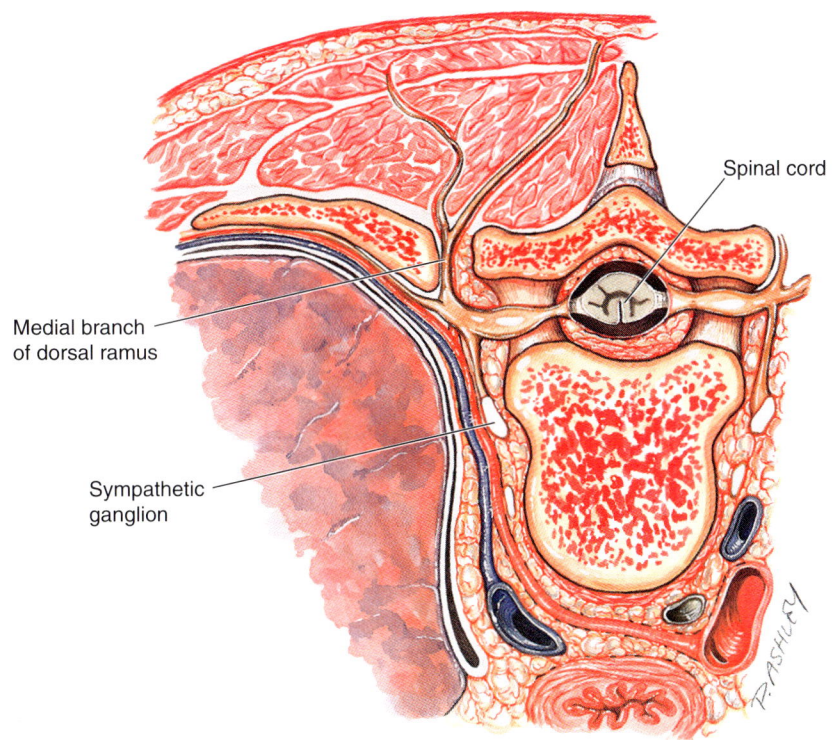

● **Figure 8-3.** The thoracic nerve root gives off a dorsal ramus, which is accompanied by dorsal branches of the posterior intercostal vessels as they course medial to the superior costotransverse ligament into the deep posterior muscular group. These structures should be identified and ligated, if necessary, to prevent excessive hemorrhage.

may be used, depending on the level of the lesion, ranging from (1) midline over the spinous processes; (2) paramedian, 2.5 inches lateral to the spinous processes; or, as I prefer, (3) curvilinear 10 to 13 cm long, starting and ending over the spinous processes with the apex approximately 6 to 8 cm from the midline over the desired rib to be accessed (Figure 8–4). Some authors perform a paramedian incision midway between the spinous processes and vertebral border of the scapula for lesions proximal to T7, with the distal limb of the incision curved obliquely laterally over the rib to be approached for lesions distal to T8.

After the skin incision, dissection is taken down through the subcutaneous fat down to the level of the posterior thoracic superficial muscular layer. The trapezius, followed by the thoracolumbar fascia or latissimus dorsi, and possibly the rhomboid musculature depending on the level, are now divided in line with their fibers close to the vertical plane of the costovertebral joints (Figure 8–5). One now is at the level of the deep paraspinal muscles, the erectae spinae and transversospinalis muscles. These are now divided over the costotransverse junction, either in line with the skin incision or in the plane between the iliocostalis laterally and the longissimus medially and sharply elevated with a Cobb instrument or elevator off the posterior surface of the transverse process and ribs (Figure 8–6). If exposure at this point is difficult, the paraspinal muscles may be divided transversely through their fibers, although this makes for a difficult closure.

The desired rib or ribs are now exposed subperiosteally with care to avoid damage to the inferiorly located neurovascular bundle and anteriorly located pleura (Figure 8–7). The rib may be sharply divided with the rib cutter 6 to 8 cm lateral to the costotransverse

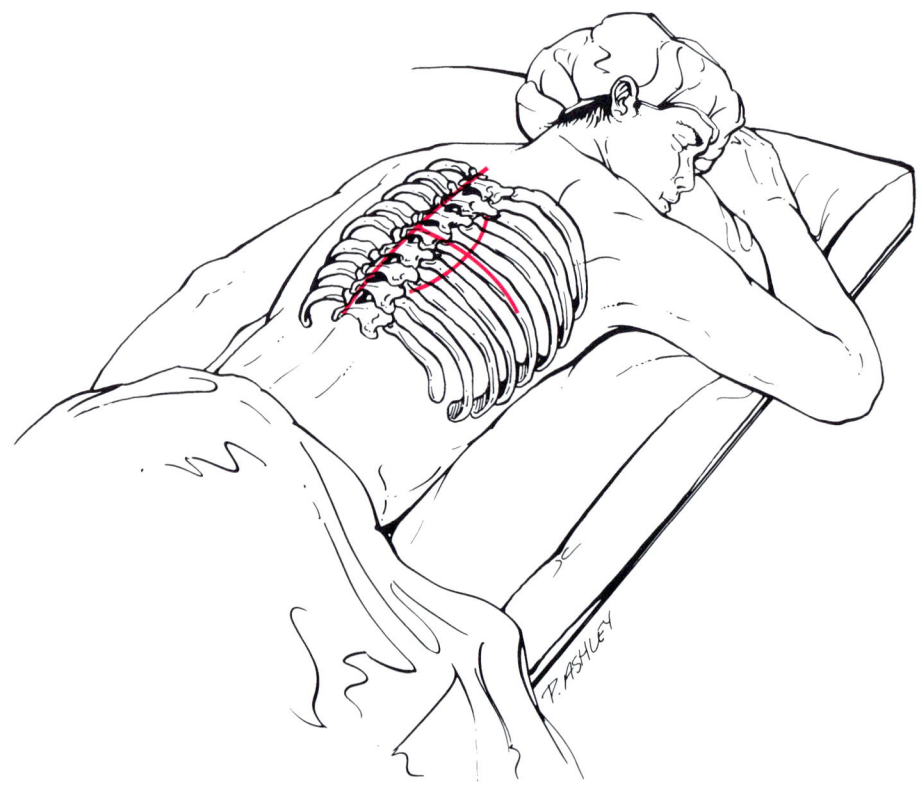

● **Figure 8-4.** The patient is placed in a prone position, as shown. A curvilinear incision is centered with its apex over the rib to be resected. Alternative incisions include an extended midline incision or an incision parallel to the rib to be resected.

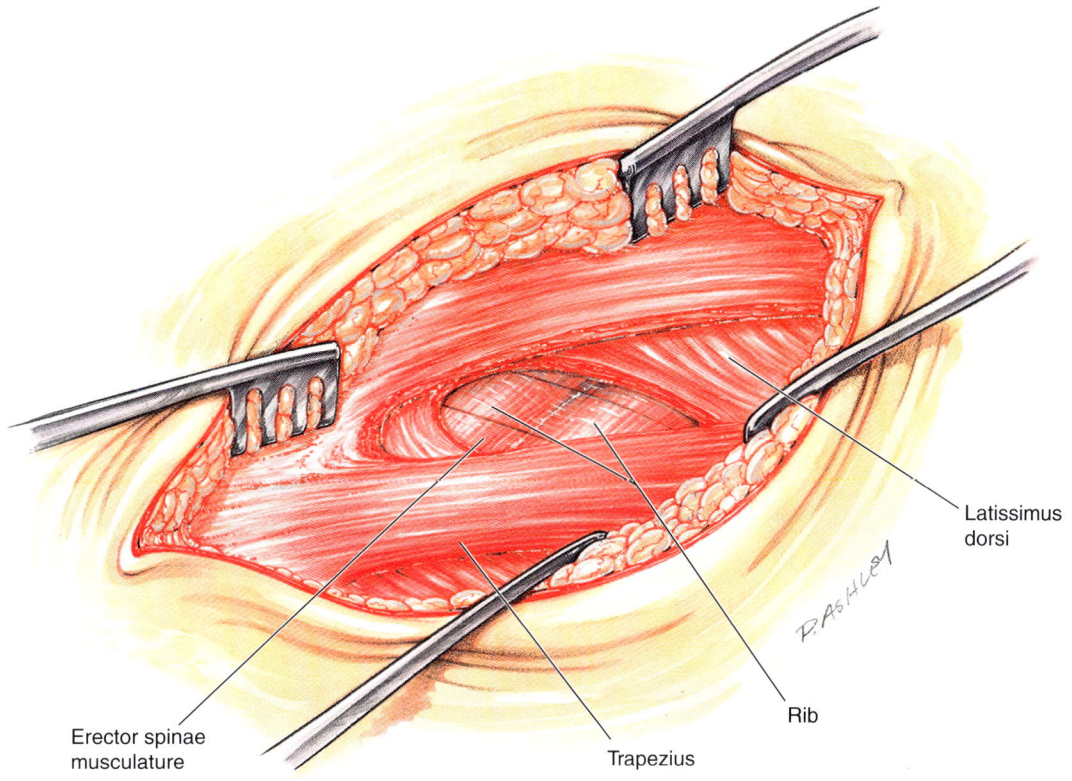

● **Figure 8-5.** The trapezius and latissimus dorsi are divided in line with their fibers, exposing the deeper paraspinal musculature, the iliocostalis, and the longissimus.

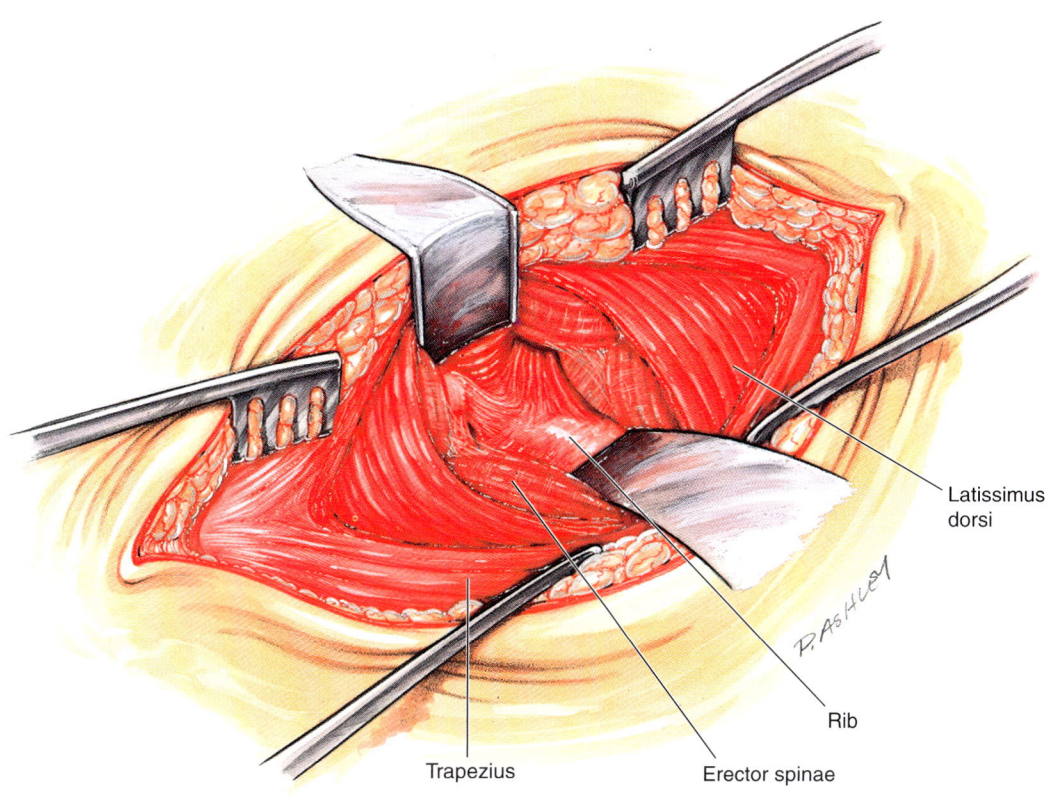

● **Figure 8-6.** The deep paraspinal musculature is divided in the interval between the iliocostalis laterally and the longissimus medially, exposing the costotransverse junction and desired rib to be resected.

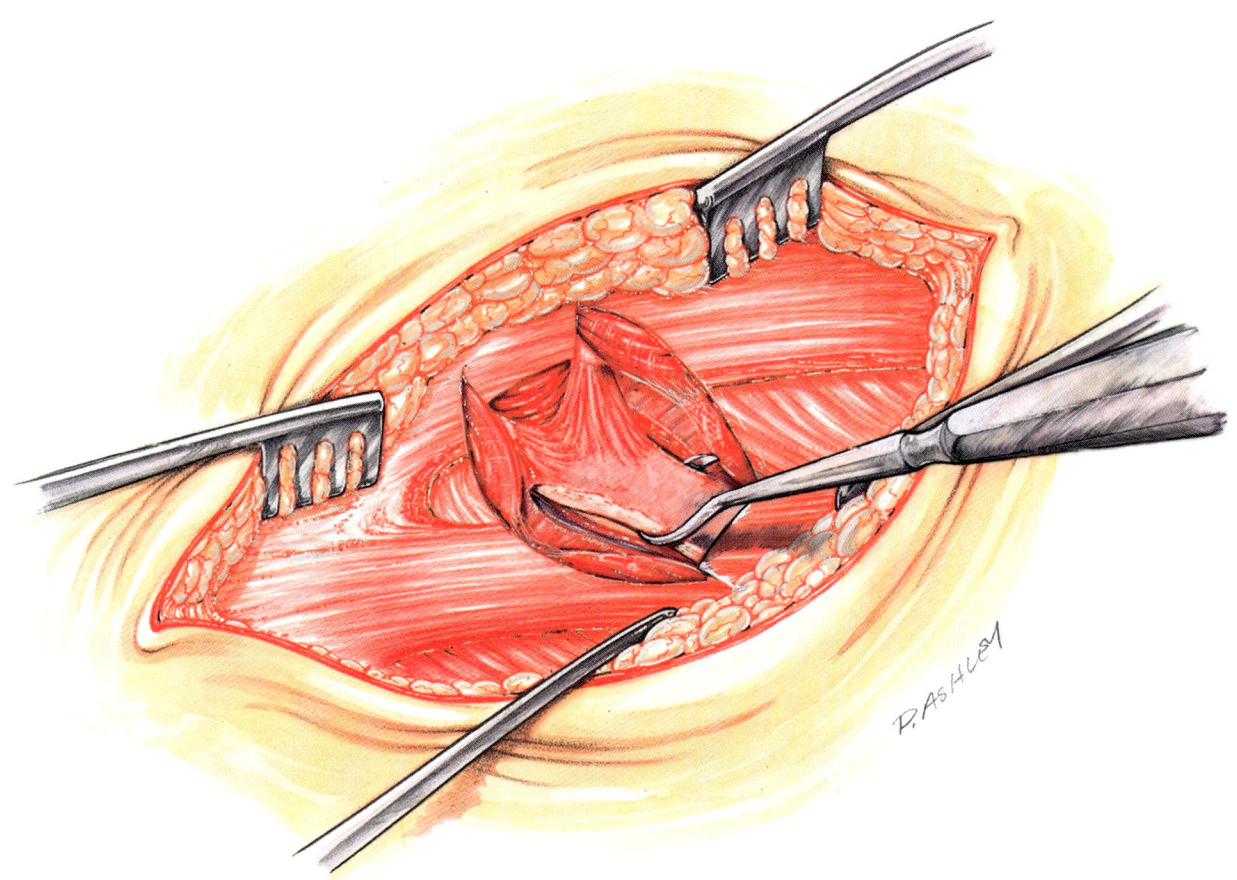

● **Figure 8-7.** The rib to be resected is freed in a subperiosteal manner with effort to protect the inferiorly located neurovascular bundle and anteriorly located pleura.

junction and carefully elevated to allow subsequent removal. The medial border of the remaining lateral rib is then beveled to protect the underlying pleura. The costotransverse ligaments (superior, medial, lateral, and radiate) can now be sharply divided with a sharp periosteal elevator or knife and ligamentum flavum rongeur as the rib is gently rotated with the bone clamp. The lateral and medial (capsular) costotransverse ligaments are easily divided under direct vision whereas the anterior or radiate ligament may need to be divided indirectly with the ligamentum flavum rongeur after reflection of the pleura from the anterolateral vertebral body surface (Figure 8–8). One may attempt to completely disarticulate the rib in its entirety or divide it at its neck with later removal of its head with the transverse process. The transverse process is now removed with a bone rongeur or osteotome down to its juncture with its superior facet and pedicle (Figure 8–9). One must always keep in mind that the articulating surface of the rib overlies the intervertebral disk at the level of the rib as well as the vertebral body cephalad to it. At this point, one may now identify the segmental vessels and thoracic nerve root.

Once the neurovascular pedicle is identified and retracted (or, if necessary, the vascular pedicle may be ligated), one may now proceed to elevate the parietal pleura and sympathetic trunk from the anterolateral surface of the vertebral body either bluntly with a finger or

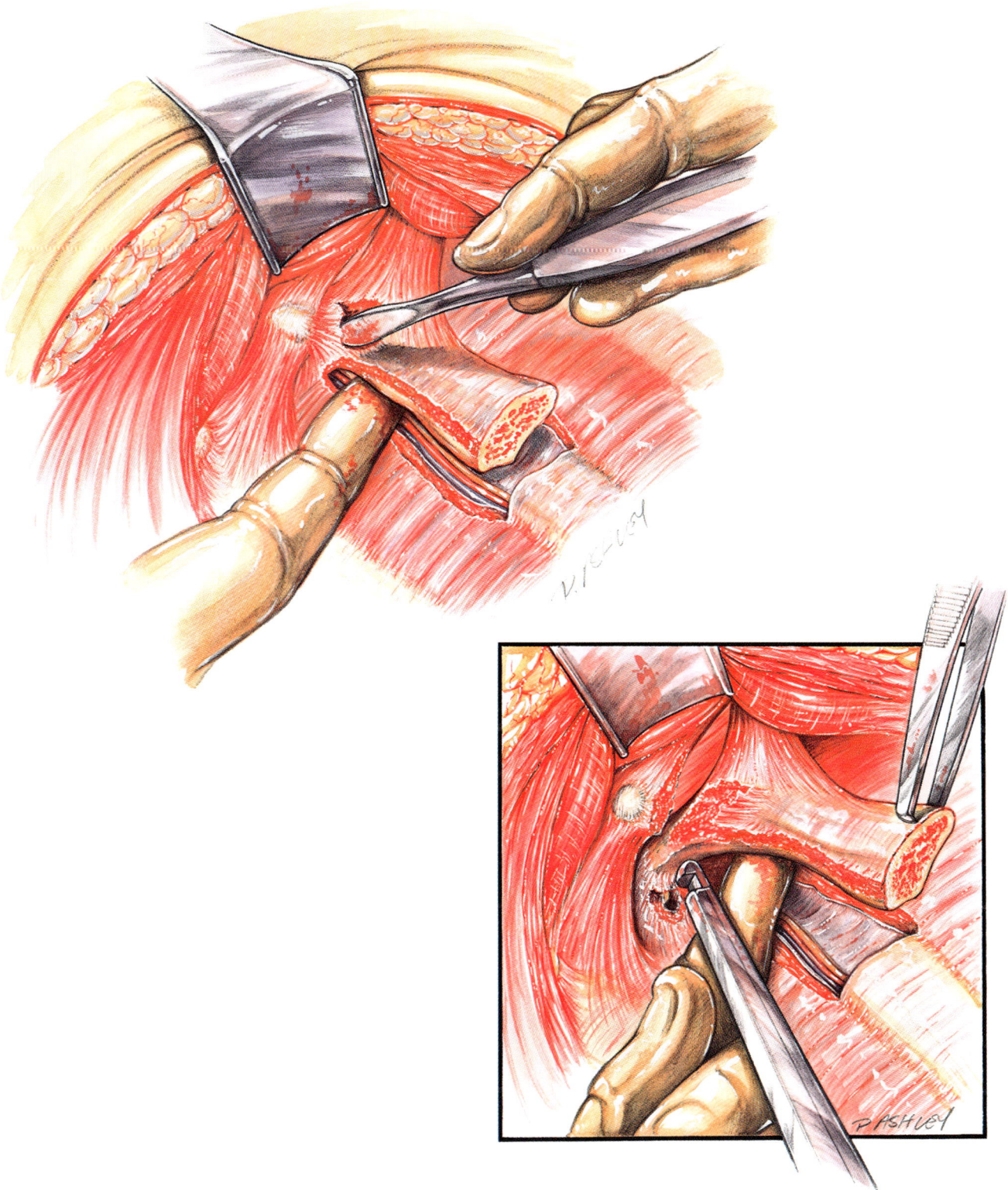

● **Figure 8-8.** The rib is resected 6 to 8 cm lateral to the costotransverse junction and gently elevated for its subsequent removal. The lateral and medial costotransverse ligaments are sharply divided under direct division with a knife or periosteal elevator. The anterior or radiate ligament securing the head of the rib with the lateral vertebral body is released sharply with a ligamentum flavum rongeur with careful protection of the underlying pleura.

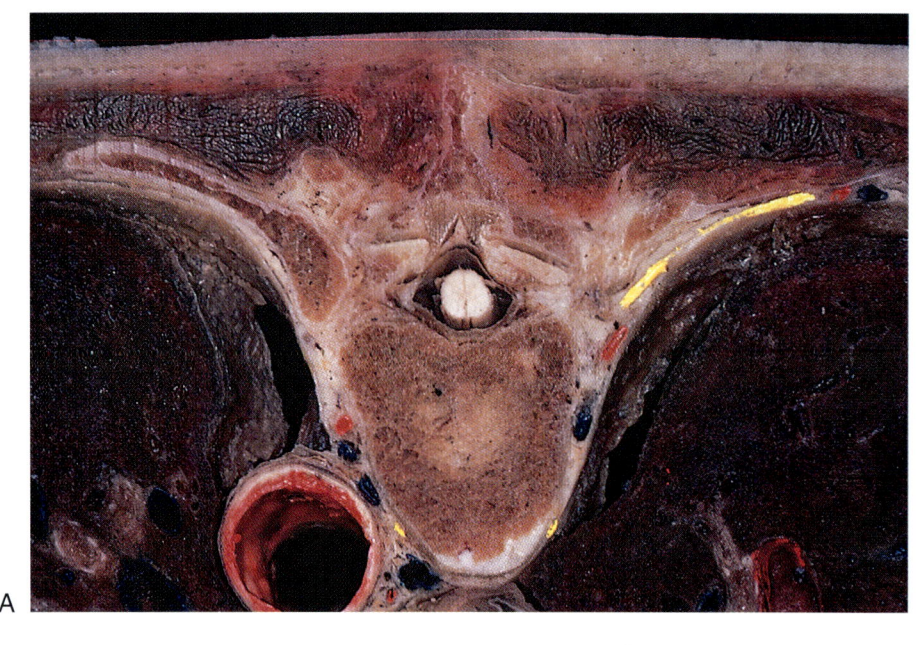

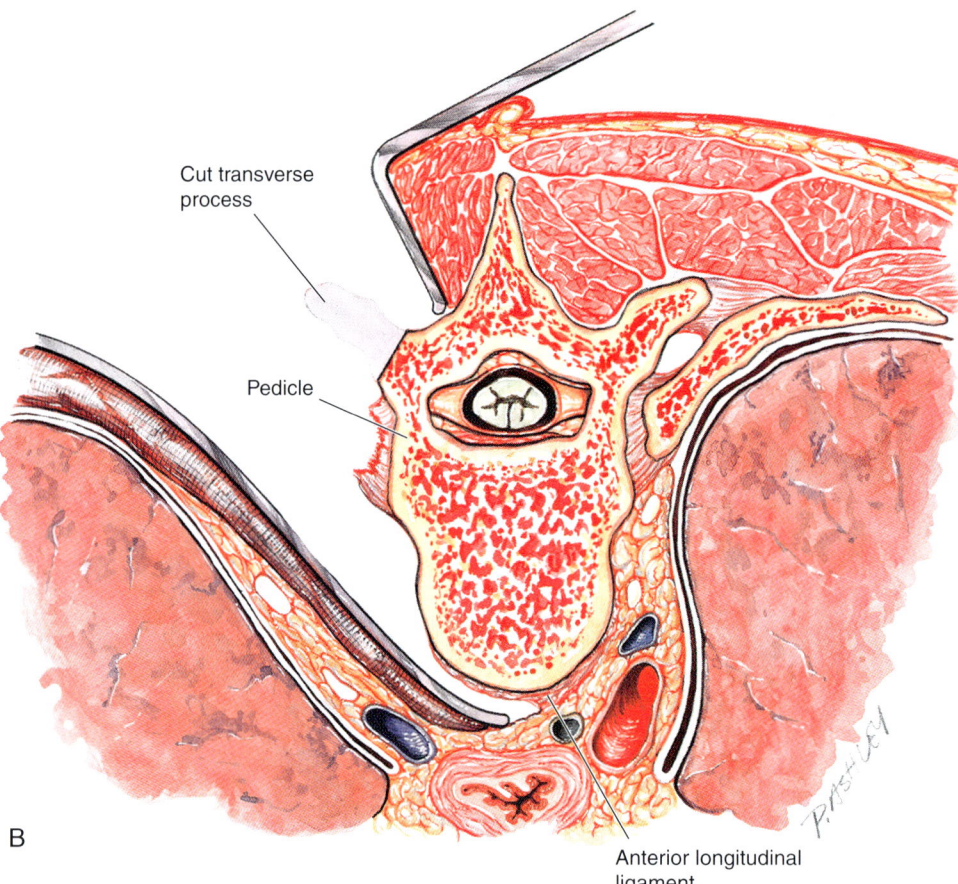

● **Figure 8-9.** A cross-sectional projection (*A*) and cross-sectional drawing (*B*) of the proposed area of bony resection. The medial 6 to 8 cm of the thoracic rib as well as the transverse process down to its juncture with its superior facet and pedicle is removed to allow access to the anterolateral vertebral body.

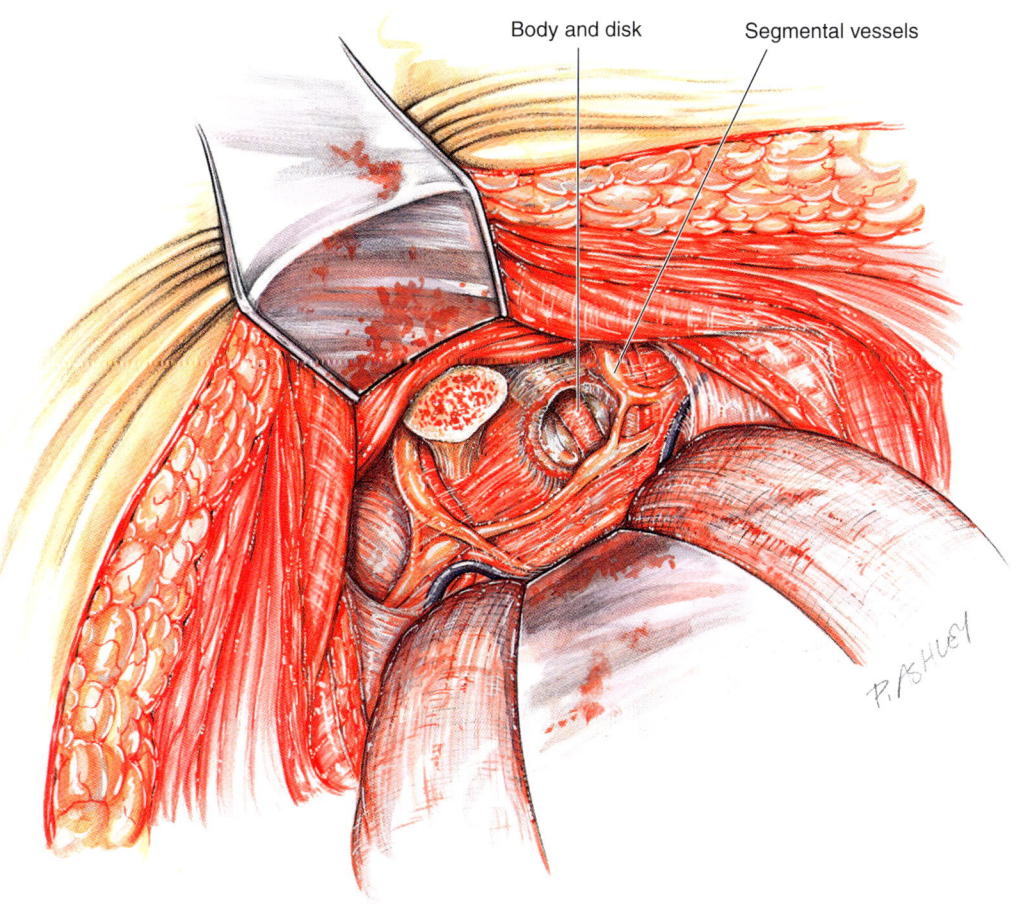

● **Figure 8-10.** The transverse process is resected with a rongeur or osteotome down to the level of its juncture with its superior facet and pedicle. The parietal pleura is then elevated either bluntly with a finger or sharply with a cob instrument off the anterolateral surface of the vertebral body with careful protection of the sympathetic trunk and segmental vessels.

sharply with a Cobb instrument (Figure 8–10). The pleura may be retracted with a padded Deaver or malleable retractor. Further dissection may proceed superiorly or inferiorly as needed, with careful avoidance of injury to the intercostal vessels. The surgical exposure may be widened by removing additional ribs and transverse processes as needed. The surgeon is now able to proceed with the desired operation as chosen.

At the completion of the procedure one must now assess the integrity of the pleural lining by requesting the anesthesiologist to inflate the lung with the wound filled with saline. If no air leak is appreciated, the wound is closed over suction drainage with each muscular and fascial layer closed separately.

Complications

The most frequent indication for the costotransversectomy approach to the thoracic spine is for decompression of a thoracic spinal or paraspinal abscess. The surrounding inflammatory environment creates significant pleural thickening, protecting the surgeon from inadvertently puncturing the pleura, especially medially, where it is at its thinnest. If a pleural tear occurs, it should be repaired if possible and a chest tube placed in the upper anterior thoracic chest cavity. Because of the close proximity of the dural sheath and vascular pedicle, injury to these structures may occur, especially in light of a small working space and the potential for obscured vision from constant oozing of blood from exposed cancellous surfaces. All dural tears should be repaired to prevent fistula formation, and any bleeding from exposed cancellous bony surfaces may be slowed or stopped by conservative application of bone wax.

An unlikely but potential intraoperative complication may be the creation of iatrogenic thoracic instability if a multilevel thoracic decompression is performed with resection of more than three ribs. Such instability may lead to a postoperative acquired scoliosis or kyphoscoliosis and, therefore, should be assessed intraoperatively through attempted manipulation of the vertebral column with appropriate performance of instrumentation and fusion if necessary. It is usually recommended that only two, or at most three, vertebral levels be approached in this procedure to avoid excessive resection of the patient's chest wall.

Conclusion

The costotransversectomy approach allows a simple, limited exposure of the anterolateral surface of the thoracic spine and is ideally suited for drainage of spinal or paraspinal abscesses, vertebral body biopsies, or limited thoracic posterolateral decompressions. The procedure is fraught with minimal complications and is especially useful in frail, debilitated patients in whom a formal transthoracic approach with its inherent risks and morbidity is contraindicated.

BIBLIOGRAPHY

Asher MA, Kraker DP: Thoracolumbosacral spine. In Reckling FW, Reckling JB, Mohn MP (eds): Orthopaedic Anatomy and Surgical Approaches, pp 207–261. St. Louis, Mosby–Year Book, 1990.

Cahill DR, Orland MJ, Reading CC (eds): Atlas of Human Cross-Sectional Anatomy with CT and MR Images, 2nd ed, pp 10–11. New York, John Wiley & Sons, 1990.

Hoppenfeld S: The spine. In Hoppenfeld S (ed): Surgical Exposures in Orthopaedics, pp 269–273. Philadelphia, JB Lippincott, 1984.

Johnson RM, Murphy MJ, Southwick WO: Surgical approaches to the thoracic spine. In Herkowitz HN, et al (eds): Spine, 3rd ed, pp 1711–1720. Philadelphia, WB Saunders, 1992.

Kostuik JP: Surgical approaches to the thoracic and thoracolumbar spine. In Frymoyer JW (ed): The Adult Spine. Principle and Practice, pp 1243–1266. New York, Raven Press, 1991.

Long DM, McAfee PC: Operations on thoracic disc. Long DM, McAfee PC (eds): Atlas of Spinal Surgery, pp 230–237. Baltimore, Williams & Wilkins, 1992.

Roy Camille R, Mazel CH: Surgical exposures and procedures. In Laurin CA, Riley LH, Roy Camille R (eds): Atlas of Orthopaedic Surgery, pp 297–356. Chicago, Year Book Medical Publishers, 1989.

Wood GW: Infections of spine. In Crenshaw AH (ed): Campbell's Operative Orthopaedics, 7th ed, pp 3323–3345. St. Louis, CV Mosby, 1987.

CHAPTER 9

ANTERIOR RETROPERITONEAL LUMBAR EXPOSURES

Sanford E. Emery, M.D.

The retroperitoneal approach is very useful for anterior exposure to the spine from T12 to L5. In reality it is an anterolateral view of the vertebrae that allows access to the segmental vessels, vertebral body, pedicle, and transverse process, as well as the spinal canal and its contents. Clinically, this approach is most commonly used in the treatment of fractures, infection, or tumors to anteriorly decompress the neural elements. It is also frequently used in scoliosis procedures in which anterior release with or without anterior interbody fusion is performed over several levels of the lumbar spine.

This approach has certain advantages over a transperitoneal approach that affords a direct anterior view of the vertebrae. The aorta and vena cava lie anterior to the spine, and access to the L4 vertebra and above requires mobilization and protection of these great vessels. The retroperitoneal approach provides an anterolateral view of the spine, and at L4 and above the great vessels are not in the way. The iliac vessels do cross over the body of L5 laterally in many patients, and access to the L5 body and L5-S1 disk space can be limited with a retroperitoneal approach. For better exposure of the L5-S1 disk space alone I prefer a transperitoneal approach or a retroperitoneal approach through the rectus abdominis.

The skin incision is an oblique one that can be made over the 12th rib or a few centimeters inferior to the 12th rib. If access to T12 or L1 is needed, I suggest making the incision over the 12th rib and removing it because this provides the best exposure in the upper lumbar area. For L2 and lower, one can either remove the 12th rib or make the incision halfway between the rib cage and the iliac crest. The illustrations in this chapter show the muscle layers traversed using an incision between the 12th rib and the iliac crest to better demonstrate the muscular layers. If one prefers the slightly higher incision, the 12th rib is simply dissected out and removed; the remaining transversalis fascia is incised and this exposes the retroperitoneal space.

Surgical Technique

The patient is placed in the lateral decubitus position, usually with the left side up (Figure 9–1). This left-sided approach is preferred because the aorta is in the field rather than the more fragile vena cava. A rolled blanket can be placed just superior to the right iliac crest,

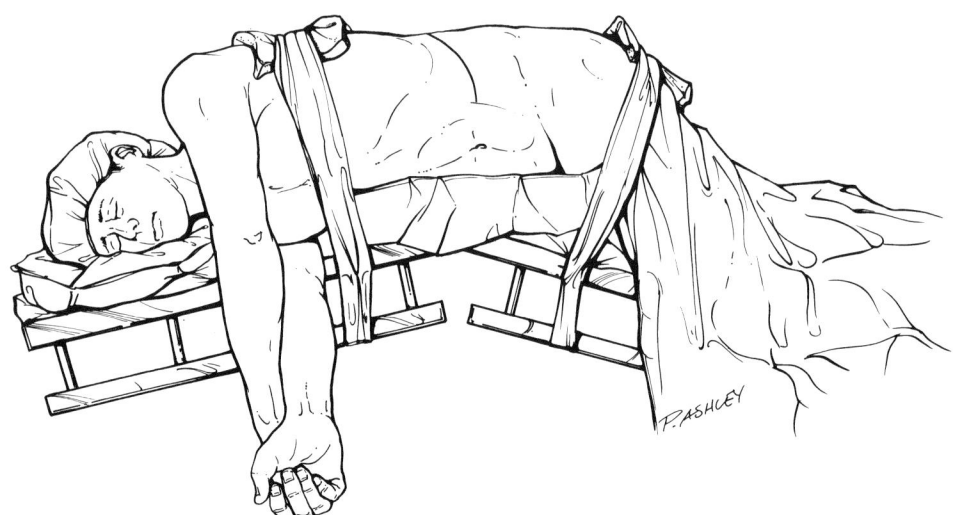

● **Figure 9-1.** Position of patient for standard retroperitoneal approach.

and the table is jackknifed. This maximizes the distance from the 12th rib to the superior aspect of the left iliac crest. This creates a lateral bend in the spine, however; and if anterior instrumentation is to be used, the table must be leveled before internal fixation to avoid securing the spine with a lateral bend deformity. I prefer to use a "bean bag" under the patient that can be deflated and subsequently reinflated if it is necessary to level the table.

The operating surgeon should be standing at the patient's abdomen. Rolling the patient 10 to 20 degrees forward toward the surgeon as opposed to a direct lateral position will assist in retraction of the peritoneal contents anteriorly to expose the retroperitoneal space. Another helpful maneuver, particularly in muscular patients, is to flex the leg at the hip to relax the iliopsoas muscle for easier retraction.

The skin incision is placed between the 12th rib and the iliac crest (Figure 9–2). To reach T12 and the uppermost lumbar vertebrae, the incision can be made directly over the 12th rib with removal of the rib. If the approach is for the midlumbar spine, then the incision can be made halfway between the 12th rib and the iliac crest. The incision begins dorsally a few centimeters from the midline and is directed parallel to the 12th rib in an oblique fashion down toward the umbilicus. The incision should end near the beginning of the rectus abdominis. A smaller incision can be used depending on the size and bulk of the patient. If a more extensile approach is needed, the dorsal origin of the incision can be extended superiorly parallel to the axis of the spine, and the ventral endpoint of the incision can be curved distally to run parallel to the rectus abdominis. The external oblique muscle is visualized and incised in line with the skin incision (Figure 9–3).

The internal oblique muscle fibers run roughly perpendicular to those of the external oblique (Figure 9–4). These are simply transected in line with the skin incision.

The transversus abdominis is the next muscle layer, and its posterior fascia is the transversalis fascia (Figure 9–5). This layer is more substantial posteriorly than anteriorly, and the thickness will also depend on the size and bulk of the patient. It is also incised in line with the skin incision.

After entering the retroperitoneum through the transversalis fascia, one sees retroperitoneal fat that is covered with a thin layer of peritoneum (Figure 9–6). The retroperitoneal fat and the peritoneal contents are carefully dissected off the lateral and posterior abdominal wall using finger or sponge dissection.

After dissection through the transversalis fascia, one sees the retroperitoneal fat anteriorly and the psoas muscle posteriorly. The patient in Figure 9–7 is a large male and the

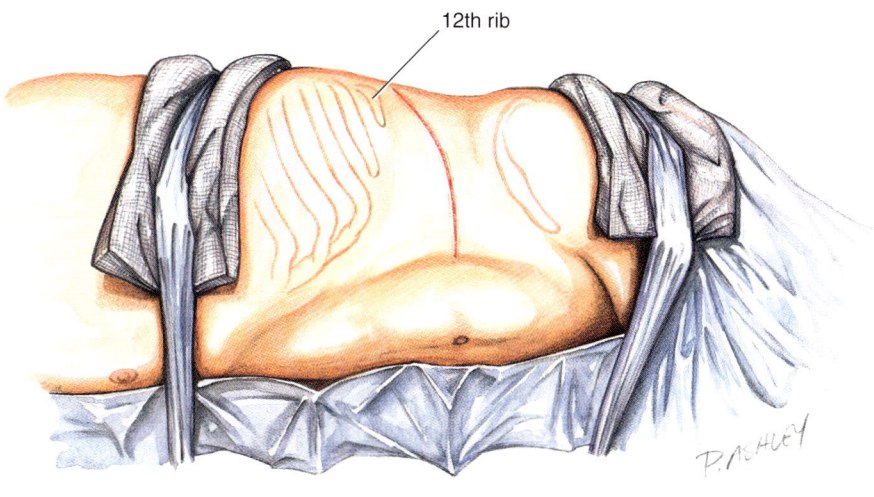

● **Figure 9–2.** Skin incision for retroperitoneal approach.

148 ● SURGICAL APPROACHES TO THE SPINE

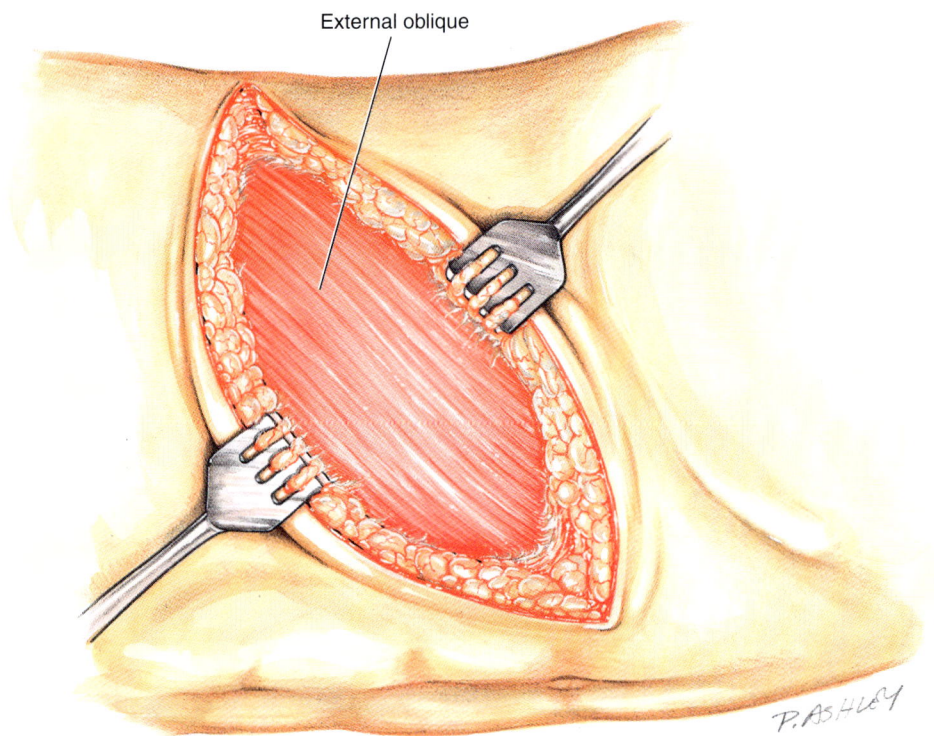

● **Figure 9-3.** External oblique muscle visualized.

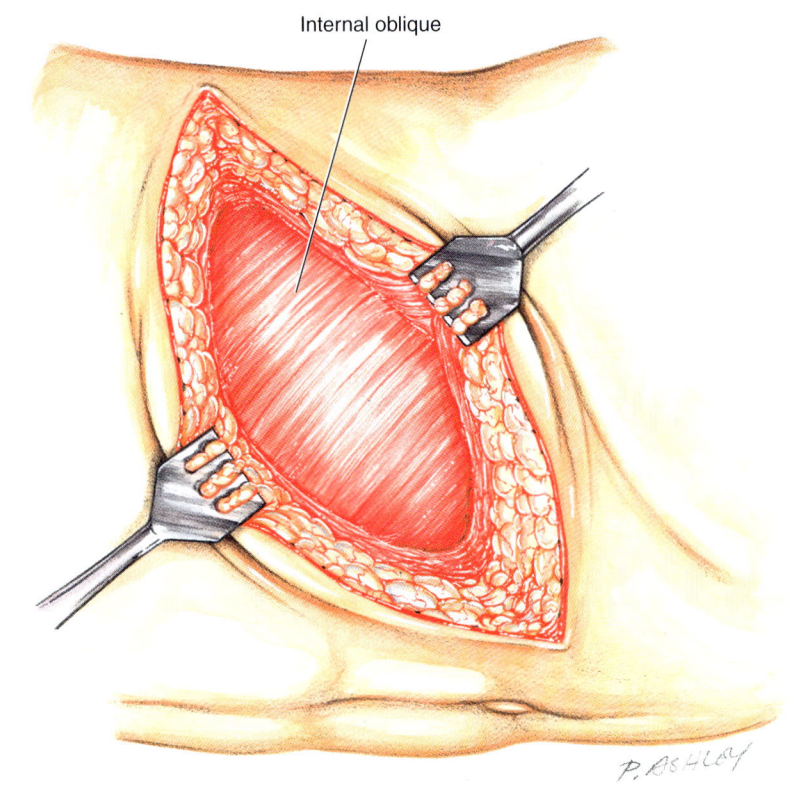

● **Figure 9-4.** Internal oblique muscle visualized.

ANTERIOR RETROPERITONEAL LUMBAR EXPOSURES • 149

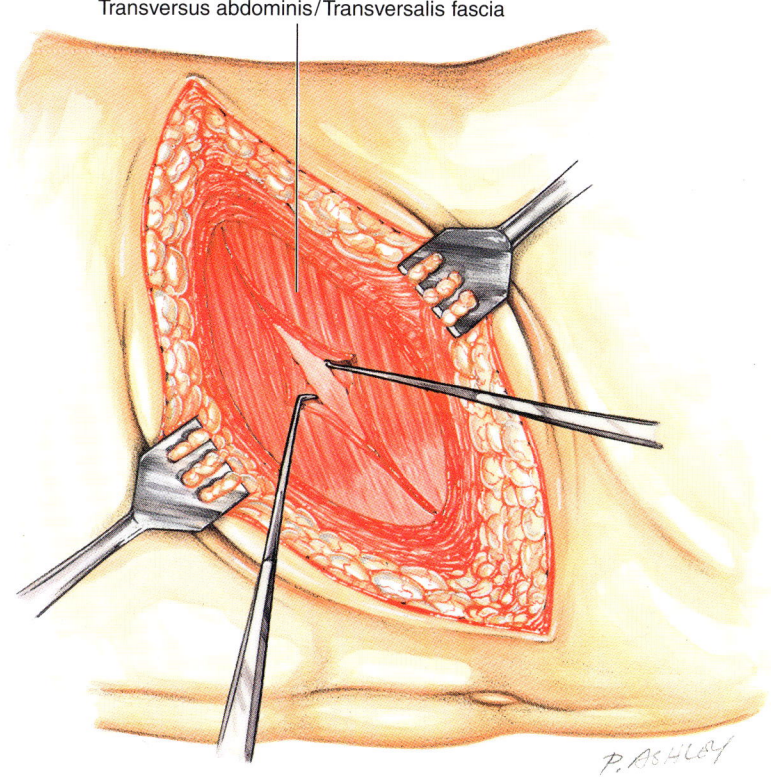

• **Figure 9-5.** Transversus abdominis layer and its posterior fascia, the transversalis fascia.

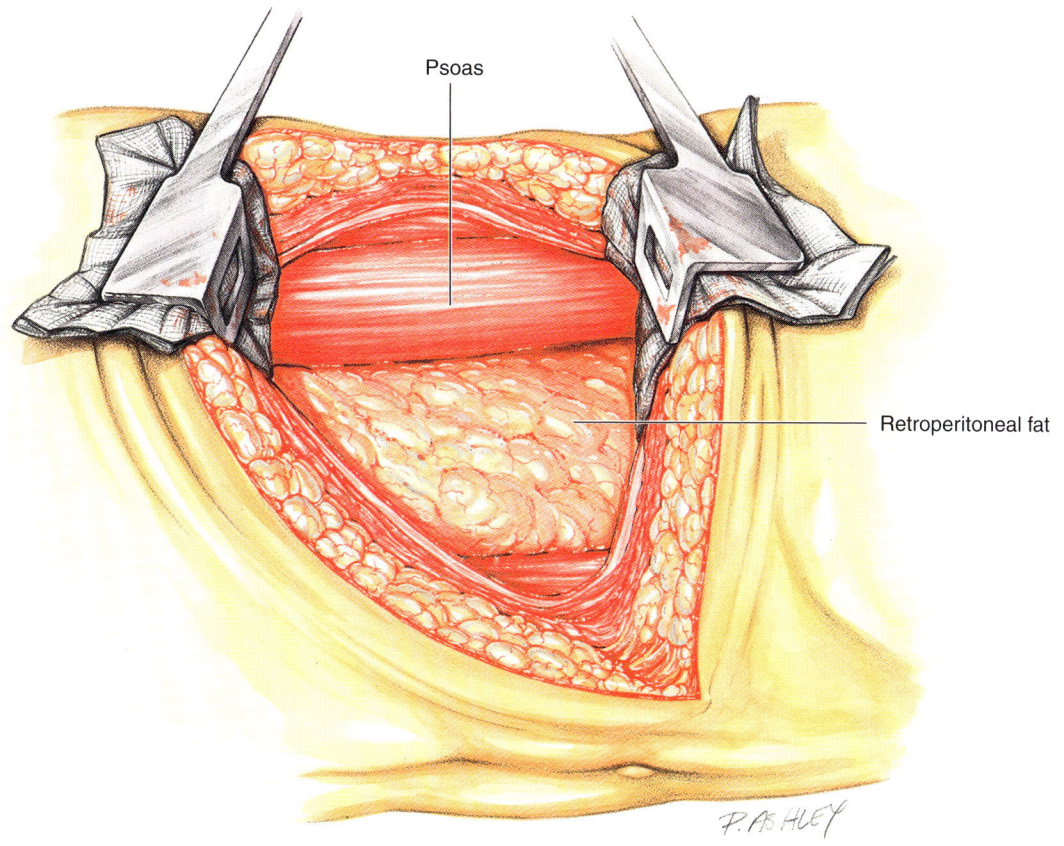

• **Figure 9-6.** View after entering the retroperitoneum.

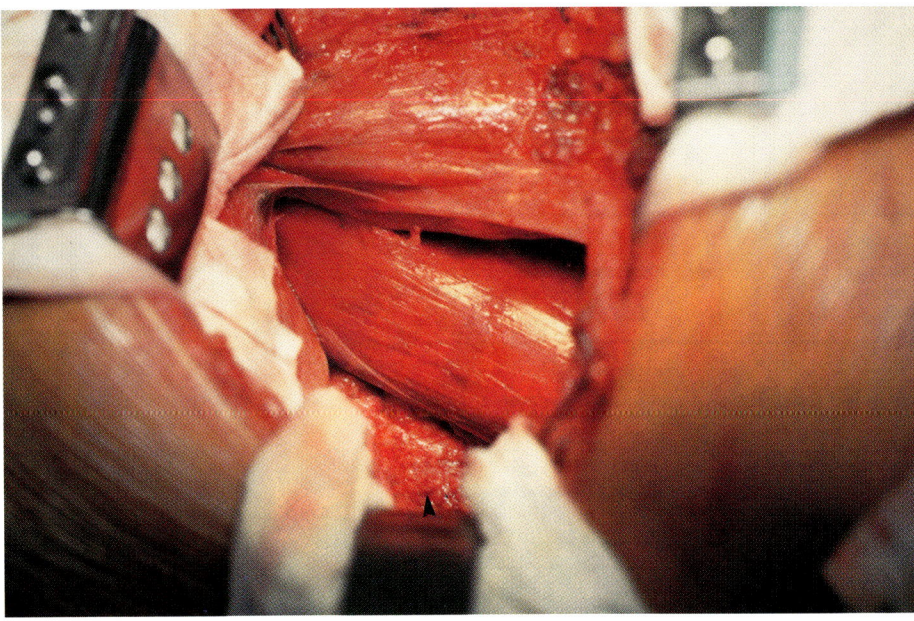

● **Figure 9-7.** Retroperitoneal fat (*arrowhead*) anteriorly with psoas muscle posteriorly.

psoas is very large. Dorsal to the psoas is the quadratus lumborum. The psoas must be mobilized from its ventral edge and retracted dorsally to expose the spinal column. The ureter usually lies on the retroperitoneal fat near the ventral border of the psoas. In the patient in Figure 9-8, a large dilated vein lies on top of the ureter.

Retraction of the peritoneal contents anteriorly can be maintained using wet laparotomy sponges held by a wide ribbon retractor (Figure 9-9). Tilting the operating table 10 to 20 degrees toward the operating surgeon also assists in anterior retraction of the peritoneal contents. The ureter may be visible in the retroperitoneal fat at this point (see Figure 9-8) and is easily retracted anteriorly with the fat and peritoneal contents. The lumbar spine is now in view, although largely covered by the psoas muscle. The aorta is easily palpable although not easily visualized because it lies anterior to the vertebrae.

For exposure of T12 and L1, the anatomy of the crus of the diaphragm and the origin of the psoas muscle are important. Most of the crus is spread over the body of T12 where it thins as one moves distally. The origin of the psoas takes off from L1 almost as a continuum of the crus. It is thus necessary to transect and elevate the attachments of the crus to expose T12 or the T12-L1 disk space. In similar fashion, the origin of the psoas is elevated to expose the body of L1. For exposure in the midlumbar spine, the psoas is to be elevated from an anterior to posterior direction. This can be done with a Cobb elevator beginning over the disk space so as not to injure segmental vessels. In positioning the patient, flexion of the ipsilateral hip allows some relaxation of the psoas and easier retraction. One or more transverse processes can also be removed using a Leksell rongeur, which can facilitate retraction of the psoas muscle. Splitting of the psoas muscle is not recommended because the iliohypogastric (T12, L1), ilioinguinal (L1), genitofemoral (L1, L2), and lateral femoral cutaneous (L2, L3) nerves travel within the substance of the muscle and would be at risk. The iliohypogastric and ilioinguinal nerves exit in the proximal part of the psoas at its lateral border. The genitofemoral nerve passes more distally through the psoas and emerges near the ventral aspect of the muscle opposite L3 or L4. The lateral femoral cutaneous nerve exits more laterally from the midportion of the psoas. Of these nerves, the

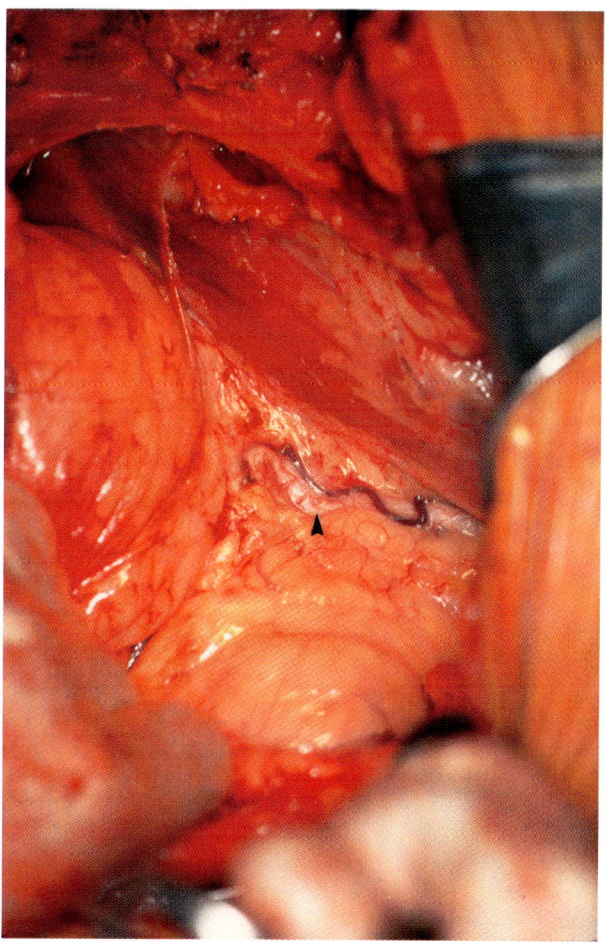

● **Figure 9-8.** Ureter (*arrowhead*) lying on retroperitoneal fat near ventral border of the psoas. Note large dilated vein on top of ureter.

one usually visualized in this approach is the genitofemoral nerve as it emerges from the psoas muscle.

The other large neural structure in the field is the sympathetic trunk (Figures 9–10 and 9–11). This lies along the ventral edge of the psoas muscle. A variable number of ganglia are present. It is often necessary to transect small branches of the sympathetic trunk for adequate exposure of the spine, but the trunk lies anterior enough that it can usually be preserved.

When the incision is over the 12th rib, the rib is removed and exposure is centered over the thoracolumbar junction (see Figure 9–10). The crus of the diaphragm inserts onto the vertebral body in this area, and the origin of the psoas muscle is also visualized here. The sympathetic chain lies ventral to the psoas muscle along the vertebrae in this plane.

To expose the disk space the psoas muscle must be elevated significantly. In Figure 9–11 note the elevation of the psoas muscle with the large retractor to expose the annulus fibrosis of the L2-3 disk.

Besides allowing visualization of the disk spaces (see Figure 9–11), elevation of the psoas muscle allows visualization of the vertebrae with the segmental vessels lying on the midportion of the vertebral body (Figure 9–12). The psoas should be elevated enough to allow good visualization of the lateral wall of the pedicle because this is a landmark for identifying the spinal canal with its neural elements, which is a critical step in operative

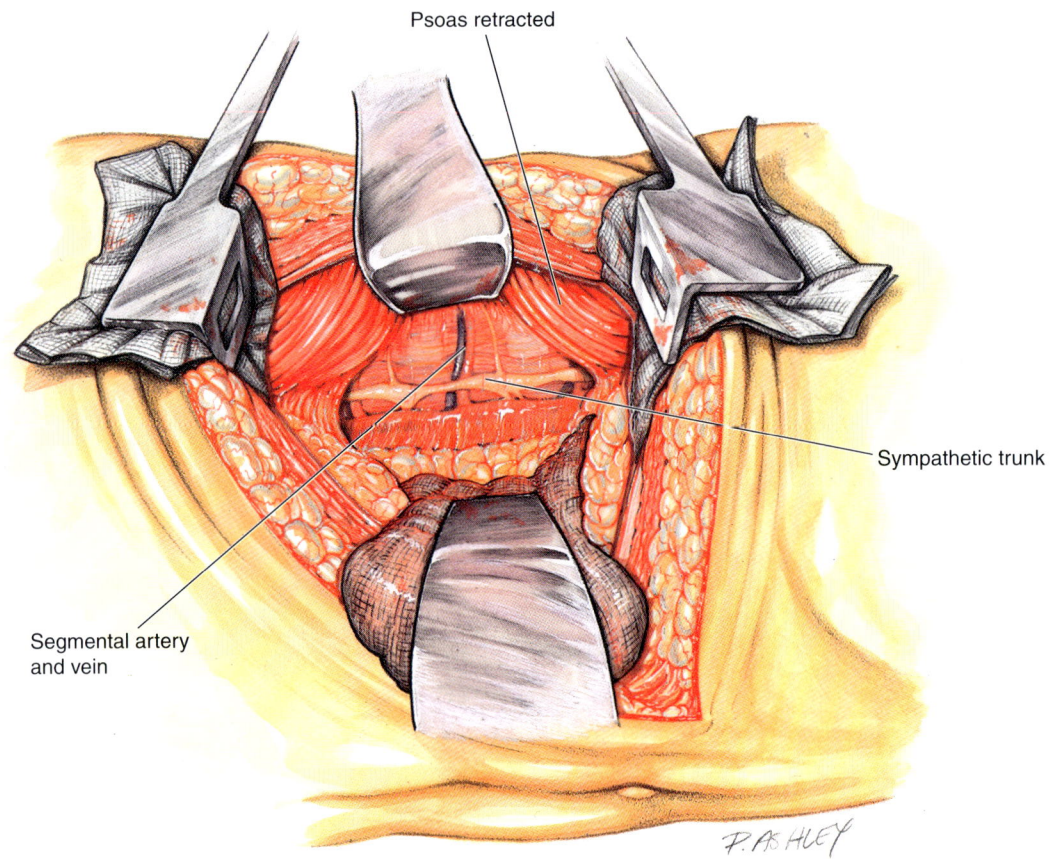

● **Figure 9-9.** Retraction of peritoneal contents anteriorly with ribbon retractor and tilting of table toward surgeon. Note view of lumbar spine after retraction of psoas. Sympathetic trunk and segmental vessels are visible.

anterior decompressions. A C-shaped ribbon retractor often can be of assistance in maintaining retraction of the retroperitoneal contents. Ligation and division of the segmental vein and artery allows for removal of the periosteum with a Cobb elevator or a large curet, exposing the vertebral bodies and adjacent disk spaces (Figures 9–13 and 9–14).

Complications

The vascular structures at risk for the retroperitoneal approach to the spine include the aorta and vena cava. Most at risk, however, are the iliac vessels when dissection is carried out to the L4-5 disk space and particularly the L5 vertebral body. The iliolumbar vein as it branches off of the vena cava lies over the L5 vertebral body and may need to be ligated as the dissection is carried distally. The iliolumbar artery arises from the internal iliac artery and turns retrograde to supply the psoas and quadratus lumborum muscles and can also be injured in the lower area of this approach.

Other complications include injury to the lumbar nerve roots and their peripheral nerves (the iliohypogastric, ilioinguinal, genitofemoral, and lateral femoral cutaneous) that traverse the psoas muscle. Injury to the sympathetic trunk results in a warmer ipsilateral lower extremity, but this usually resolves, as documented by the general surgical experience with sympathectomy. The sympathetic hypogastric plexus lies directly anterior to the spine over the body of L5 and the sacrum. This plexus provides the sympathetic innervation to the

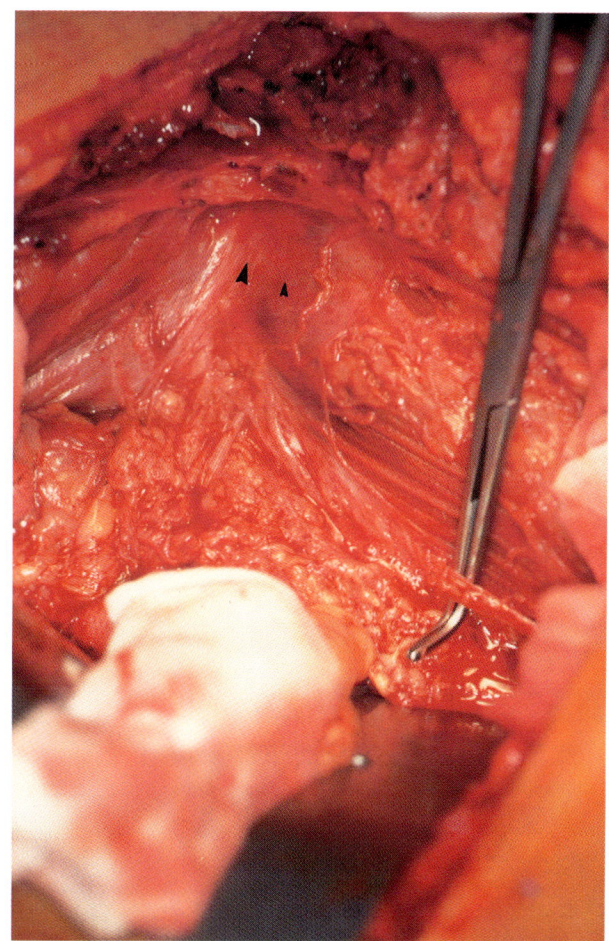

● **Figure 9-10.** Exposure after removal of 12th rib centering view on thoracolumbar junction. Large arrowhead (crus of diaphragm) indicates vertebral body. Smaller arrowhead identifies the origin of the psoas muscle. Instrument is elevating sympathetic chain lying ventral to the psoas muscle along the vertebrae.

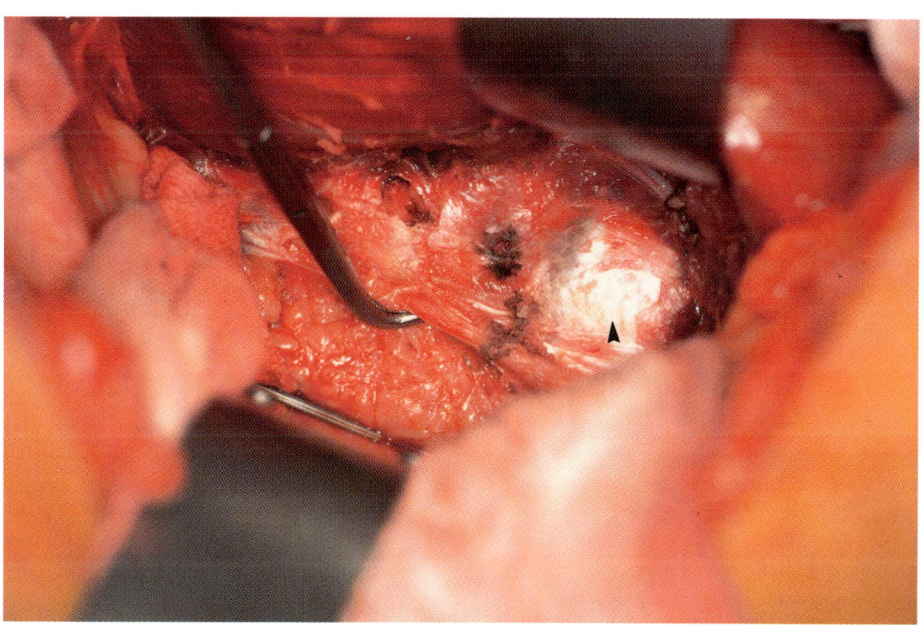

● **Figure 9-11.** Elevation of psoas demonstrating annulus fibrosis of L2-3 (*arrowhead*). Instrument is identifying sympathetic trunk.

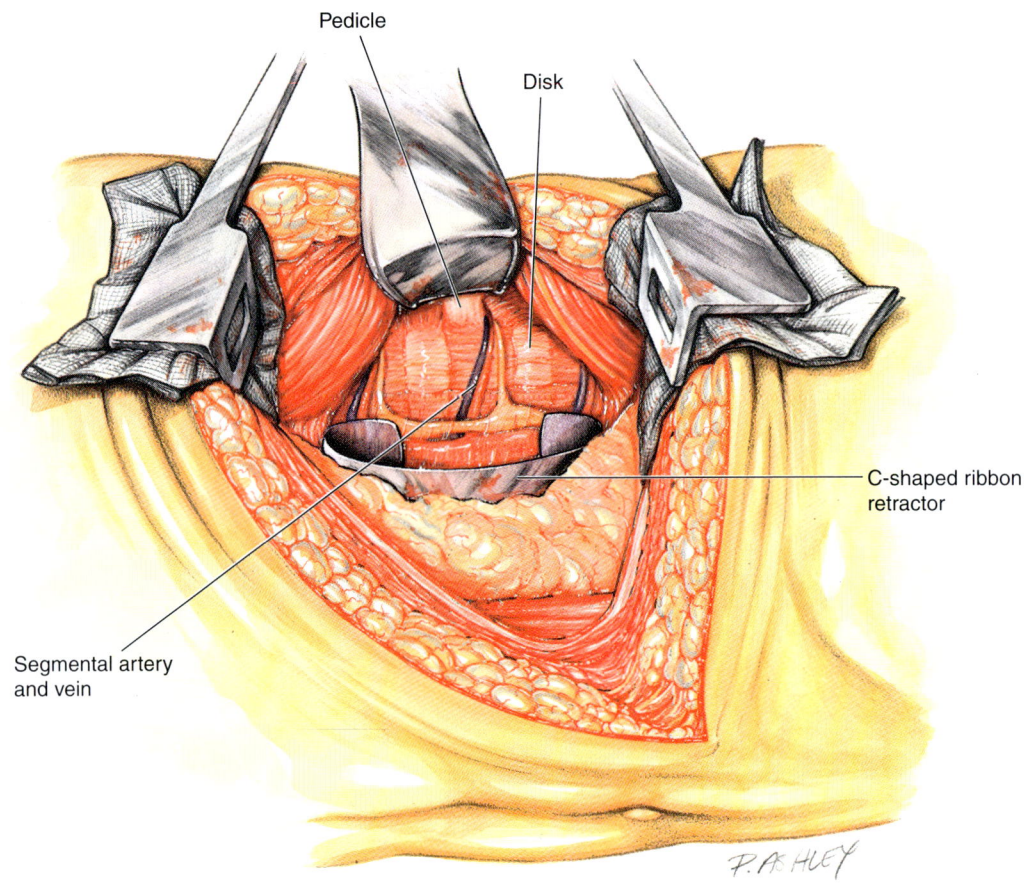

● **Figure 9-12.** Visualization of disks, vertebrae, and segmental vessels, lying in midportion of vertebral body. Note visualization of pedicle by adequate psoas retraction (allowing identification of landmark for spinal canal).

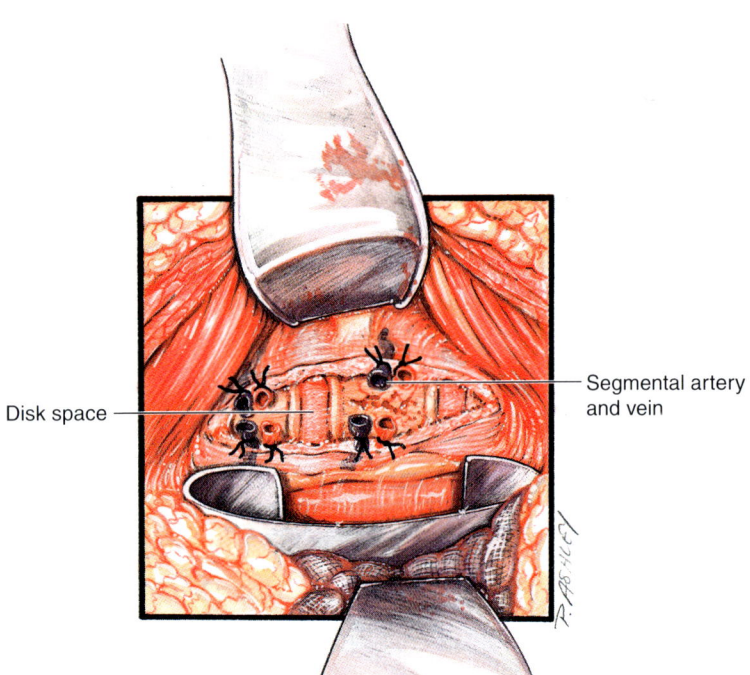

● **Figure 9-13.** Removal of periosteum of vertebral body can only be performed after ligation of segmental vessels. This allows exposure of vertebral bodies and disk spaces.

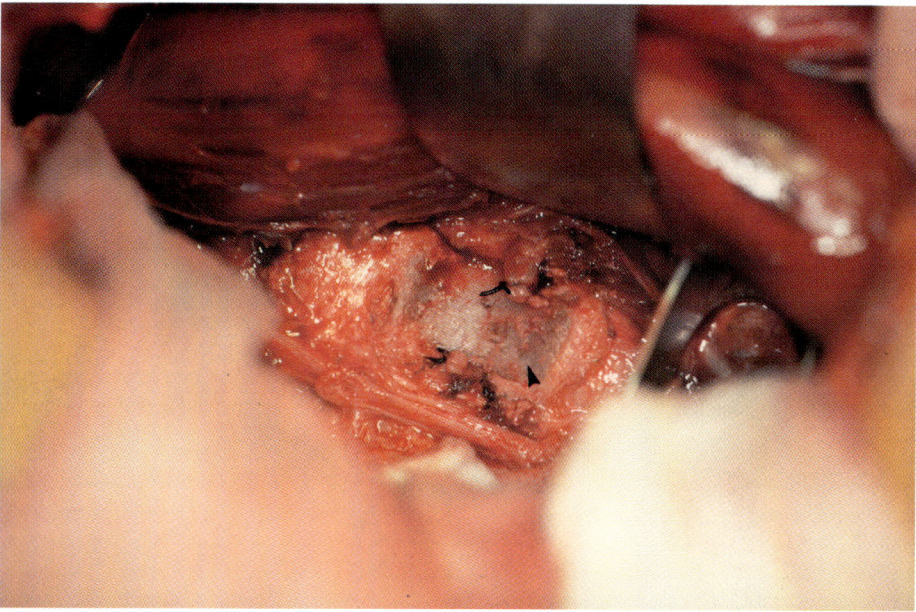

● **Figure 9-14.** L2 vertebral body after ligation of segmental artery and vein. Periosteum has been elevated to expose the lateral cortex of the vertebral body (*arrowhead*).

urogenital system. An injury to it results in retrograde ejaculation; however, because it lies directly anterior to the vertebra, it is at minimal risk from the retroperitoneal approach.

Care must be taken when entering the retroperitoneal space and blunt dissection used to minimize the risk of tearing the peritoneal layer. Any rent in the peritoneum should be closed with absorbable suture if at all possible. When dissecting off the crus of the diaphragm to expose the body of T12, one must be aware of the retropleural space; it is not uncommon to have a small rent in the pleura at this corner that should be repaired. Immediate postoperative radiographs should be obtained to rule out a pneumothorax. Careful closure of the muscle layers should be performed, because incisional hernias can develop and may be difficult to repair at a later date.

Conclusion

The retroperitoneal approach to the spine is generally considered to be a safe and utilitarian approach to the anterior lumbar spine. As in any surgical approach, training and experience are essential for its safe and effective use. In a young, healthy person, the anatomy is often quite straightforward; however, in cases of vertebral osteomyelitis, tumor, or late fractures, the exposure of the vertebrae and spinal canal can be a more difficult undertaking.

BIBLIOGRAPHY

Anderson JE (ed): Grant's Atlas of Anatomy, 7th ed. Baltimore, Williams & Wilkins, 1978.
Garfin SR (ed): Complications of Spine Surgery, Baltimore, Williams & Wilkins, 1989.
Gray Anatomy of the Human Body, 29th American ed. CM Goss (ed). Philadelphia, Lea & Febiger, 1973.
Hoppenfeld S, de Boer P: Surgical Exposures in Orthopaedics: The Anatomic Approach. Philadelphia, JB Lippincott, 1984.

CHAPTER 10

ALTERNATIVE ANTERIOR LUMBAR EXPOSURES

Phillip R. Adams, M.D.
Howard B. Cotler, M.D.

The introduction of the anterior approach to the lumbar spine was initially designed for treatment of tuberculosis. In 1934, Ito and associates[1] reported on the replacement of a diseased vertebral body by using either tibial or rib autograft. Hodgson and colleagues[2-4] obtained international recognition when they described the anterior surgical approaches to the spine and reported on Potts' disease using anterior spinal fusion surgery. Subsequently, Kelly and Whitesides,[5] Fountain,[6] and Bohlman and Eismont[7] have applied the surgical principles to the management of trauma to the spine. Other authors have described anterior spinal surgery for various other conditions.[8-10]

Indications

The anterior approach to the lumbar spine is indicated when anterior spinal pathology requires directed treatment. Anterior approaches to the lumbar spine may be either transperitoneal or retroperitoneal. The anterior transperitoneal approach to the lumbar spine has historical background in the treatment of spondylolisthesis[11-13] and tuberculosis.[14] This approach requires knowledge of the abdominal cavity and may be complicated by injury to the intra-abdominal contents. The retroperitoneal approach to the lumbar spine affords a plane of dissection that is lateral to the peritoneum that is relatively avascular. By avoiding the formal abdominal cavity, complications associated with transperitoneal surgery may be avoided. The current indications for the use of anterior lumbar surgery are primarily for débridement and stabilization operations. Thus, the indications are as follows:

1. Spinal trauma and spinal cord injury
2. Spinal infections
3. Correction of selected spinal deformities
4. Vertebral body tumors
5. Failed spinal operations (posterior nonunions)
6. Disk lesions
   - Internal disk disruption syndrome
   - Isolated disk reabsorption syndrome
   - Central disk herniation

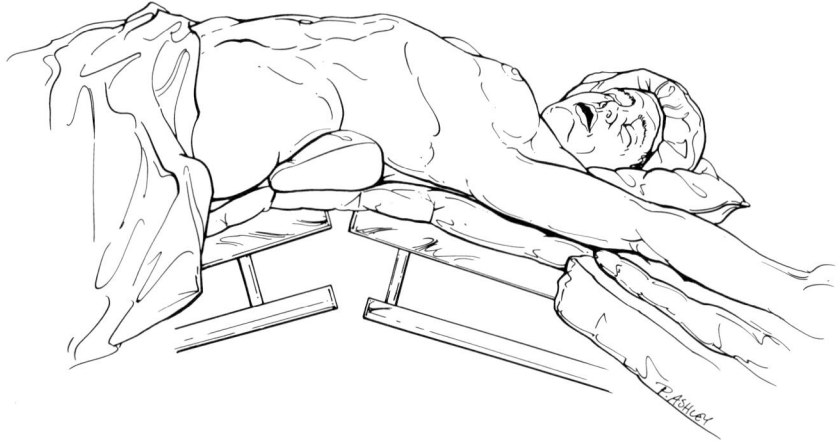

- **Figure 10-1.** For the anterior approach to the lower three lumbar segments, a roll is placed in the small of the patient's back and the table is "jackknifed."

Positioning

For upper lumbar surgery (T12-L2), the patient is placed in the right lateral decubitus position with the left flank up. A rolled sheet is usually placed between the pelvis and chest cavity to prevent upper and midlumbar sag and the patient may be jackknifed on the table.

For approaches to the lower three lumbar segments, the patient is placed supine on the operating table with a rolled sheet, blanket, or pillow in the small of the patient's back. We have found the use of an electric hydraulic radiolucent table (Quantum #3080 RL, AMSCO, Erie, PA) to be of immense help during the procedure (Figure 10–1).

General Considerations

The lumbar and lumbosacral spine is most easily approached through the extraperitoneal route. This relatively avascular plane permits easy mobilization of the intraperitoneal contents and the ureter, which (unless dissected free) generally remains attached to the mobile peritoneum. The upper lumbar (thoracolumbar) vertebral bodies are always approached through the patient's left side whereas the lower lumbar (and lumbosacral) vertebral bodies may be approached from either side.

Approach to the Upper Lumbar Spine (T12-L1-L2)

Exposure of the T12-L1-L2 vertebral levels is carried out by a thoracotomy over the 10th, 11th, or 12th rib (Figure 10–2). As a general rule, it is always easier to go one or two levels above the intended vertebral body level of surgery, because it is easier to work down.

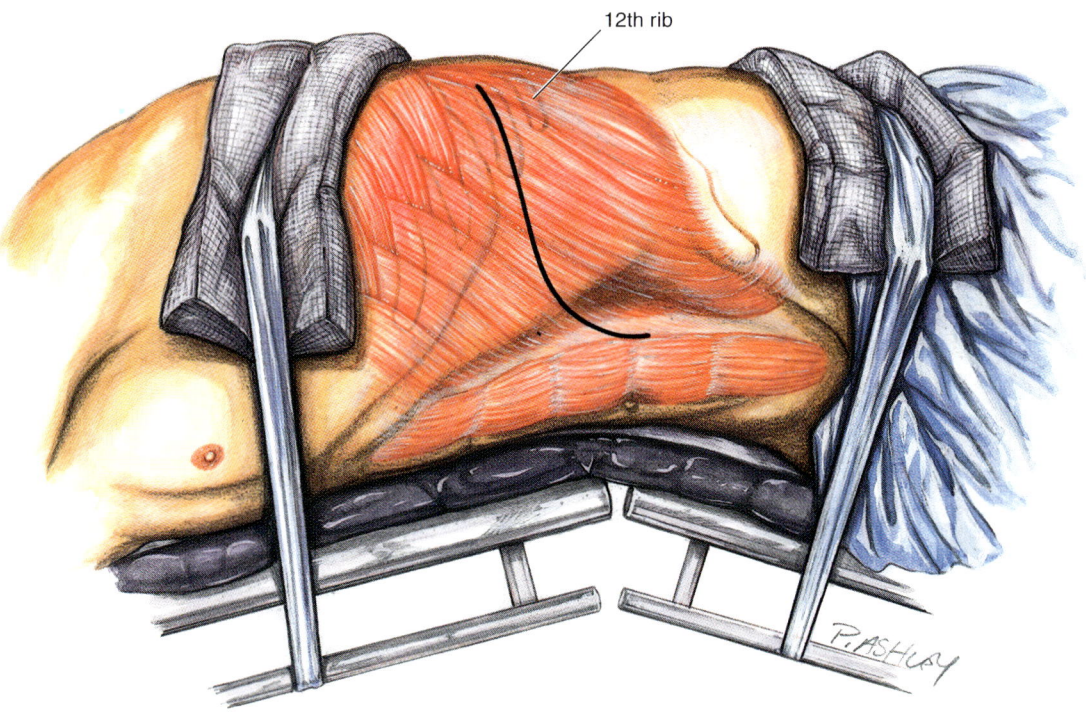

● **Figure 10–2.** Thoracoabdominal approach. Incision is made overlying the 10th, 11th, or 12th rib.

This approach allows exposure to thoracic and abdominal cavities. The skin is incised from the posterior paraspinal region on the 10th, 11th, or 12th rib extending anteriorly along the lateral border of the rectus abdominis muscle. The dissection is carried through the subcutaneous and muscular layers. The thoracic musculature is sharply incised or more usually cut with electrocautery. The periosteum of the rib is incised and elevated, allowing resection of the rib for bone grafting if it is needed. The pleura along the rib bed is incised. The costal cartilage is used as landmark for retroperitoneal exposure and repair of the diaphragm (Figure 10–3). The peritoneum is bluntly dissected off the diaphragm and vertebral column. The abdominal extension of the approach is then completed by incising the external oblique, internal oblique, and transversus abdominis muscles. Lumbar (thoracolumbar) L1-L3 surgery often requires detachment of the hemidiaphragm from its lateral insertions in the thoracoabdominal wall (Figure 10–4). Along the lateral and anterior aspects of these upper lumbar vertebrae are the insertion of the iliopsoas, quadratus lumborum, and crus of the diaphragm. Dissection following the orientation along the fibers of these large skeletal muscles permits access to the anterior longitudinal ligament. The diaphragmatic crus insertion on the anterolateral vertebral column is incised to allow exposure of the T12-L1 level. The psoas muscle may also be detached from its origin for further exposure. The parietal pleura is incised at the thoracic level, and exposure of the vertebral column is completed after ligation of the intercostal vessels. Possible complications from this approach may be either pulmonary, hemorrhagic, neurologic, an injury to major organs, or from a hernia.

Approach to the Lower Lumbar Spine (L3-L4-L5-S1)

The anterior retroperitoneal approach with the patient in the supine position has been described by Hodgson and Stock,[2,3] Crock,[15] and Selby and coworkers.[16] Some surgeons prefer positioning the patient in the right lateral decubitus position because it decreases the

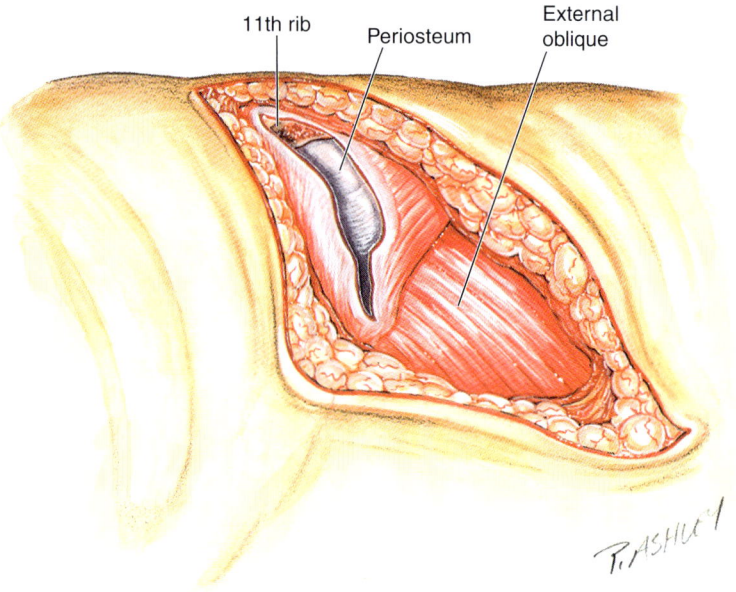

● **Figure 10–3.** Thoracoabdominal approach, depicted here through the 11th rib. The extrapleural-extraperitoneal space is encountered beneath the bed of the rib.

ALTERNATIVE ANTERIOR LUMBAR EXPOSURES • **161**

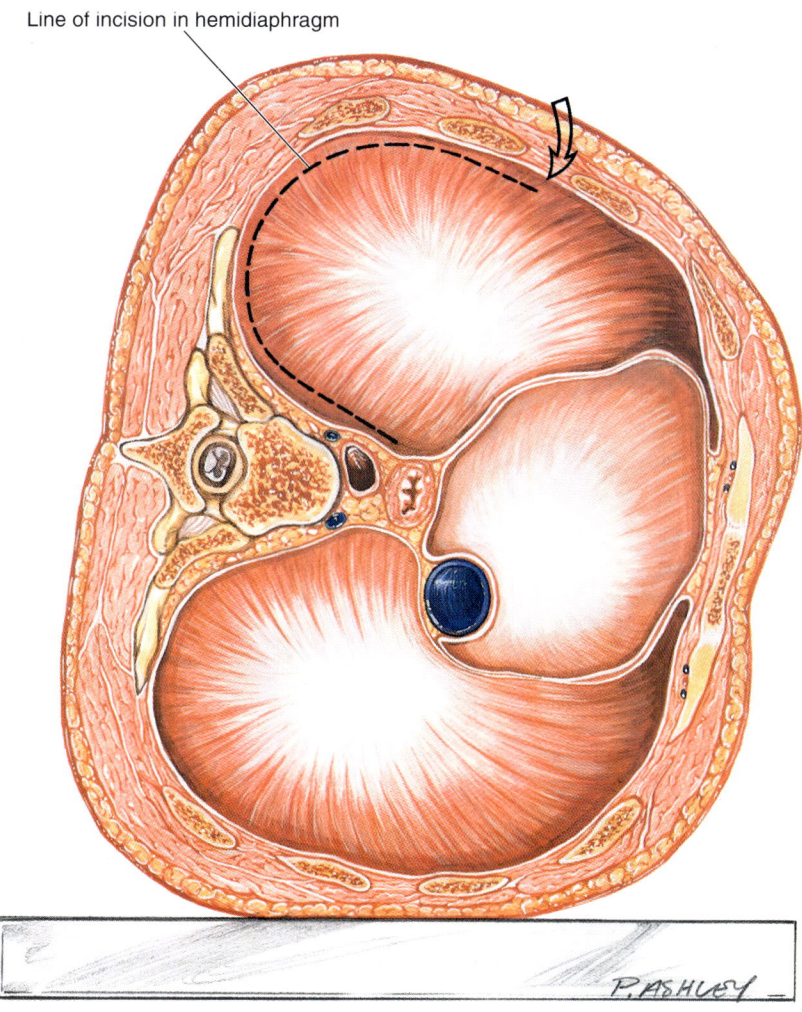

• **Figure 10-4.** Detachment of the left hemidiaphragm from its lateral insertions in the thoracoabdominal wall.

need for retraction as the viscera fall away from the operative field and also allows for the harvesting of iliac crest bone graft (Figure 10-5).[17,18] We favor the supine position for exposure of the lower three lumbar segments because it allows for better visualization of the spinal canal and restoration of a lumbar lordosis (Figure 10-6). To initiate the approach, the skin incision is key. First, one must evaluate the anteroposterior lumbar radiographs to determine the anatomic relationships between the highest and lowest interspaces to be approached and the superior iliac crest. Generally, the intercrestal line is at the L4-5 level. The L5-S1 level can usually be found halfway between the umbilicus and the symphysis pubis, whereas the L3-4 level is usually at the level of the umbilicus. If two levels require exposure, then the incision is placed halfway between the appropriate levels. In those patients requiring more than two sequential levels or a fusion above the L3-4 level, then a left paramedian vertical incision is made. The transverse incision is placed as described to permit exposure of the desired spinal segments. With the vertical incision the rectus sheath is entered through a paramedian skin incision and the rectus is retracted laterally.

Then the posterior rectus sheath is carefully incised to identify the preperitoneal space and this space is carefully developed laterally and horizontally.

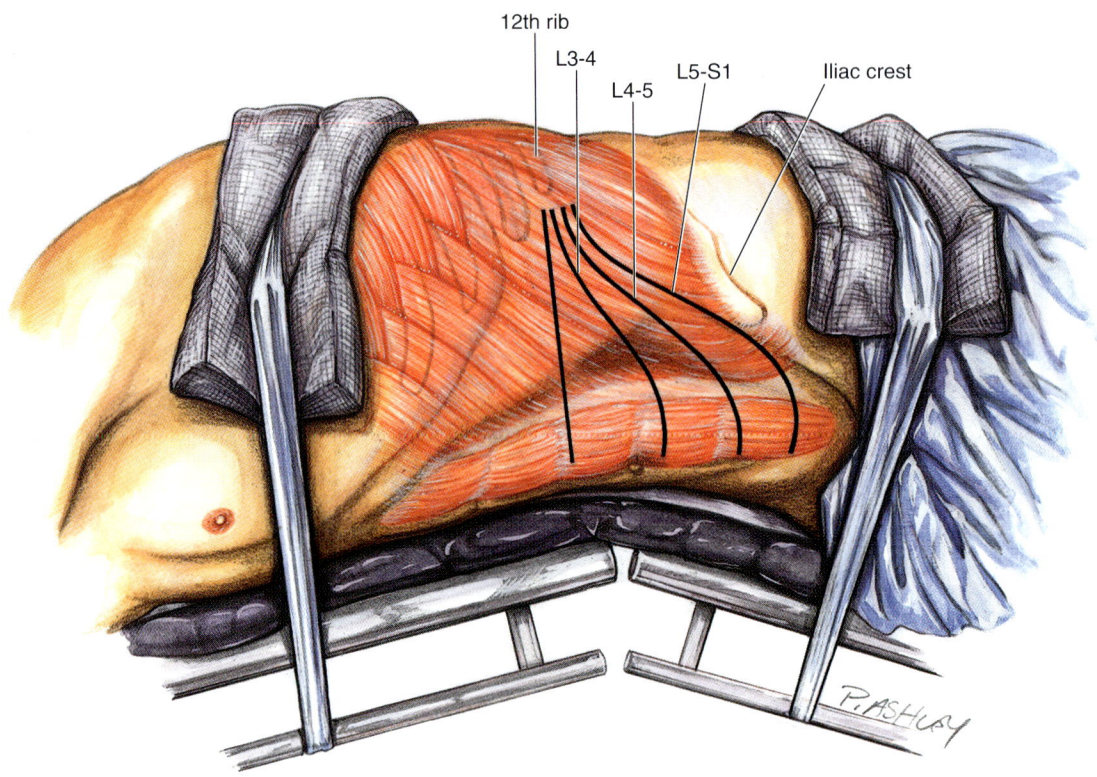

● **Figure 10-5.** Lateral retroperitoneal approach to the lumbosacral spine.

After the incision has been made, the muscle fibers may be divided along their lines or electrocautery may be used to divide the muscles of the abdominal wall in line with the incision. This includes the external oblique muscle, internal oblique muscle, and transversus abdominis muscle. Medially, the incision is carried into the anterior and posterior rectus sheaths. The rectus muscle may be partially divided, but total division is not required and should be avoided (Figure 10–7). The thin transversalis fascia is then carefully incised posterior to allow exposure of the extraperitoneal space. The peritoneum is bluntly dissected off the transversalis fascia and interposing retroperitoneal fat toward the midline (Figure 10–8). Any violation of the peritoneum should be repaired. The dissection is carried down to the psoas muscle. The psoas muscle is far lateral to the spine, and the peritoneal contents must be retracted medially. The ureter can be identified on the inferior surface of the peritoneal reflection. If the location of the ureter is unknown, either the suspected structure may be pinched to observe for peristalsis or a urologic consultation is obtained preoperatively for passage of a ureteral catheter to aid in the identification of the structure. The lateral cutaneous nerve is lateral to the psoas muscle. The genitofemoral nerve with its lateral femoral and medial genital branches lies on the surface of the psoas muscle. The dissection is subsequently carried medial to the psoas for exposure of the aorta, vena cava, sympathetic chain, iliac vessels, and spine (Figure 10–9). Caution should be used when evaluating the venous anatomy of the lower lumbar spine because there may be wide variation in structure.

Exposure of the L4, L5 (and transitional), or sacral vertebral bodies requires mobilization of the common iliac vein (or veins). It is unnecessary to dissect the vein on its medial aspect. Lateral and posteriorly located tributaries must be identified, secured, and divided (Figure 10–10). The vein can then be easily elevated and retracted medially beyond the midline to permit the desired exposure of the spine. If an unrecognized tributary is avulsed

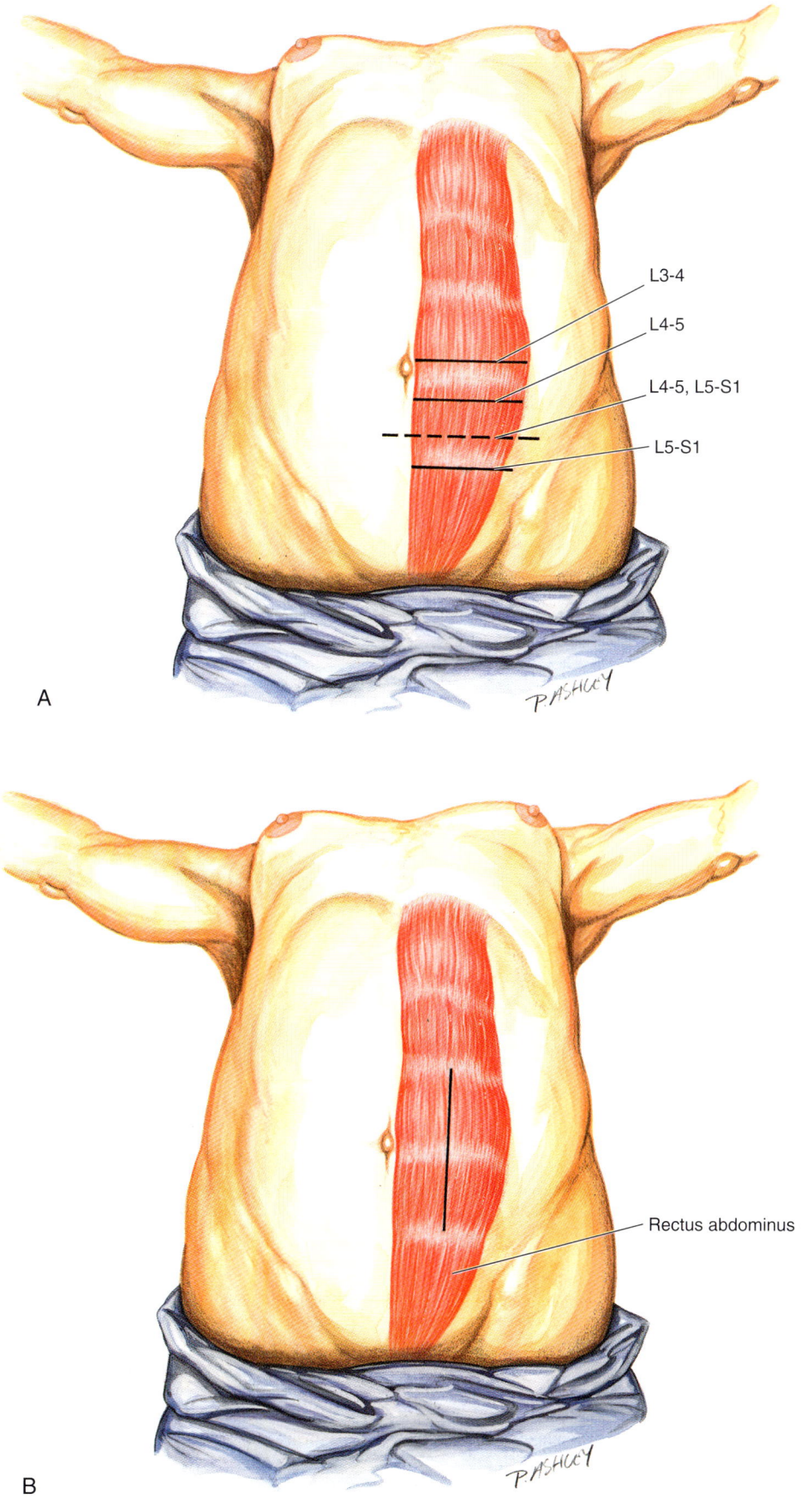

- **Figure 10-6.** *A*, Transverse incisions for one- or two-level lumbar disease. *B*, Vertical paramedian incision for multisegment lower-lumbar disease.

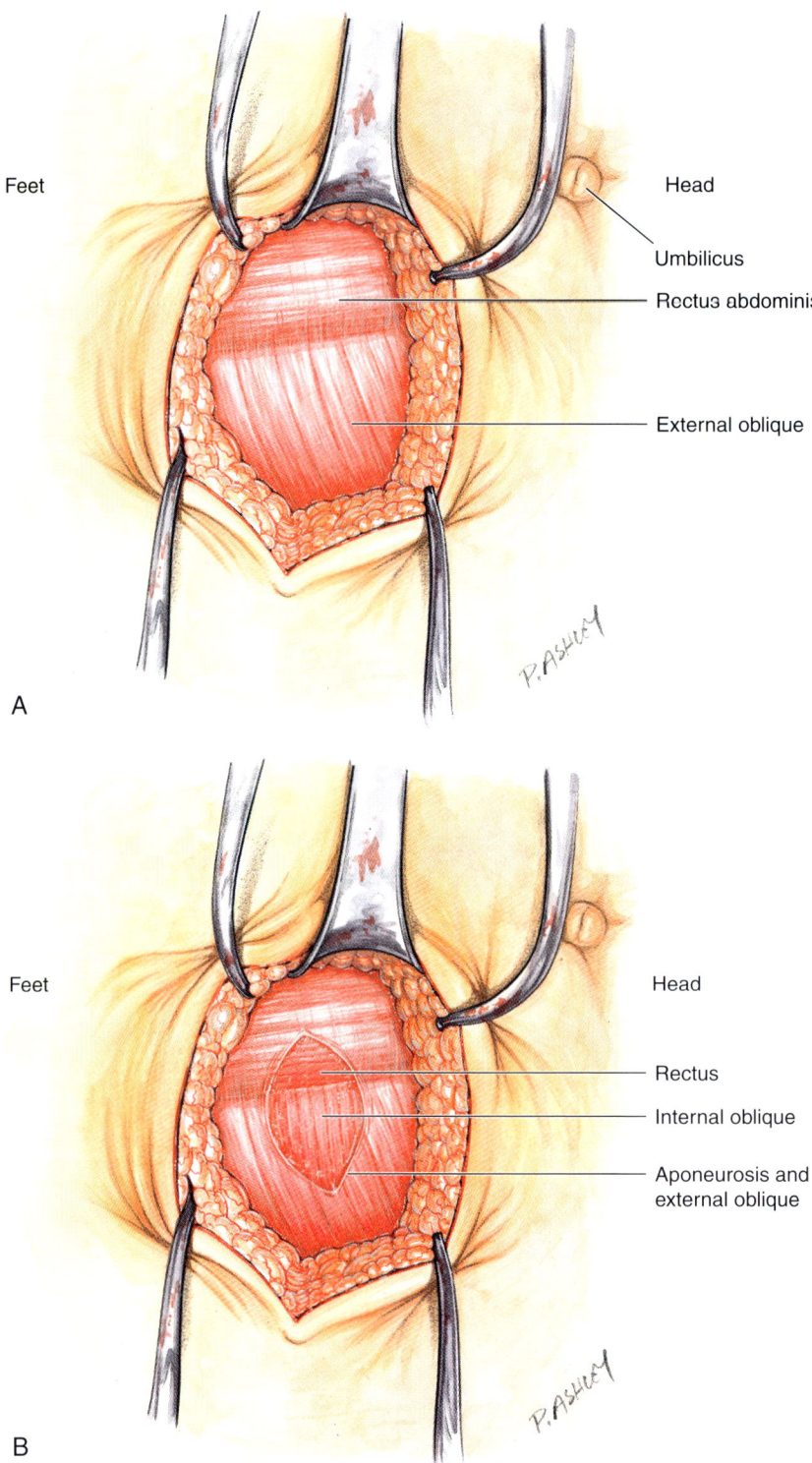

● **Figure 10-7.** *A*, Division of anterior rectus sheath and external oblique muscle. *B*, Division of lateral edge of rectus muscle; divided external and internal oblique muscles exposing the transversalis fascia.

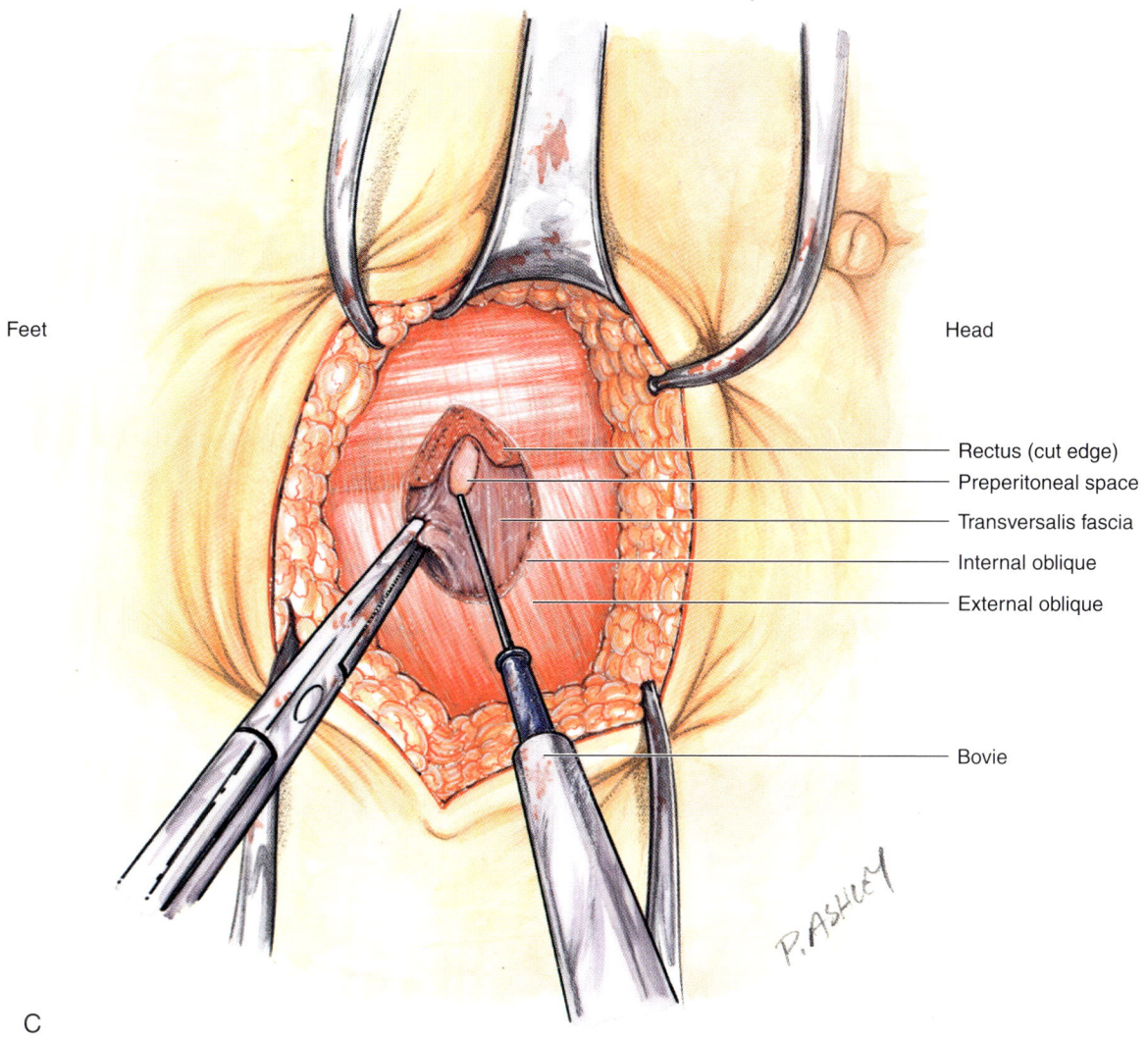

● **Figure 10-7** *Continued C*, Division of transversalis fascia exposes the peritoneum and preperitoneal space.

during the mobilization, it is most important to complete the mobilization of the common iliac vein, elevating that area into view and permitting accurate venorrhaphy. If the adventitia of the vein is preserved, bleeding from small tributaries encountered on the posterior aspect of the vein will not necessitate repair when the vein is returned to its anatomic location because the bleeding is controlled by tamponade against the spinal column. Also, small vessels on the anterior aspect of the spine should not be electrocauterized because the heat transmission may injure the sympathetic nerves and result in retrograde ejaculation. It is unnecessary to dissect lateral to the sympathetic chain (Figure 10–11). Variation in venous anatomy is the rule. Arterial injury can occur by disruption of the intima or an existing atherosclerotic plaque. If any arterial injury occurs, it should be recognizable and immediately addressed by exploring the injured segment, excising it, and restoring distal flow by primary end-to-end repair or use of a prosthetic (interposition) graft. Delayed recognition can have catastrophic consequences.

After the orthopaedic procedure is completed, the vessels and viscera are allowed to return to their anatomic position and the abdominal wound is closed in layers using 1-0

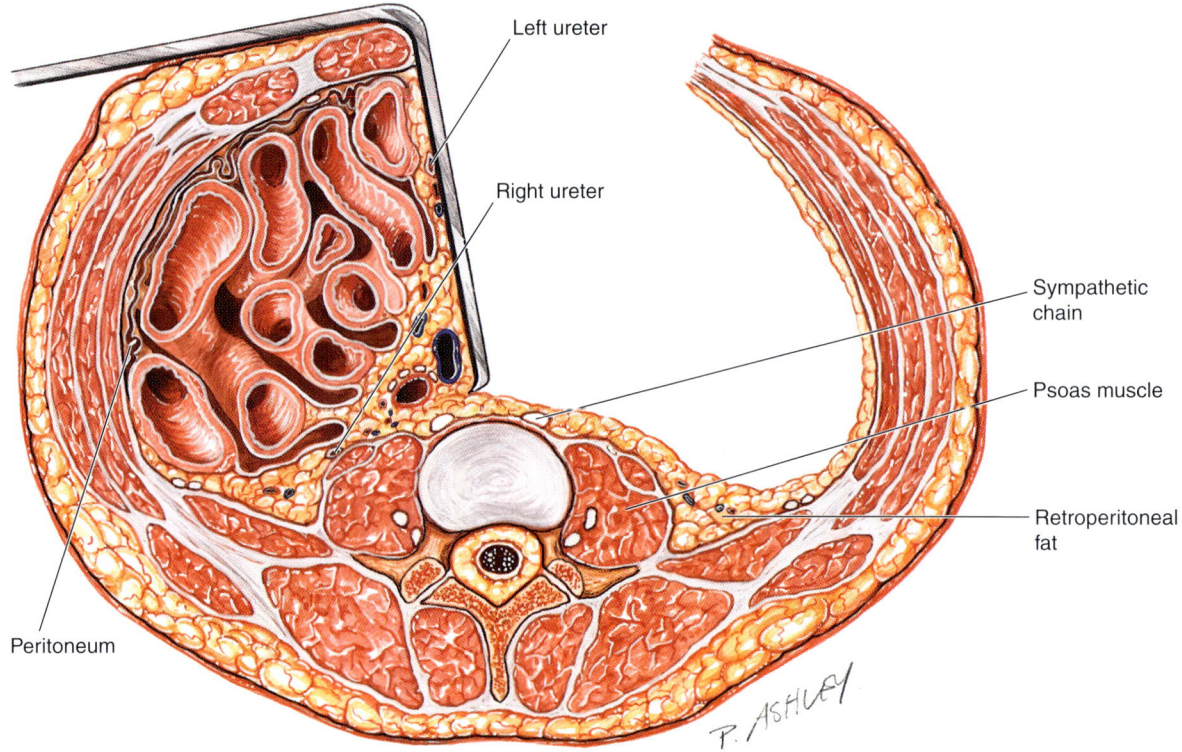

● **Figure 10-8.** Entering the retroperitoneal space. The peritoneum and its contents are retracted beyond the midline. The ureter will remain attached and the vessels will be able to be mobilized after dividing the lateral and posterior tributaries and branches.

polyglycolic acid suture material. The subcutaneous tissue is loosely reapproximated, and a stapling device is used to reapproximate the skin. This approach may be made more difficult by pre-existing conditions. These include inflammation in the left lower quadrant or retroperitoneum as a consequence of previous surgery or infection. Perhaps the most common and most difficult of these pre-existing conditions to treat is acute or chronic inflammation of the intervertebral disk. This can result in scarification with fusion of the posterior wall of the common iliac vein and the anterior longitudinal ligament. It is our practice to mobilize the anterior longitudinal ligament, preserving its intimate relationship with the vein.

The vascular surgeon can play a significant role in providing a consistent, safe approach, permitting excellent exposure of the spine, further enhancing operative results, and perhaps extending the application of procedures directed at the anterior spinal column.

Conclusion

The anterior retroperitoneal approach to the lumbar spine is a safe, efficient technique for managing various pathologic conditions of the lumbar spine. This approach, when employed by a surgical team (vascular and orthopaedic spine surgeons), may be performed in less than 1 hour with minimal loss of blood.

The orthopaedic spine surgeon would be wise to work with a vascular surgeon until such time that the orthopaedic surgeon is thoroughly familiar with every aspect of the

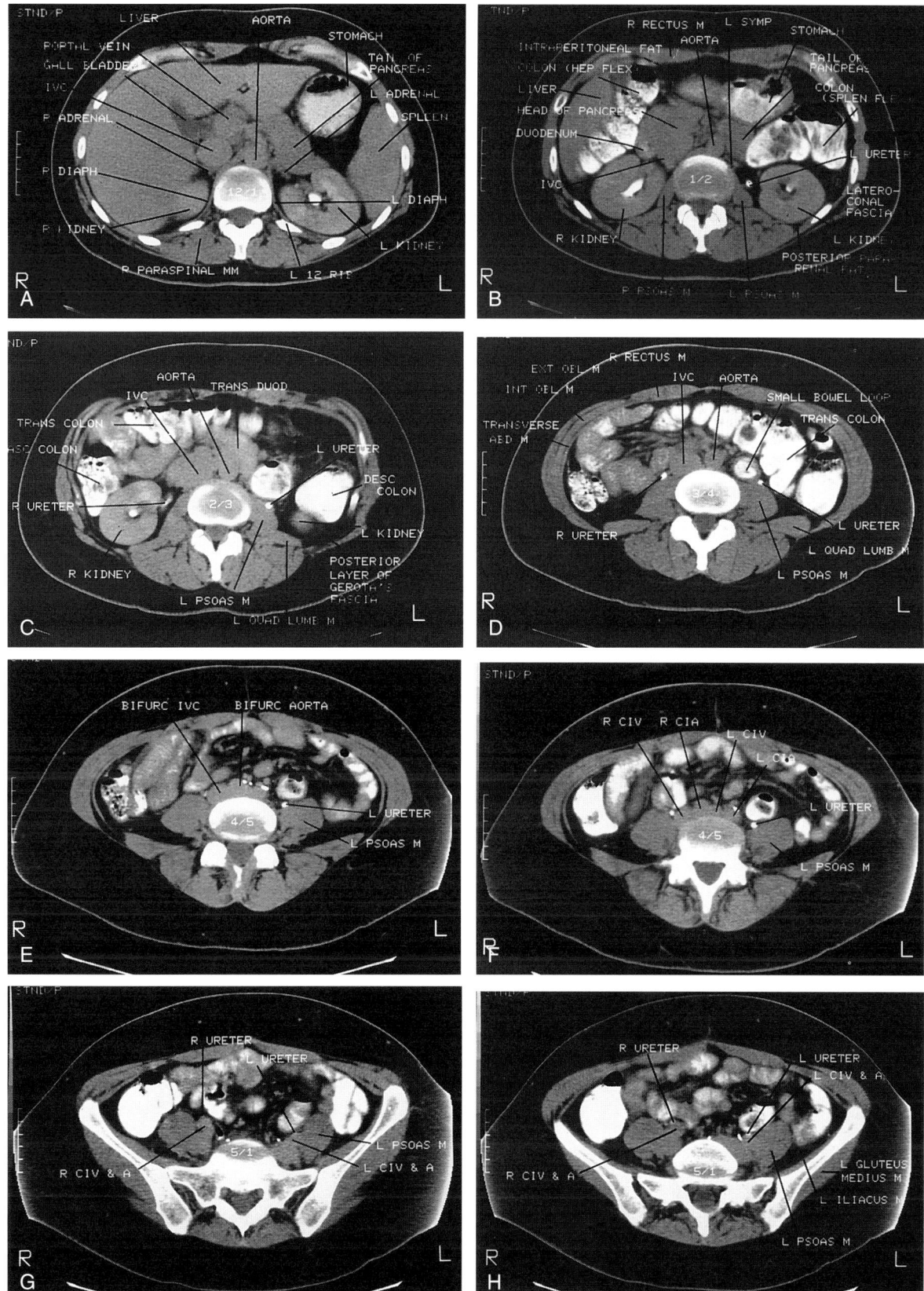

● **Figure 10-9.** Computed tomographic scans of abdomen demonstrating the cross-sectional anatomy at each level. *A,* T12-L1 disk space level. *B,* L1-2 disk space level. *C,* L2-3 disk space level. *D,* L3-4 disk space level. *E,* L4-5 disk space level. *F,* L4-5 disk space level. *G,* L5-S1 disk space level. *H,* L5-S1 disk space level.

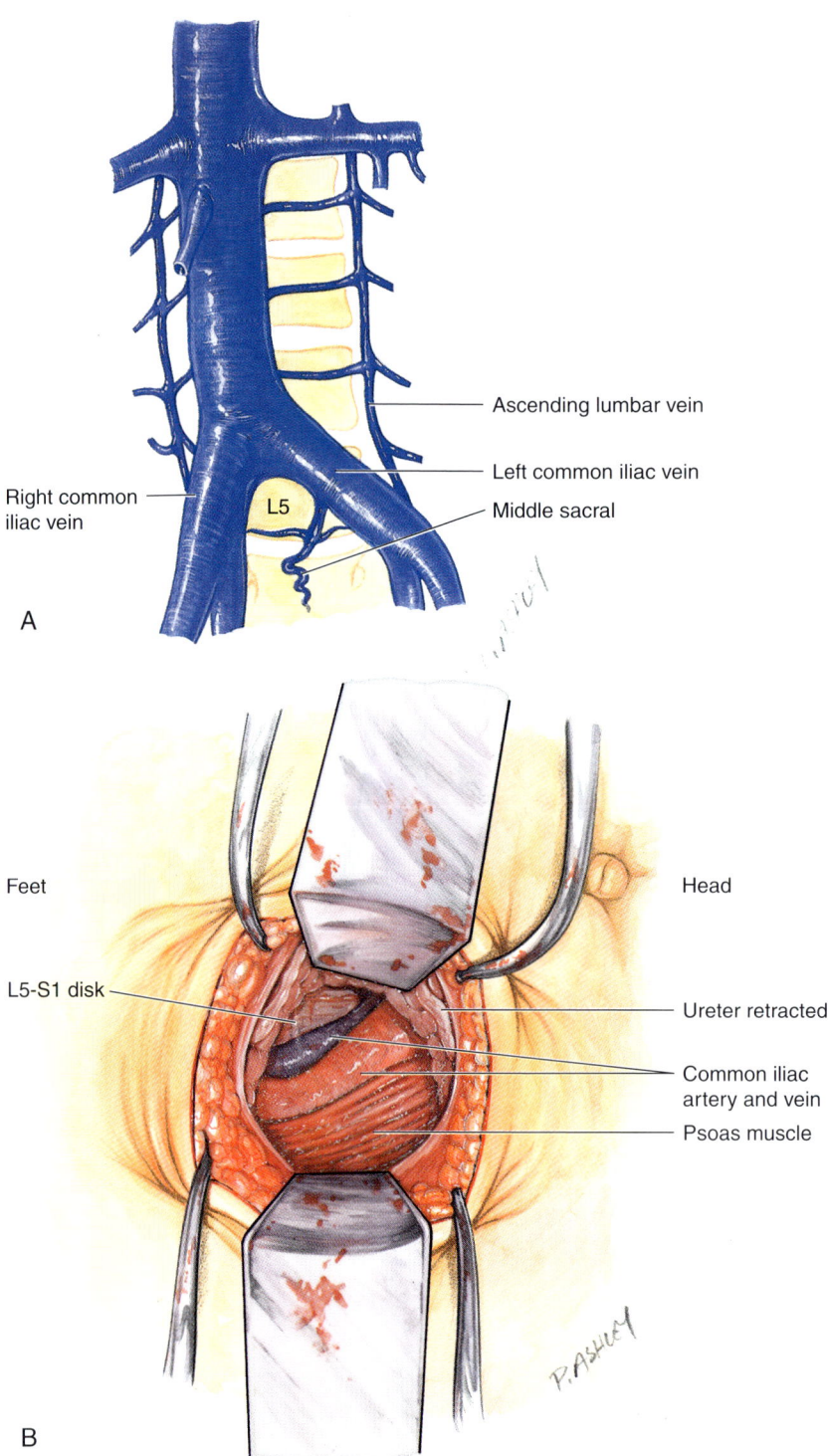

- **Figure 10-10.** *A,* Venous tributaries entering the common iliac vein are best ligated and divided to avoid avulsion when vein is retracted. Variation in these tributaries is the rule not the exception. *B,* Exposure of L5-S1 disc, necessitating retraction of common iliac artery and vein.

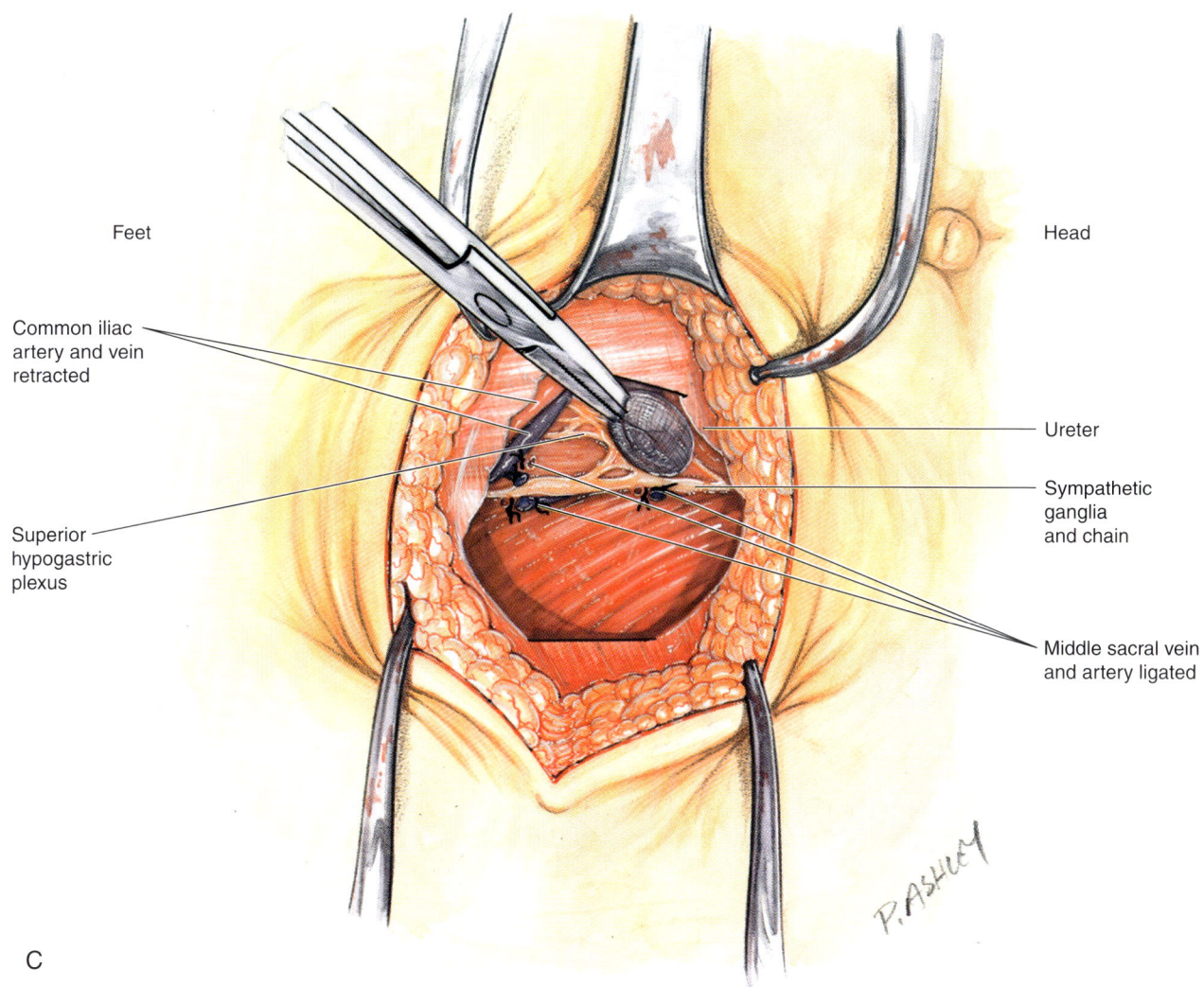

● **Figure 10-10** Continued *C,* The sympathetic plexus is preserved to prevent retrograde ejaculation. Ligation of the middle sacral artery and vein.

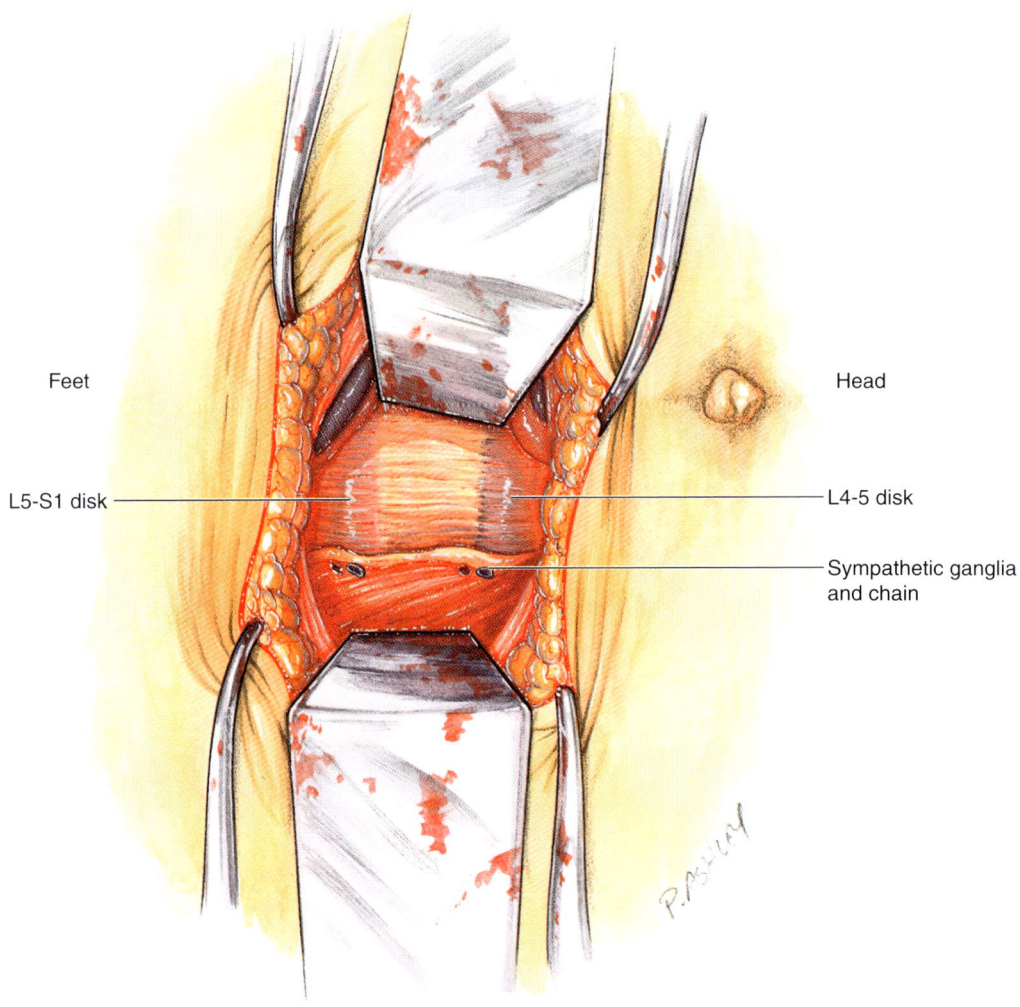

● **Figure 10-11.** The sympathetic chain and ganglia are preserved. They are the limits of the lateral extent of the diskectomy or corpectomy on the anterior surface of the spinal column.

procedure. Crock warns, "when anterior lumbar interbody fusion is attempted by surgeons who are not specially trained, the results can be devastating and the patient may lose his life."[15]

REFERENCES

1. Ito H, Tsuchya J, Asami G: A new radical operation for Pott's disease. J Bone Joint Surg 16:499, 1934.
2. Hodgson AR, Stock FE: Anterior spine fusion: A preliminary communication on the radical treatment of Pott's disease and Pott's paraplegia. Br J Surg 44:266, 1956.
3. Hodgson AR, Stock FE: Anterior spine fusion for the treatment of tuberculosis of the spine. J Bone Joint Surg Am 42:295, 1960.
4. Hodgson AR, Stock FE, Tany HSY, et al: Anterior spine fusion: Operative approach and pathologic findings in 412 patients with Pott's disease of the spine. Br J Surg 44:172, 1960.
5. Kelly RP, Whitesides TE Jr: Treatment of lumbodorsal fracture-dislocations. Ann Surg 167:705, 1968.
6. Fountain SS: A single-stage combined surgical approach for vertebral resections. J Bone Joint Surg Am 61: 1011, 1979.

7. Bohlman HK, Eismont FJ: Surgical techniques of anterior decompression and fusion for spinal care injuries. Clin Orthop 154:57, 1981.
8. Cotler HB, Cotler JM, Stoloff A, et al: The use of autografts for vertebral body replacement of the thoracic and lumbar spine. Spine 10:748, 1985.
9. Flynn JC, Hogue MA: Anterior fusion of the lumbar spine. J Bone Joint Surg 61:1143, 1979.
10. Kozak JA, O'Brien JP: Simultaneous combined anterior and posterior fusions: An independent analysis of a treatment for the disabled low-back pain patient. Spine 15:322, 1990.
11. Capener V: Spondylolisthesis. Br J Surg 19:374, 1932.
12. Burns BH: An operation for spondylolisthesis. Lancet 1:1233, 1933.
13. Mercer W: Spondylolisthesis. Edinburgh Med J 43:545, 1936.
14. Kirkaldy-Willis WH, Allen PB, Rostrup O, et al: Surgical approaches to the anterior elements of the spine: Indications and technique. Can J Surg 9:294, 1966.
15. Crock HV: Practice of Spinal Surgery. New York, Springer-Verlag, 1983.
16. Selby DK, Henderson RJ, et al: Anterior lumbar fusion. In White AH, Rothman RH, Ray CD (eds): Lumbar Spine Surgery, pp 383–402. St. Louis, CV Mosby, 1987.
17. Fraser RD, Gogan NJ: A modified muscle-splitting approach to the lumbosacral spine. Spine 17:943, 1992.
18. Fraser RD: A wide muscle splitting approach to the lumbosacral spine. J Bone Joint Surg Br 64:44, 1982.

CHAPTER 11

POSTERIOR LUMBAR APPROACH

David L. Kramer, M.D.
Robert E. Booth, Jr., M.D.
Todd J. Albert, M.D.
Richard A. Balderston, M.D.

The posterior midline approach to the lumbar spine is the most frequently used approach in surgery of the spine. It is an extensile approach that provides access to the posterior bony arch and pedicles of the spine, the underlying spinal cord, and the intervertebral disks. Accordingly, it is an approach well suited for posterior decompression of the spinal cord and exploration of exiting nerve roots in degenerative conditions of central and foraminal spinal stenosis. It allows unilateral or bilateral access to herniated disks. Intradural and extradural tumors may be exposed. When indicated, this approach may provide lateral exposure of the transverse processes for onlay in-situ bone grafting, as well as identification of the dorsal entry site of the cortical cylinder of the pedicle for biopsy of the vertebral body or for placement of bone screws used with instrumentation for posterior lumbar fusion.

Anatomy

The anatomy of the lumbar spine is well established. The lumbar vertebrae consist of relatively large vertebral bodies with blunt posterior arch structures. The superior articular facets are directed dorsomedially and lie anterolateral to the inferior articular facets of the more cephalad lumbar vertebra. As such, in degenerative conditions of the spine, it is primarily the superior articular facet that is responsible for lateral foraminal stenosis and the inferior articular facet that is responsible for central spinal stenosis (Figure 11–1).

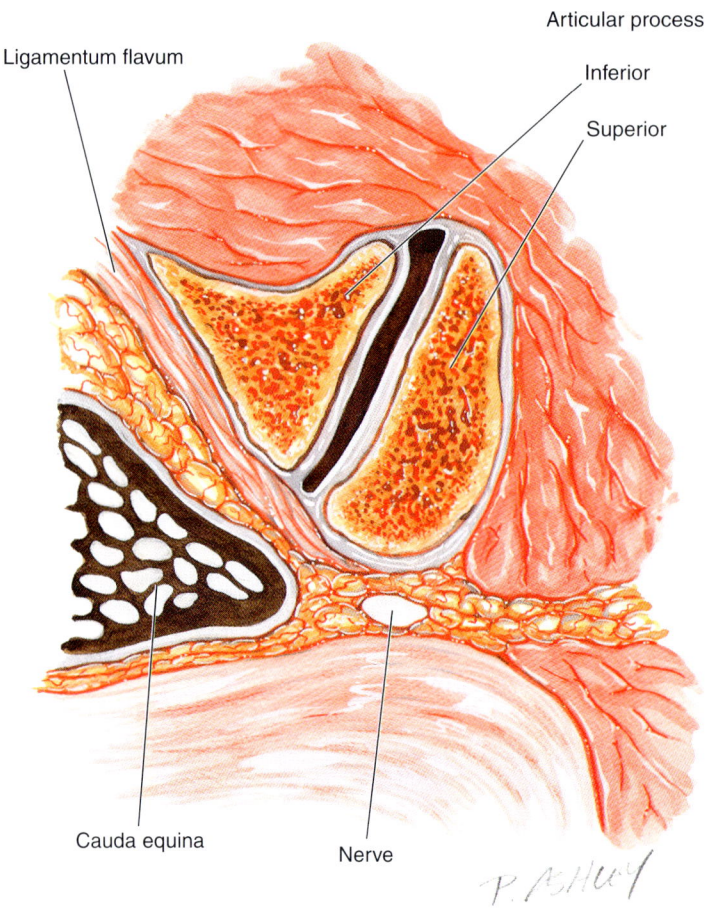

● **Figure 11-1.** Inferior and superior articular process. The anterior margin of the superior articular process lies just posterior to the neuroforamen.

The pedicle is the cortical cylinder that connects the anterior vertebral body to its posterior bony arch. These cortical cylinders increase in diameter from L1 through L5. The axis of the pedicle creates an angle with the midline that also increases from approximately 7 degrees at L1 to 17 degrees at L5. The sagittal intervals between the pedicles, the intervertebral foramen, are elliptical conduits with vertical diameter 12 to 19 mm in height, through which pass the spinal nerve, artery, vein, and branches of the sinuvertebral nerve (Figure 11–2).

Several ligaments support and stabilize the bony contour of the lumbar spine (Figure 11–3). The supraspinous ligament is a continuous collection of collagen fibers running along the dorsal aspect of the spinous processes that add posterior column support and stabilize the cantilevered vertebral bodies anteriorly. The spinous processes are further stabilized to one another by the segmentally developed interspinous ligaments. The intertransverse ligament is also a segmental structure that is best developed in the lumbar spine and creates a fibrous sling between the transverse processes. The ligamentum flavum is a strong, elastic structure that originates on the ventral surface of a cephalad lamina and inserts on the superior lip of the next caudal lamina. Its resilient and elastic nature allows it to remain taut with lumbar extension and thereby avoid infolding with subsequent compression on the cord. The anterior longitudinal ligament consists of longitudinal bands of collagen fibers that run along the

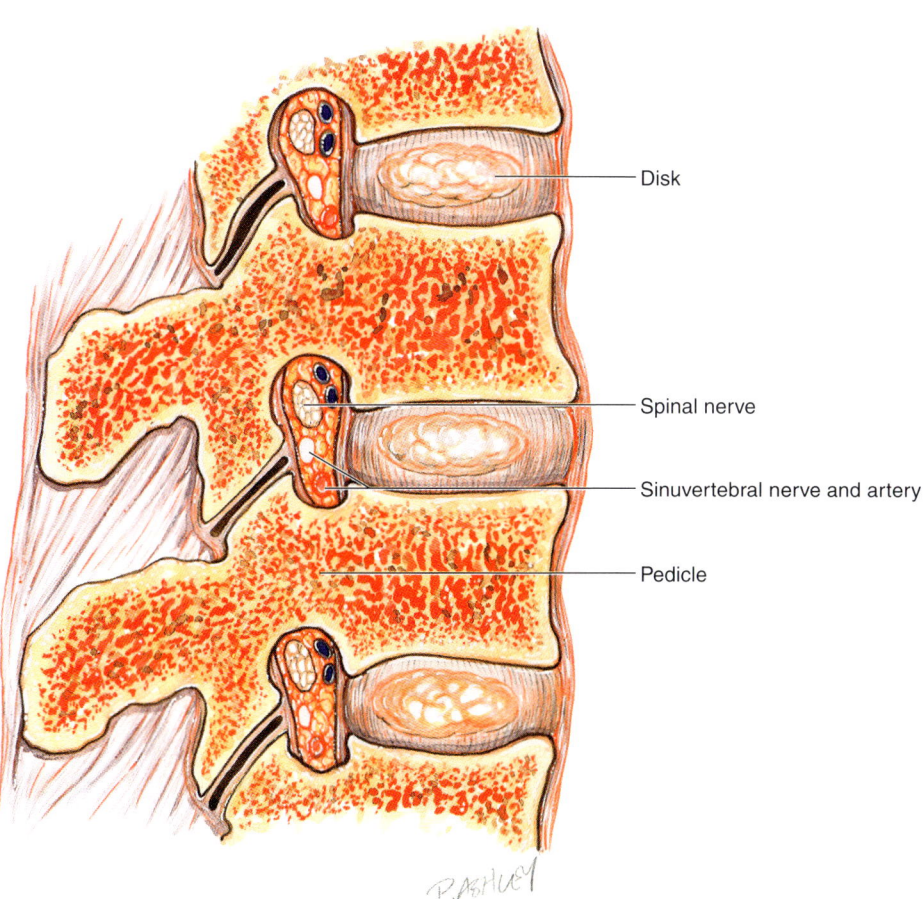

● **Figure 11-2.** Anatomy of the intervertebral foramen in relation to the disk and pedicles. The two structures passing ventral to the spinal nerve are the sinuvertebral nerve and the artery. The other vessels are veins.

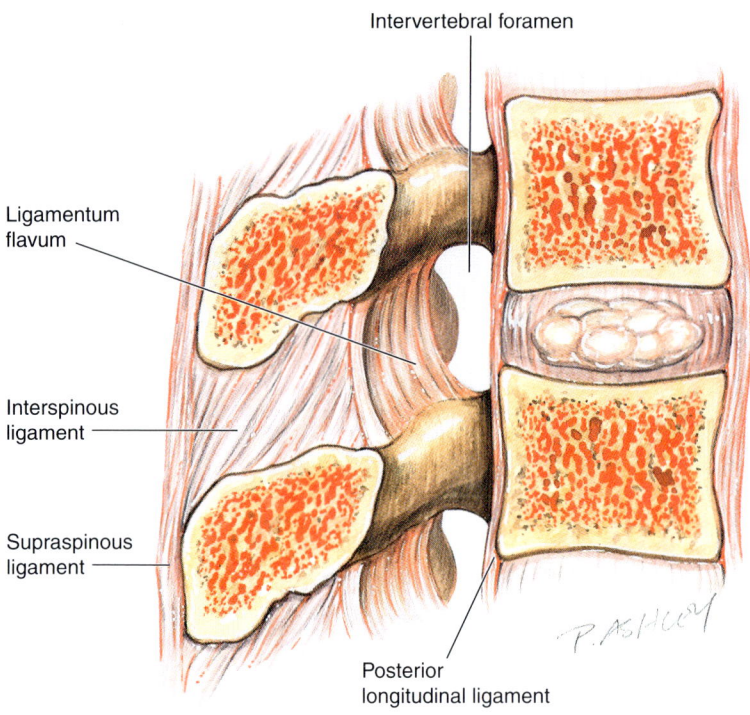

● **Figure 11-3.** Ligaments of the lumbar spine.

ventral surface of the spine from the skull to the sacrum. This broad anterior ligament is intimately related to the periosteum of the anterior vertebral bodies and loosely adherent to the intervening intervertebral disks. In contrast to this, the posterior longitudinal ligament is a thick but narrow band of fibrous tissue that runs along the posterior aspect of the vertebral bodies. Unlike the anterior longitudinal ligament, this ligament actually bowstrings over the vertebral bodies and has its strongest attachments at the level of the disk as it extends out laterally through the intervertebral foramen. This cruciform pattern may account for the observation that most disk herniations are lateral to this strong midline strap.

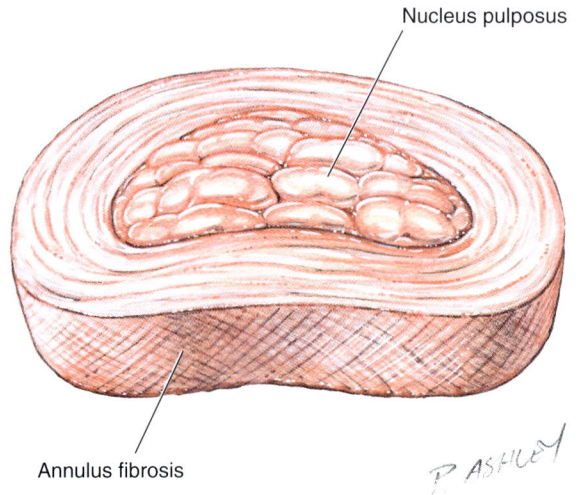

● **Figure 11-4.** Disk showing annulus fibrosis and nucleus pulposus.

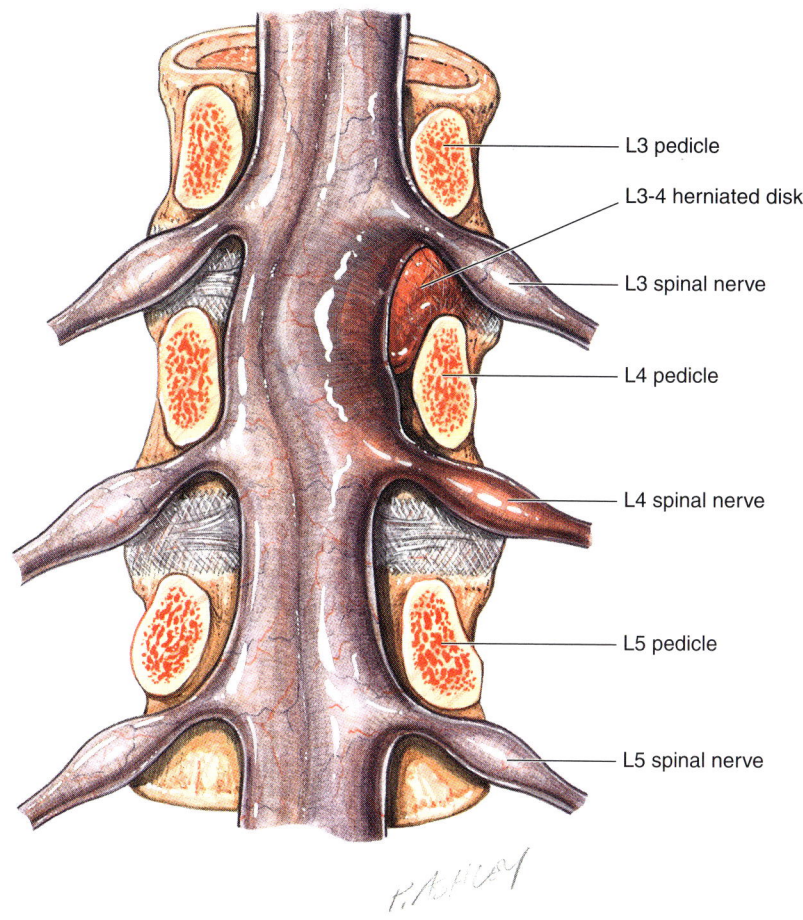

● **Figure 11-5.** Lumbar nerve roots with L3-4 herniated disk.

The intervertebral disk comprises the outer annulus fibrosis, a series of concentric fibrous lamellae running oblique to the long axis, and the inner nucleus pulposus, composed primarily of water, type II collagen, and proteoglycan. The nucleus pulposus responds as a viscous fluid under pressure and as such acts to resist and redistribute axial compressive forces within the spine. In contrast, the annulus functions to resist tension from horizontal pressure that has been redirected by the nucleus in response to axial load (Figure 11-4). The annulus also resists torsional stress as well as stress created by the angular vertebral separation that permits lumbar flexion and extension.

Neural structures in the lumbar spine follow fairly consistent anatomic patterns. The conus medularis is usually found between L1 and L2, below which the spinal cord continues as a collection of nerve roots collectively referred to as the cauda equina. The nerve roots of the cauda equina descend within the canal to exit beneath their respectively named pedicles (Figure 11-5). For example, the L4 nerve root descends posteriorly over the L3-4 disk before it turns laterally to exit beneath the L4 pedicle through the L4-5 foramen.

Blood supply to the lumbar vertebral elements and muscles is derived from a modified segmental system of vessels called the iliolumbar system. As opposed to the thoracic spine, where segmental blood flow comes off the aorta (which ends at L4), the segmental blood flow in the lumbar spine originates from branches of the fourth lumbar artery, the middle sacral artery, the internal iliac artery, and the iliolumbar artery (Figure 11-6). Dorsal

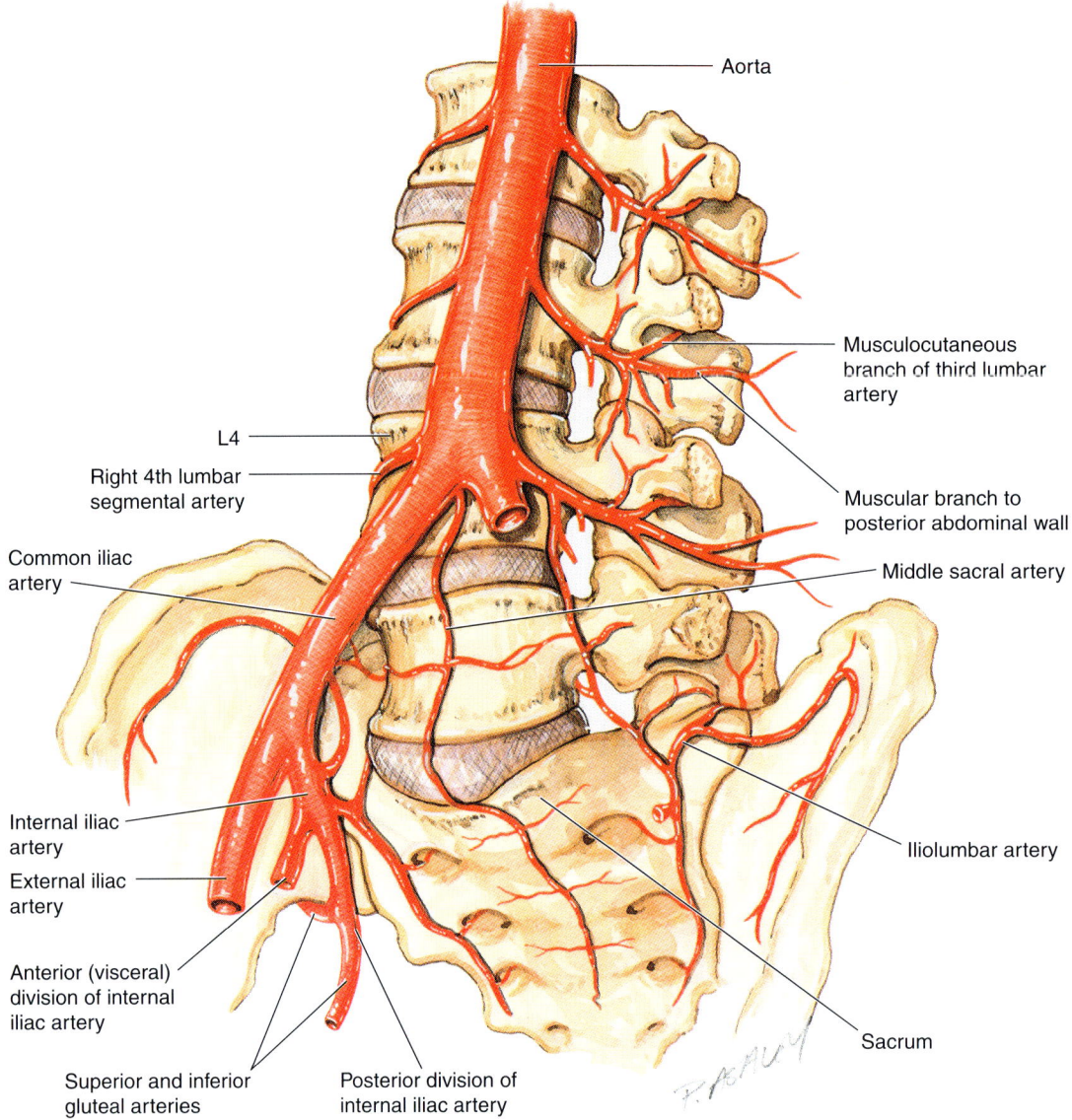

● **Figure 11-6.** Drawing of the distribution and major variations of the sacroiliolumbar system of arteries that supply the vertebrae and their associated structures inferior to the fourth lumbar vertebra.

branches of this system reach the paraspinal muscles by ascending in the interval between the facet joints, just lateral to the pars interarticularis. It is this segmental vessel that is often encountered while dissecting within the soft tissue lateral to the pars (Figure 11-7).

The muscles of the lumbar spine may be divided into three layers: superficial, middle, and deep (Figure 11-8). The superficial layer consists primarily of muscles related to the shoulder girdle: the latissimus dorsi, trapezius, and serratus posterior. As such, these muscles are innervated by peripheral nerves taking their origin within the brachial plexus. The intermediate layer consists of long, longitudinal muscle masses extending over several motion segments. Taken together, these are referred to as the erector spinae (from lateral to medial: iliocostalis, longissimus, spinalis). The deep layer is the only layer composed of true spinal muscles, in that they are innervated and have origins and insertions at each spinal

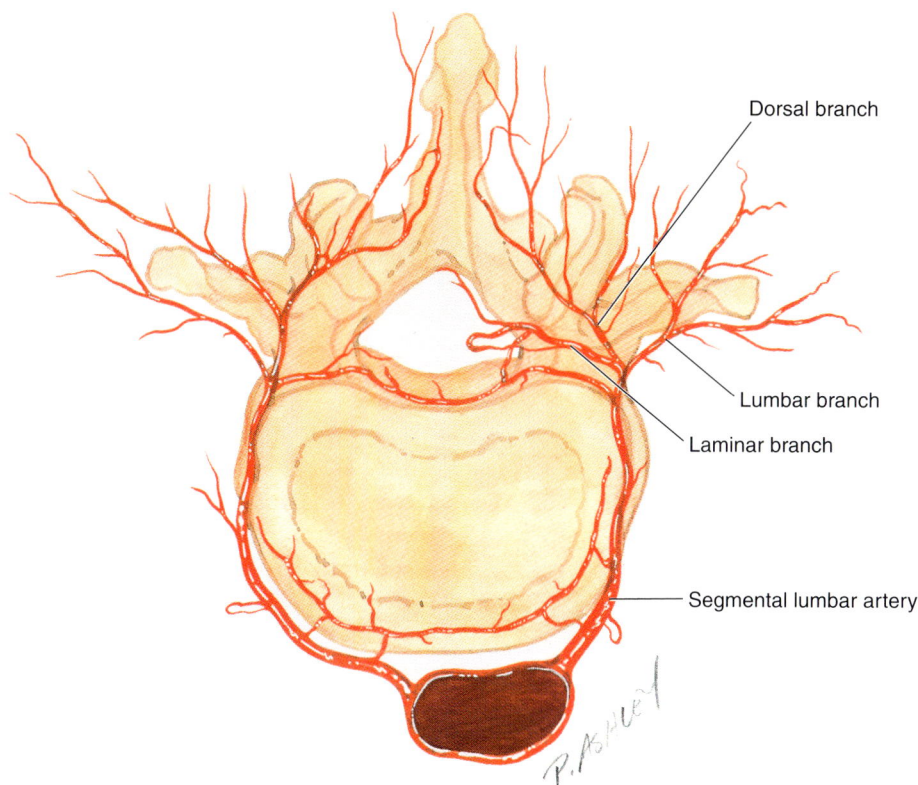

● **Figure 11-7.** Distribution of segmental artery as it passes near the facet joint and the pars interarticularis.

level. The muscles that make up this layer are the multifidi, rotatores, levatores, and intertransversarii.

Surgical Approach

Proper positioning of the patient is the crucial first step in minimizing total blood loss during the posterior lumbar approach. By ensuring that the abdomen is allowed to hang free, intra-abdominal pressure is kept at a minimum, thereby reducing spinal venous pressure and decreasing subsequent bleeding. Several frames exist that allow such decompression of the abdomen and free excursion of the chest (Figure 11–9). The criticism of these frames is that they tend to increase lumbar lordosis, making laminotomy and lateral recess decompression somewhat more difficult. This position of relative hyperextension, however, reproduces the axial compression of the neural elements. If the spine is effectively decompressed in this extended position, relief of radicular symptoms may be expected when the patient is erect. When kneeling frames are used, care should be taken to thoroughly pad all bony prominences (knees, anterior tibiae, elbows) and abduction of the arms should not exceed 90 degrees to the trunk axis.

The length of the incision is determined by palpation of the spinous processes of the appropriate levels. The skin incision is made in the midline directly over these spinous

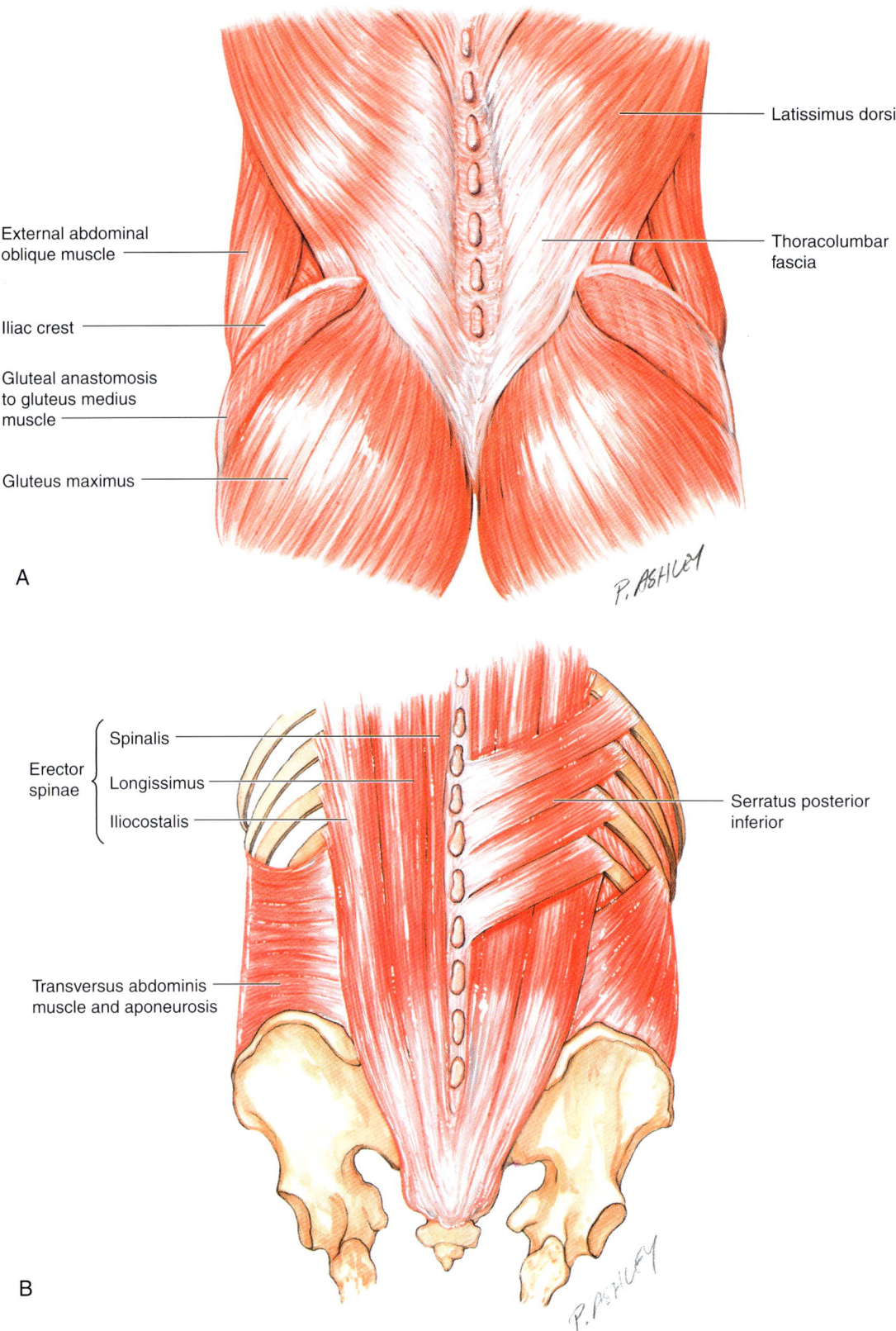

● **Figure 11-8.** Muscle layers of lumbar spine. *A,* Superficial layer. *B,* Intermediate layer.

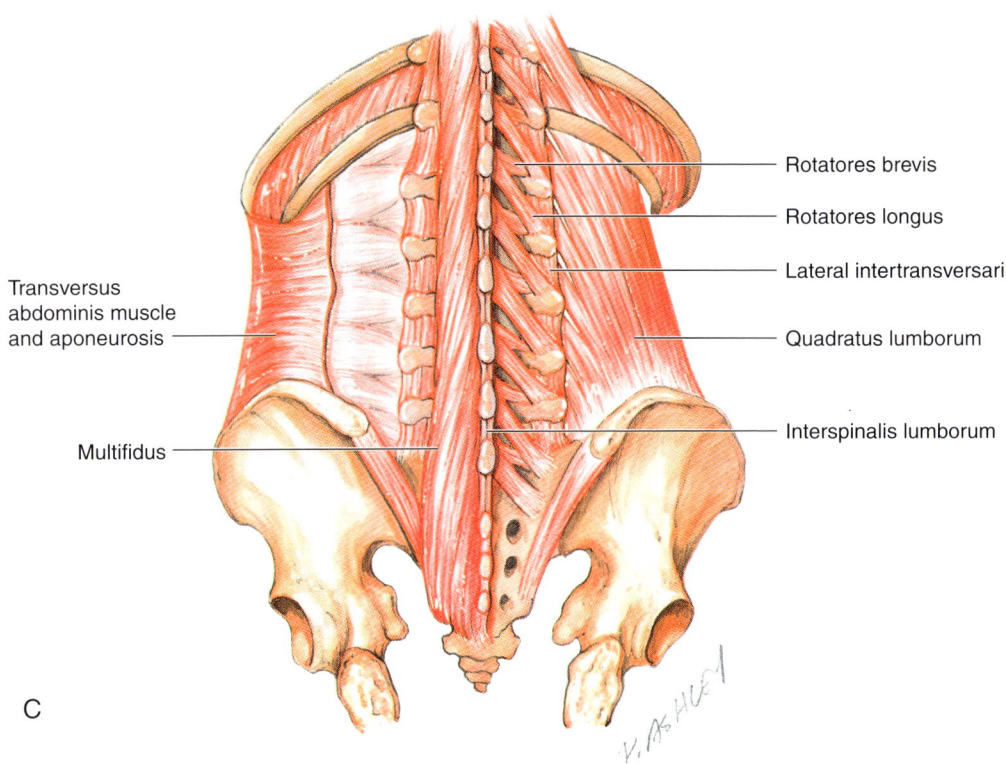

● **Figure 11–8 Continued** C, Deep layer.

processes after infiltrating the skin with 1:100,000 epinephrine solution (usually with 0.25% Marcaine). Dissection is carried down through the subcutaneous adipose tissue, either sharply or with electrocautery, to the level of the lumbodorsal fascia. This thick fascial layer, clearly seen in the anatomic specimen (Figure 11–10), is composed of the fascial extension of the latissimus dorsi, the quadratus lumborum, and the trapezius and envelops the underlying erector spinae muscles. The deep fibers of the lumbodorsal fascia coalesce with the periosteum of the spinous processes and laminae medially and with the fascia of the psoas anteriorly. By performing a subperiosteal dissection along the spinous processes, one can, for the most part, preserve this muscle envelope and avoid violation of the intramuscular vessels. The tip of the spinous processes has a bulbous shape. Accordingly, dissection with the elevator or cautery must be directed initially dorsally to go under the edge and thus avoid dissecting into the paraspinous musculature. This is the first obstacle to be addressed in the posterior approach, because meticulous hemostasis is required to prevent the slow, persistent bleeding, pooling within the depths of the wound, that may plague the surgeon for the remainder of the surgical procedure. Avoidance of straying into the muscles may be facilitated by gentle lateral retraction of the erector spinae muscles with a Cobb elevator, thereby delineating under tension the origin of the deeper segmental muscles (i.e., multifidi) as they originate off the interspinous ligaments (Figure 11–11). This subperiosteal dissection is carried in a distal to proximal direction as the paraspinous muscles originate obliquely on the midline interspinous ligament. Instruments passed from caudad to cephalad will stay in the subperiosteal plane, thus avoiding further muscle bleeding.

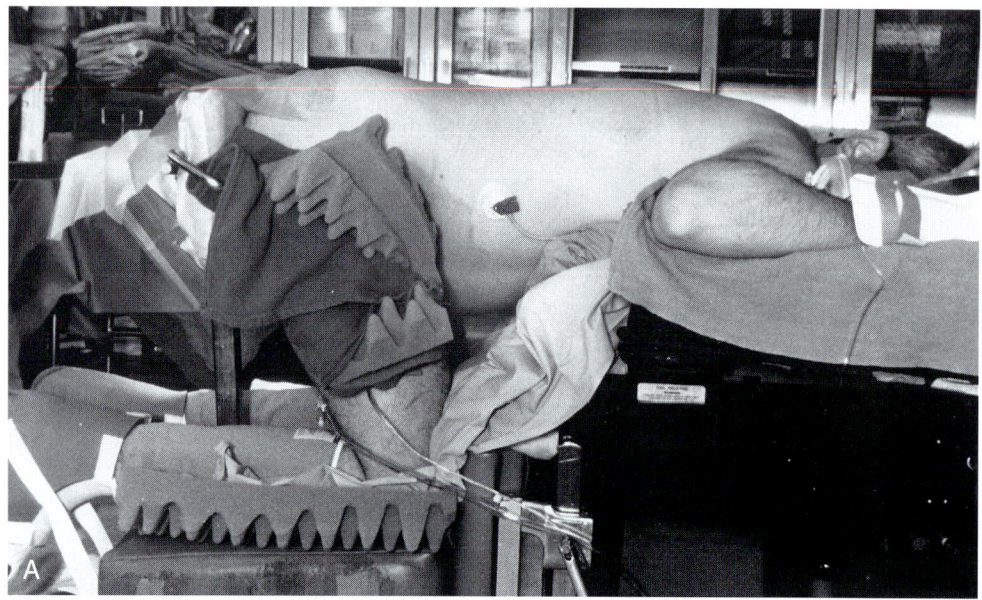

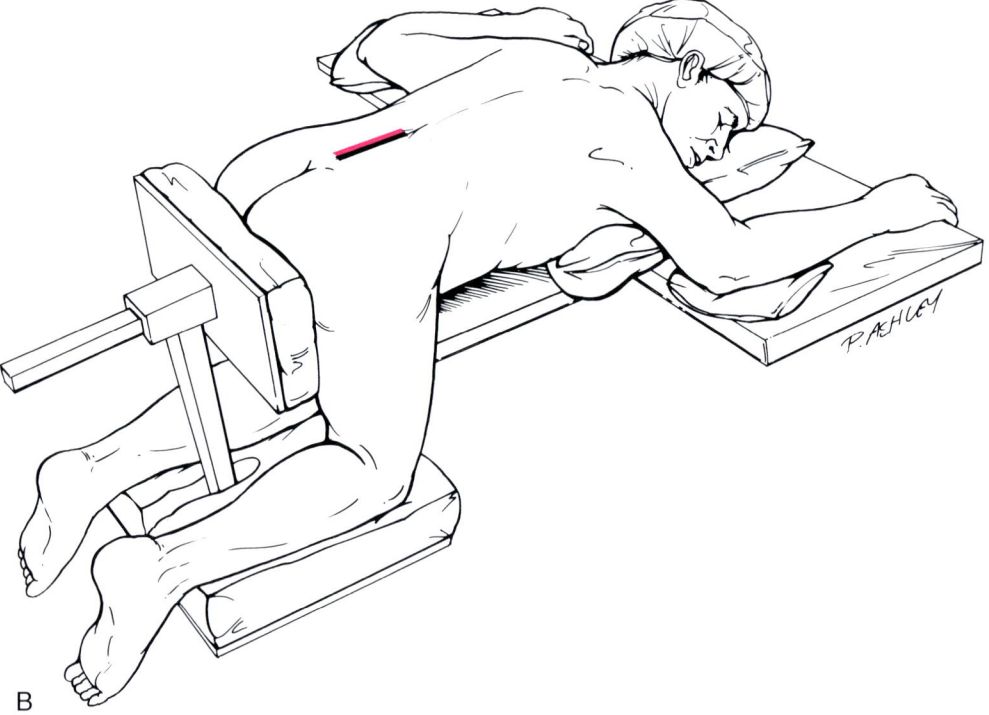

● **Figure 11-9.** Patient on Andrews frame. *A,* Note abdominal decompression preventing pressure on inferior vena cava. *B,* Incision line.

The second obstacle encountered during the posterior approach is the dissection carried out lateral to the facet joints. As mentioned, this lateral extension is usually required only during the approach for fusion using posterolateral bone graft or pedicle instrumentation. Once the subperiosteal dissection has been carried down to the level of the lamina, care must be taken to avoid inadvertent subperiosteal dissection into the facet joint. This may be difficult in spondylarthritic spines where facet osteophytes cause medial overhang of the

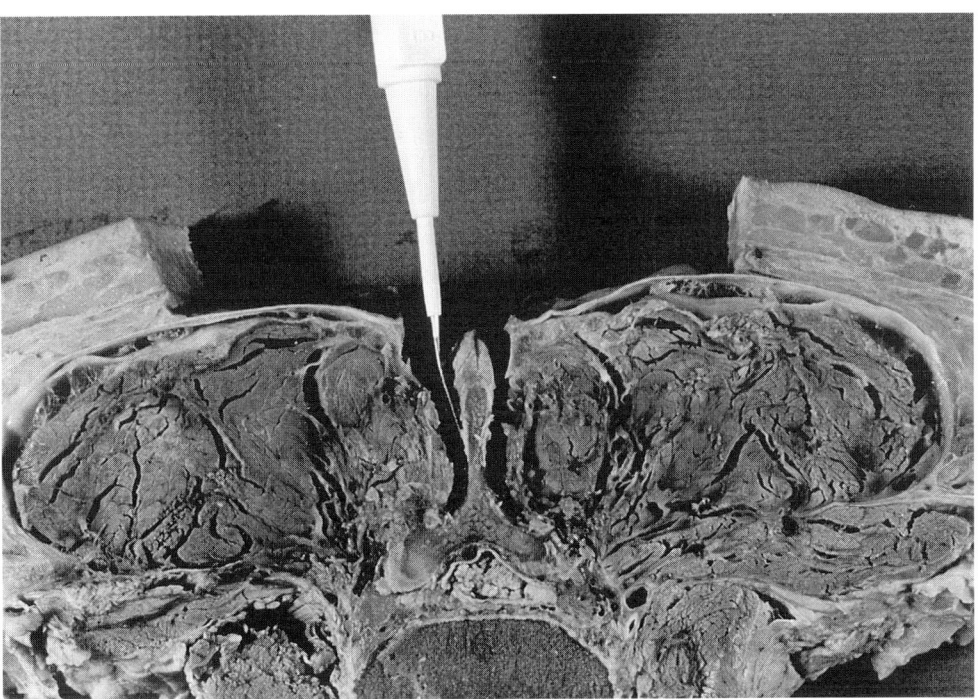

● **Figure 11-10.** The lumbosacral fascia envelops the underlying erector spinae muscles. The deep fibers of the fascia coalesce with the periosteum of the spinous processes and lamina medially and with the fascia of the psoas anteriorly.

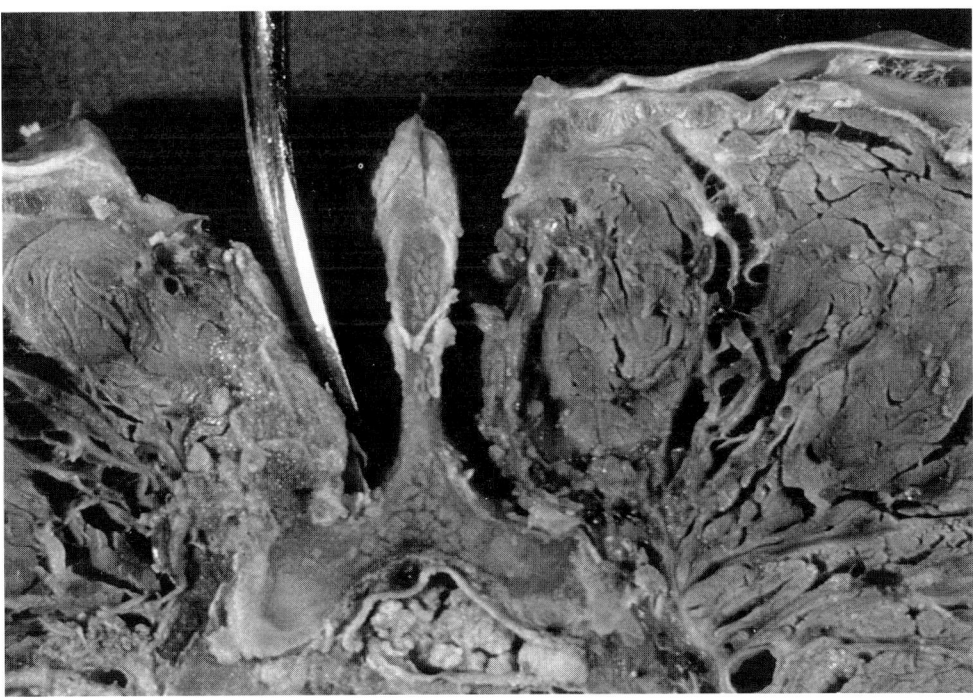

● **Figure 11-11.** Subperiosteal dissection of paraspinal muscles off the spinous process and laminae.

inferior articular process. Once the medial margin of the facet joint is encountered, self-retaining retractors may be placed to enlarge the operative field and to compress the intramuscular vasculature to reduce hemorrhage. Delineation of the pars interarticularis is an extremely helpful maneuver as it defines the lateralmost margin of the canal between the pedicles. Subperiosteal removal of soft tissue overlying the pars is facilitated by carefully cutting down to the bone with a Cobb elevator perpendicular to the axis of the pars and then gently rotating the elevator laterally against the bone, sweeping the soft tissue lateral to the pars. Electrocautery can be used with this maneuver to facilitate the removal of the soft tissue. In cases of spondylolisthesis or spondylolysis, one must exercise extreme caution to avoid penetration through a fibrous or dysplastic pars defect. Additional brisk bleeding is often encountered immediately lateral to the pars, between the facet joints. This arises from inadvertent and planned interruption of the segmental facetal artery previously described. These vessels may be safely controlled with electocautery as the neural elements pass deep to the transverse processes and intervening intertransverse ligament. Dissection of the paraspinal muscles off the facet joints is facilitated by gently retracting the muscle mass up and over the intact facet joint capsule. By applying lateral tension to the muscle, muscle fiber origins arising from the joint capsule are more clearly delineated and may be dissected off under direct visualization, thereby preserving the facet joint capsule (Figure 11–12). Preservation of the intact facet joint is necessary if the surgeon wishes to preserve stability of the spine while avoiding fusion of the motion segment.

The last obstacle to be overcome during this approach is the exposure of the transverse processes. These may be palpated lateral and just caudad to each facet joint. Each facet joint is composed of the superior articular process of the caudal vertebra and the inferior articular process of the cephalad vertebra. As described earlier, the superior articular process of the caudal vertebra lies anterolateral to the inferior articular process of the cephalad vertebra. The transverse process may be identified by following the base of the superior articular process out laterally. The pedicle may also be located directly anterior to the base of the superior articular process. One can easily see how the anatomy of the facet joint serves as an important guide for understanding the three-dimensional anatomy of the spine (Figure 11–13). A Cobb elevator may then be gently applied to the dorsomedial aspect of the transverse process, and a gentle lateral sweeping motion will facilitate definition of the upper and lower borders of the process. Electrocautery may then be used to subperiosteally dissect the segmentally arising muscles (intertransversarii, rotatores, levatores) off the bony process. Care must be taken to avoid excessive downward force against the process because it is easily fractured. All attempts must be made to preserve the intertransverse ligament, because it serves to define the safe boundary anterior to which injury to the nerve roots, vascular structures, and retroperitoneal space may take place. This ligament also serves as a fibrous sling on which to place bone graft for an intertransverse process fusion (Figure 11–14). Once sufficient lateral exposure has been obtained, the lateral gutters may be tamponaded with thrombin-moistened sponges and attention may be turned to carrying out the procedure at hand.

In the case of decompressive laminectomy, attention is directed to the midline interval between the ligamentum flavum and the superior edge of the lamina defining the caudal extent of the decompression. This is most readily accomplished using a medium-sized (2 mm) curved curet with a gentle sweeping motion against the superior laminar edge (Figure 11–15). The curet must be supported with two hands to avoid inadvertent penetration of the ligamentum, which, owing to its segmental origin, may be quite thin where it meets (but does not fuse) with its homologue in the midline. Once the caudal insertion of the ligamentum has been taken down and entry into the canal has been accomplished, Kerrison rongeurs may be placed carefully within the canal, taking care to maintain contact of the boot of the instrument with the undersurface of the lamina. In the event that any resistance is encountered with the Kerrison rongeur, a Penfield dissector may be used to

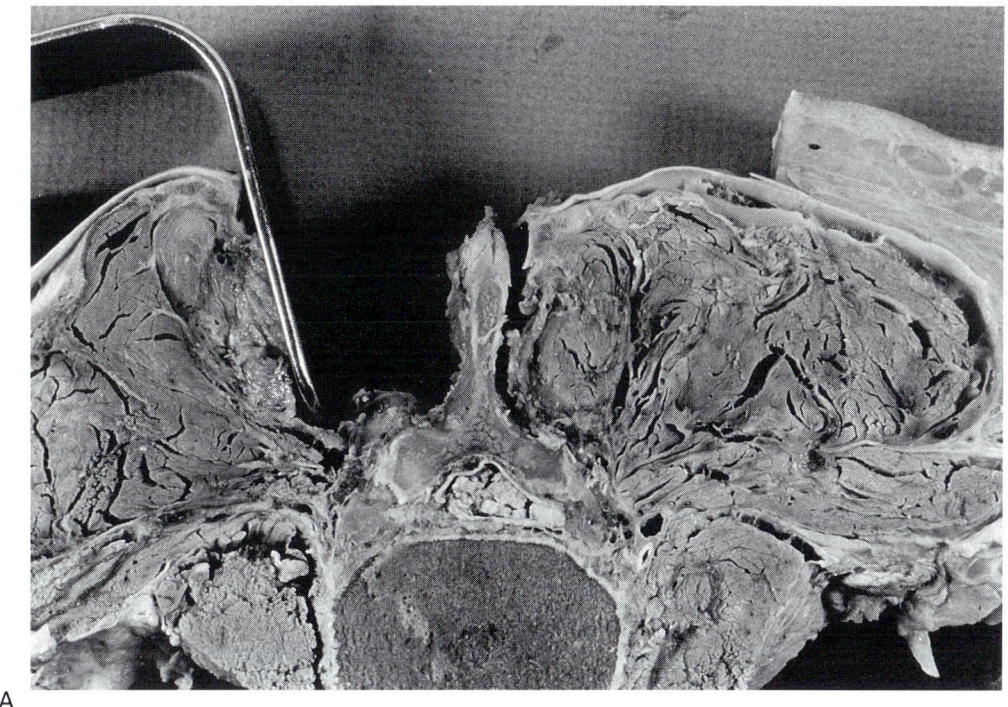
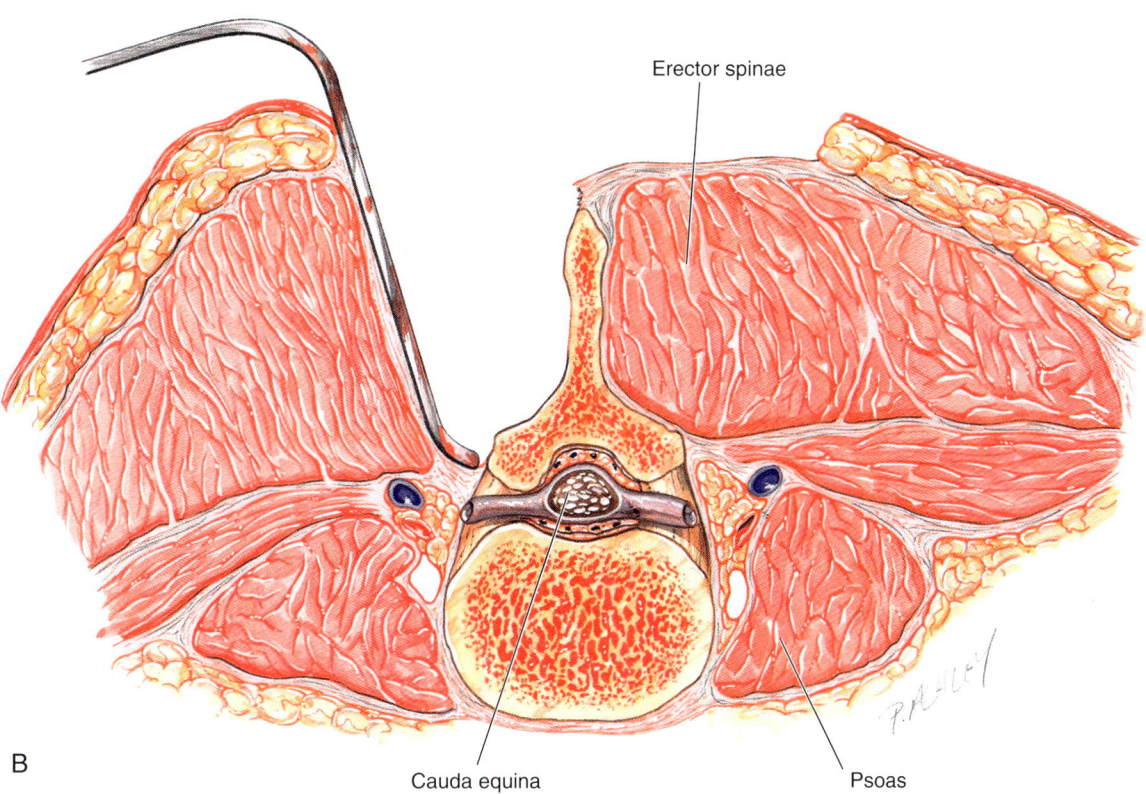

- **Figure 11-12.** *A* and *B*, The paraspinal musculature is dissected off the facet capsules under tension, thereby exposing the transverse processes laterally.

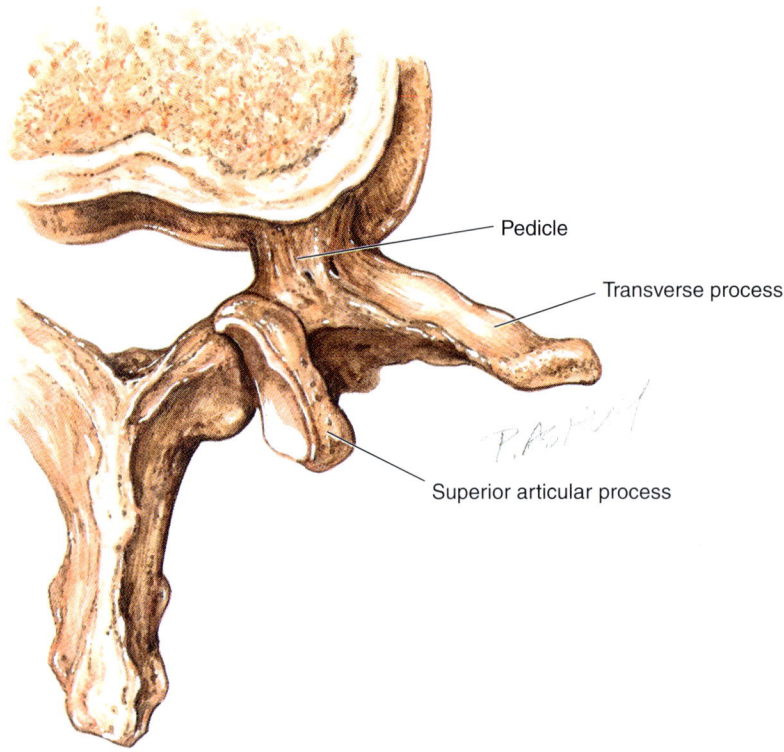

● **Figure 11-13.** Three-dimensional model of superior articular process in relationship to the transverse process, the pedicle, the disk, and the exiting nerve root.

gently release any sublaminar adhesions. In this fashion, a central trough may be created across the levels to be excised in a caudad to cephalad direction (Figure 11–16). This trough may then be widened using Kerrison rongeurs angled caudad and laterally toward the lateral recess. Care must always be taken to keep the angle of the Kerrison rongeur parallel with the dura to avoid inadvertent trapping of the dura within the teeth of the instrument. By proceeding in this fashion, the lateral recesses may be decompressed of facetal osteophytes and hypertrophy of the ligamentum as it extends out laterally toward the foramen.

If fusion with pedicle instrumentation is desired, one must first identify the axis of the pedicle. The dorsal entry site to the cortical cylinder of the pedicle is identified at a point formed by the intersection of a line bisecting the transverse process in the coronal plane with a perpendicular line just lateral to the base of the superior articular process in the parasagittal plane (Figure 11–17). Entry to the pedicle is made with a bur or awl. As described, the angle created by the axis of the pedicle relative to the midline increases as one proceeds from L1 to L5.

Unilateral laminotomy for diskectomy is carried out with an approach similar to that used for lumbar laminectomy, although the dissection is carried out only on one side of the interspinous ligament. With this approach, one can limit the size of the initial skin incision. Dissection proceeds to the level of the lumbodorsal fascia. At this point, sharp dissection through this fascial layer proceeds between the spinous processes above and below the affected level only on the side of the pathology. By subperiosteally sweeping the paraspinal musculature off of the spinous processes and intervening interspinous ligament with a Cobb elevator, one can gain access to the laminae overlying the disk herniation. The paraspinal

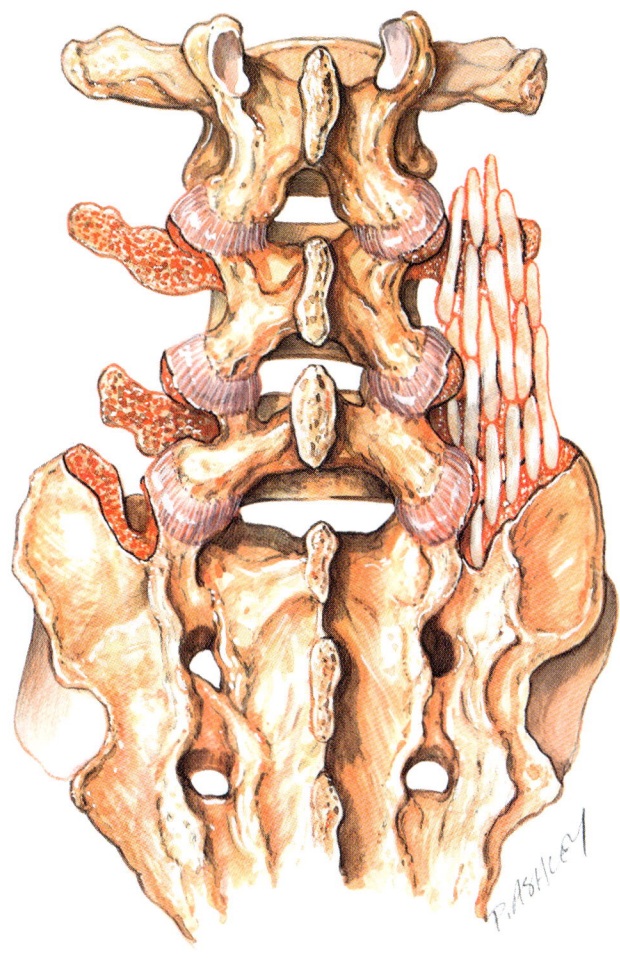

● **Figure 11-14.** Intertransverse process fusion with autogenous bone graft.

musculature is held lateral to the facet joint with a Taylor retractor. As in the case of decompression for spinal stenosis, the interval between the superior edge of the caudal lamina and the ligamentum flavum is exploited with a small curved curet. Kerrison rongeurs are then used to create a laminotomy overlying the disk herniation by resecting a portion of the superior edge of the caudal lamina and the inferior edge of the cephalad lamina (Figure 11–18). One must keep in mind that the L5-S1 disk is at the level of the interlaminar space; yet as one progresses in a cephalad direction, the disk space proportionately is in a more cephalad position than the interlaminar space. Exposure of the L2-L3 disk space therefore requires more removal of the L2 lamina because the disk is in a more cephalad position compared with the interlaminar space. Removal of some bone from the medial aspect of the pars interarticularis may be necessary to gain enough lateral exposure to the underlying disk, although at least 8 mm of the pars should be left intact to preserve stability. Once again, preserving the facet capsule is paramount to preserving stability of the motion segment. Once the laminotomy is created, the dura and affected nerve root may be identified and gently retracted toward the midline, exposing the underlying disk herniation (Figure 11–19).

Closure of the posterior lumbar approach involves reapproximating the paraspinal musculature with interrupted absorbable sutures in an attempt to close the potential space created

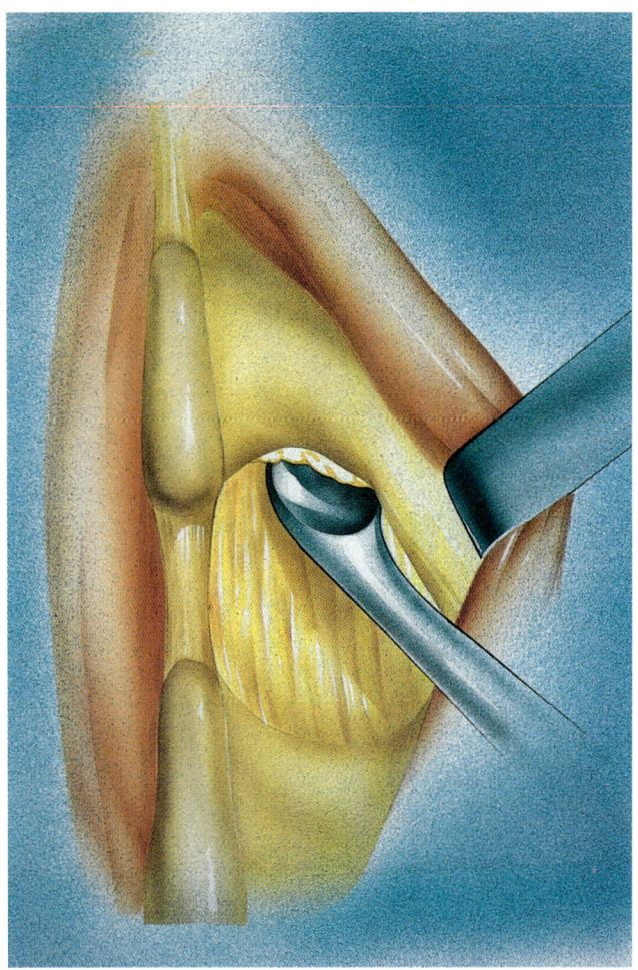

● **Figure 11-15.** Taking down ligamentum flavum with curet.

by the lateral dissection. The lumbodorsal fascia is then reapproximated to itself as the strength layer in the closure, using interrupted or running absorbable sutures. The subcutaneous layers and skin are then closed in a standard fashion of the surgeon's choosing.

Complications

Complications encountered with this approach include (1) identification of the wrong level, (2) injury to neural elements, (3) excessive bleeding, and (4) destabilizing the motion segment. Prevention is the key to avoiding each of these complications.

Identification of the appropriate level can be ensured by several means. The most important step is to carefully evaluate the preoperative films. One should determine if there are any "sacralized" or "lumbarized" vertebrae. Significant anterolistheses or retrolistheses must also be identified. Evaluation of spinal dysraphism such as spina bifida occulta is critical to avoid penetration of the canal and injury to the neural elements. The sacrum is usually easily identifiable. No motion between spinous processes is detected when one sacral spinous process is moved with a Kocher clamp. Tapping on a sacral lamina also tends to

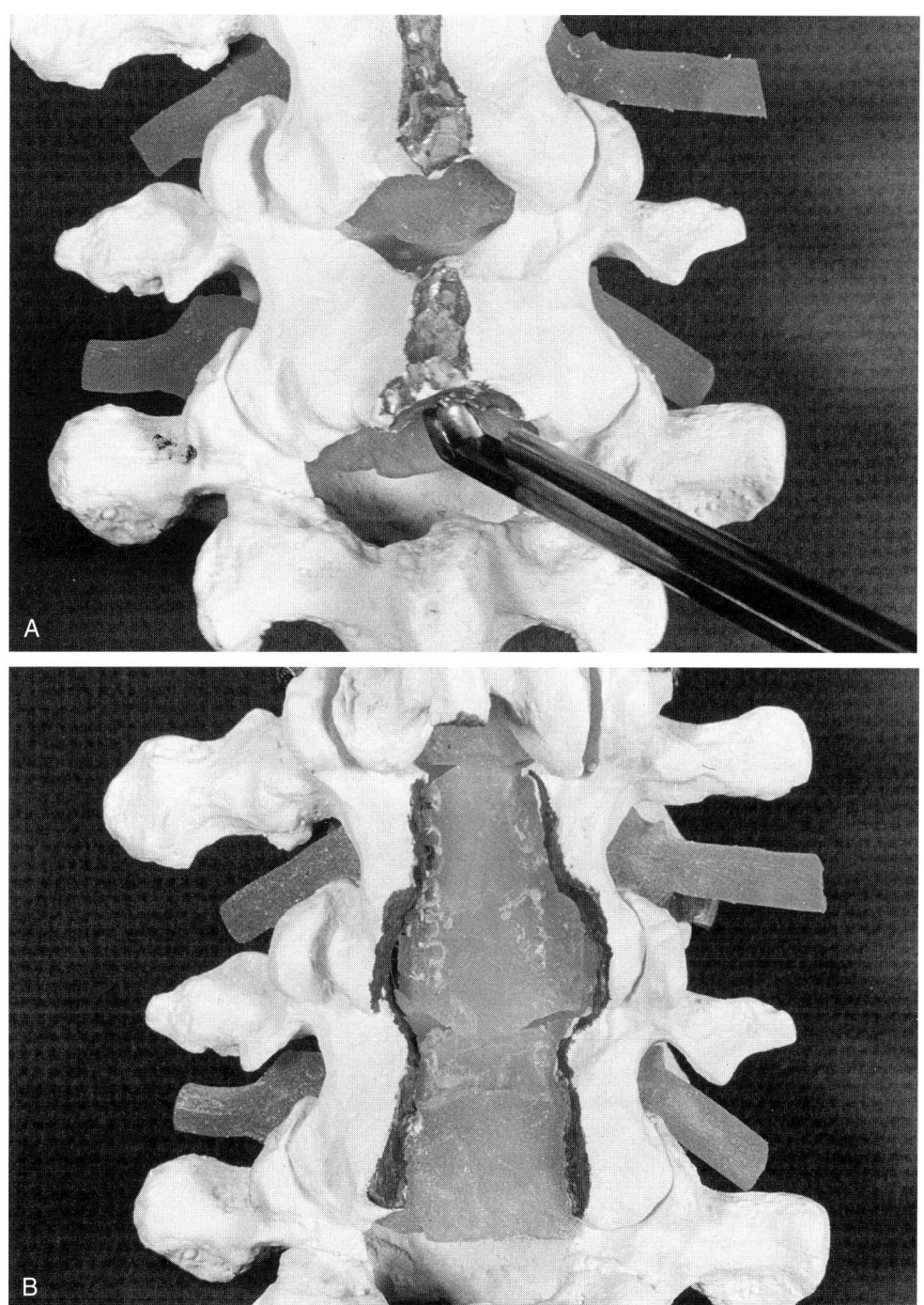

● **Figure 11-16.** During the laminectomy, a central trough is created in a caudad to cephalad direction (A). The trough is then widened (B) with the Kerrison rongeur toward the lateral recesses.

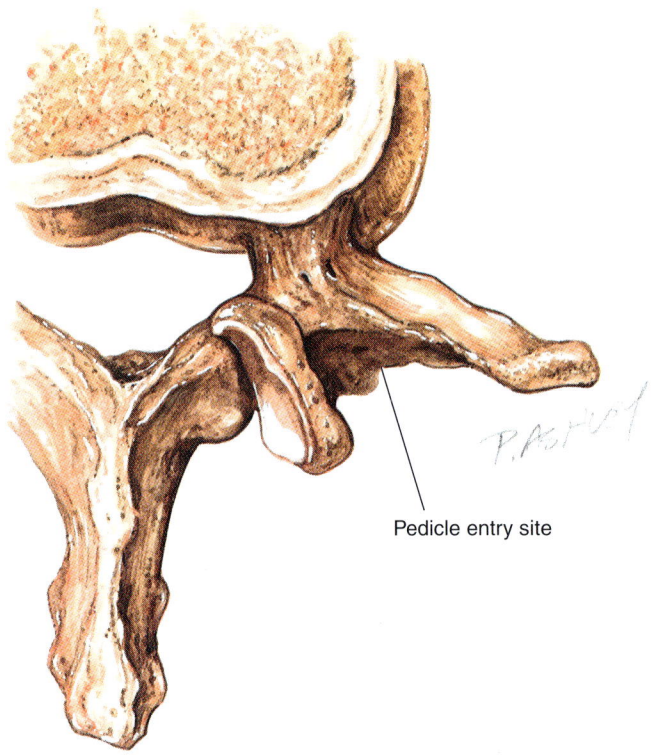

● **Figure 11-17.** Pedicle entry site.

produce a relatively dull sound when compared with nonfused lumbar segments. An intraoperative lateral radiograph should always be obtained with a Kocher clamp on the cephalad portion of the spinous process at the level of the pathologic process. A Kocher clamp in this position tends to be directly posterior to the pedicle at that level and may allow more clear identification of the marked level.

Neural elements, especially nerve roots, must be identified individually and protected. The more lateral the dissection, the easier it is to identify the nerve root and retract it so that the disk may be seen. Realization that the dura may be closely applied, and at times adherent to, the undersurface of the ligamentum flavum inspires the surgeon to exercise extreme caution and meticulous handling of this soft tissue plane.

Excessive bleeding may be avoided by taking several preventive measures throughout the procedure. Staying strictly subperiosteal during the initial approach through the paraspinal muscles should ensure a relatively dry exposure of the posterior bony elements. Identifying the pars interarticularis early in the dissection followed by cauterization of the segmental facetal artery just lateral to the pars will assist in maintaining a dry field during exposure of the transverse processes. A branch of the posterior primary ramus of the lumbar nerve root tends to run with the segmental vessel as it passes adjacent to the facet joint and pars interarticularis. As it supplies the paraspinal musculature in a segmental fashion, loss of some of these nerve branches tends not to significantly denervate the muscle. Care must be taken to avoid penetration of the coronal plane between the transverse processes, because significant bleeding may arise in the retroperitoneal space. Excessive bleeding may also be encountered during blunt dissection through the epidural venous plexus en route to the disk.

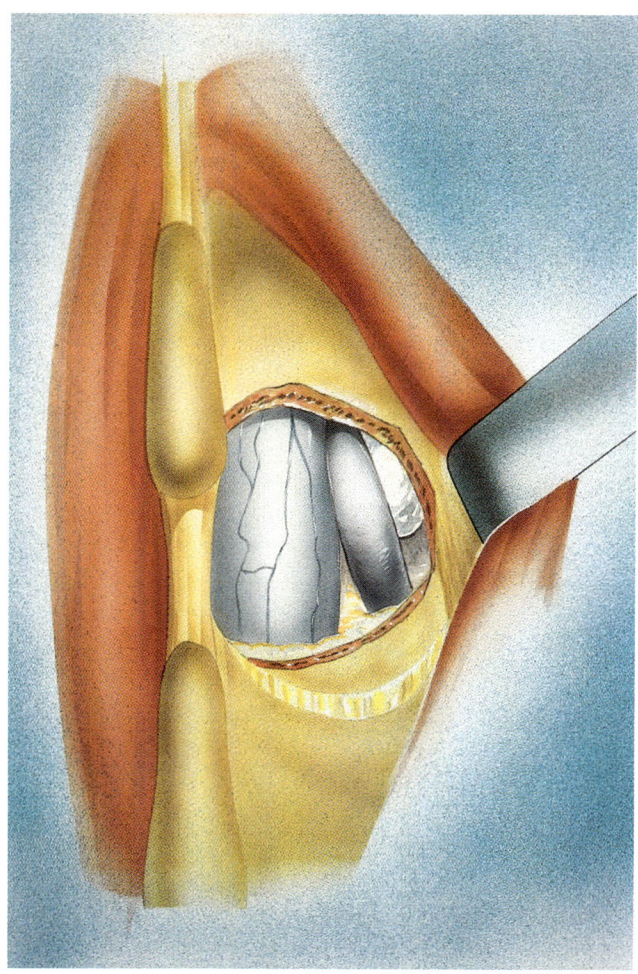

● **Figure 11-18.** Laminotomy with Kerrison rongeur.

This bleeding may be lessened with proper positioning on a laminectomy frame and with the use of a spinal anesthetic. If encountered, it may be controlled with Gelfoam and thrombin-soaked cottonoid patties. Bipolar Malis electrocautery may also be used with caution to coagulate identifiable venous bleeding vessels. Lastly, penetration of the anterior annulus fibrosus with an open pituitary rongeur during overzealous resection of the intervertebral disk may also lead to devastating consequences, such as injury to the adjacent iliac vessels.

Unless a fusion is part of the preoperative plan, no posterior surgical approach to the lumbar spine is likely to improve stability. Accordingly, the surgeon must rely on technique to preserve stabilizing structures wherever possible. As emphasized, facet joint capsules must be identified and protected. If a unilateral approach to the spine is used, the supraspinous and interspinous ligaments should also be preserved. The pars interarticularis imparts bony stability between the facet joints. Excessive resection of the pars during laminectomy (i.e., less than 5 to 8 mm of pars remaining) may result in subsequent fracture, predisposing the motion segment to a state of instability. If significant resection of the pars is required to achieve a complete decompression of the nerve root, one should incorporate a fusion across the involved motion segment.

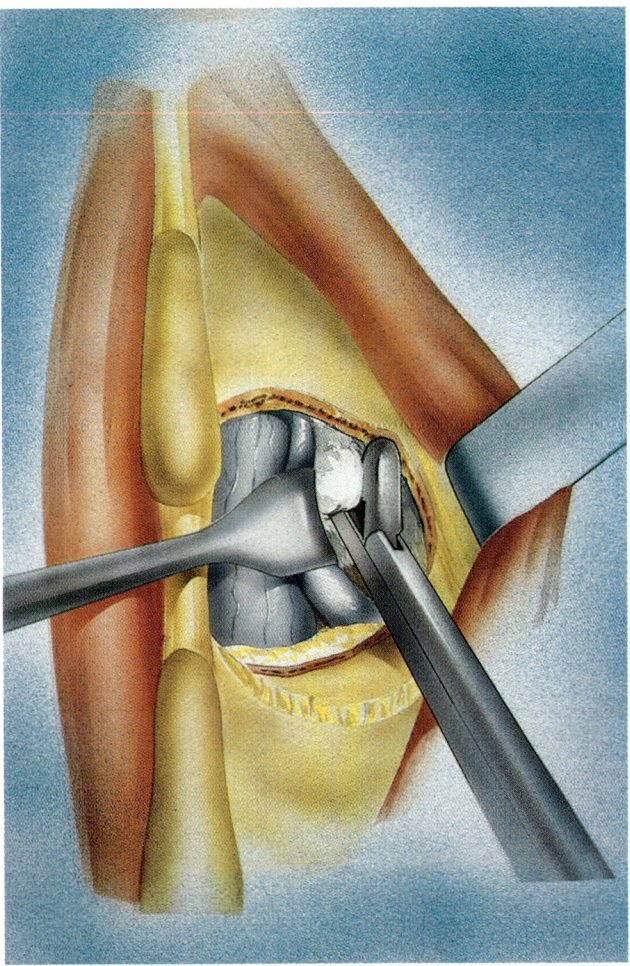

● **Figure 11-19.** Medially retracted dura with exposure of disk herniation.

Conclusion

The three-dimensional anatomy of the lumbar spine must be clearly understood to be able to locate anterior structures when looking at the posterior aspect of the spine. The key to the posterior topographic anatomy of the spine is the facet joint. By identifying this structure, one can identify the location of the transverse process as well as the underlying pedicle. The key to the anatomy within the canal is the pedicle. Identification of the pedicle orients the surgeon to the level of the disk and the position of the exiting nerve root through its foramen. Respect for those soft tissue and bony elements that contribute to spinal stability is necessary if one is to successfully approach the posterior aspect of the spine without doing harm to the patient.

BIBLIOGRAPHY

Hollingshead WH: Anatomy for Surgeons, 3rd ed, vol 3. Philadelphia, Harper & Row, 1982.
Rauschning, W: Normal and pathologic anatomy of the lumbar root canals. Spine 12:1008, 1987.
Rothman RH, Simeone FA: The Spine, 3rd ed. Philadelphia, WB Saunders, 1992.
Watkins MB: Posterolateral fusion of the lumbar and lumbosacral spine, J Bone Joint Surg 35A:1014, 1953.

CHAPTER 12

WILTSE PARAVERTEBRAL MUSCLE POSTEROLATERAL EXPOSURES

Srdjan Mirkovic, M.D.
Steven R. Garfin, M.D.

The paraspinal Wiltse approach to the lumbar spine involves splitting the sacrospinalis muscle in the sagittal plane, two to three fingerbreadths from the midline.[1,2] It allows direct access to the transverse processes and the lateral masses and can extend medially as far as the base of the spinous processes.

The classic Wiltse approach entails two skin incisions (Figure 12–1) about 1¾ inches, or three fingerbreadths, lateral to the midline and medial to the posterior-superior iliac spine. These incisions curve toward the midline at their ends, thus allowing a transverse cut through the underlying fascia.

Clinical Anatomy

See discussion of anatomy for posterior lumbar approach in Chapter 11.

Surgical Technique

The patient is placed in a prone position on an Andrews table. A Wilson frame or chest rolls may also be used, based on the type of surgery and on the surgeon's preference to perform the procedure with the spine in flexion or extension. Support hose and compression boots are applied to the lower extremities, and a Foley catheter is inserted if the procedure is expected to last longer than 2 to 3 hours.

A midline, utilitarian skin incision is made from L3 to the sacrum (Figure 12–2), allowing easy access to a paravertebral approach through the fascia, as well as the posterior iliac crest, for bone graft harvesting. Although this incision is somewhat longer than the classic Wiltse incision, the patient's cosmetic appearance is more acceptable.

The skin and dermis are incised to the subcutaneous tissues with a blade. Dermal bleeding vessels are controlled using bayonet forceps and Bovie cautery. To minimize bleeding, Bovie dissection is carried to the paravertebral fascia in the midline. With Cobb elevators, the subcutaneous tissues are then reflected off the paravertebral fascia, stripping about four fingerbreaths lateral to the midline, thus exposing the lateral edge of the sacrospinalis muscles (Figure 12–3). The paravertebral fascia is then incised bilaterally over the

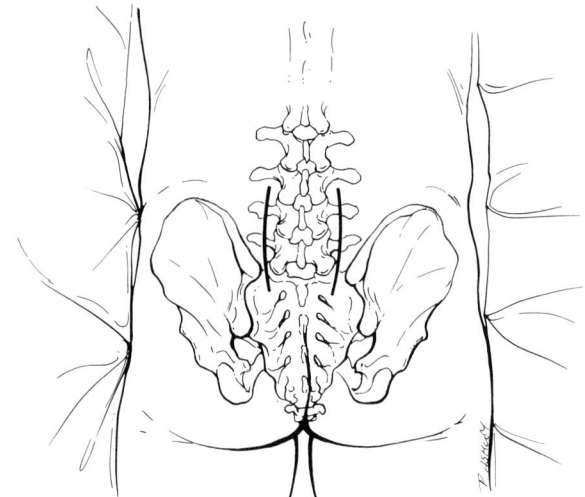

● **Figure 12-1.** The classic Wiltse approach. Two paravertebral skin incisions are made three fingerbreadths lateral to the midline. The incisions curve slightly toward the midline at their ends.

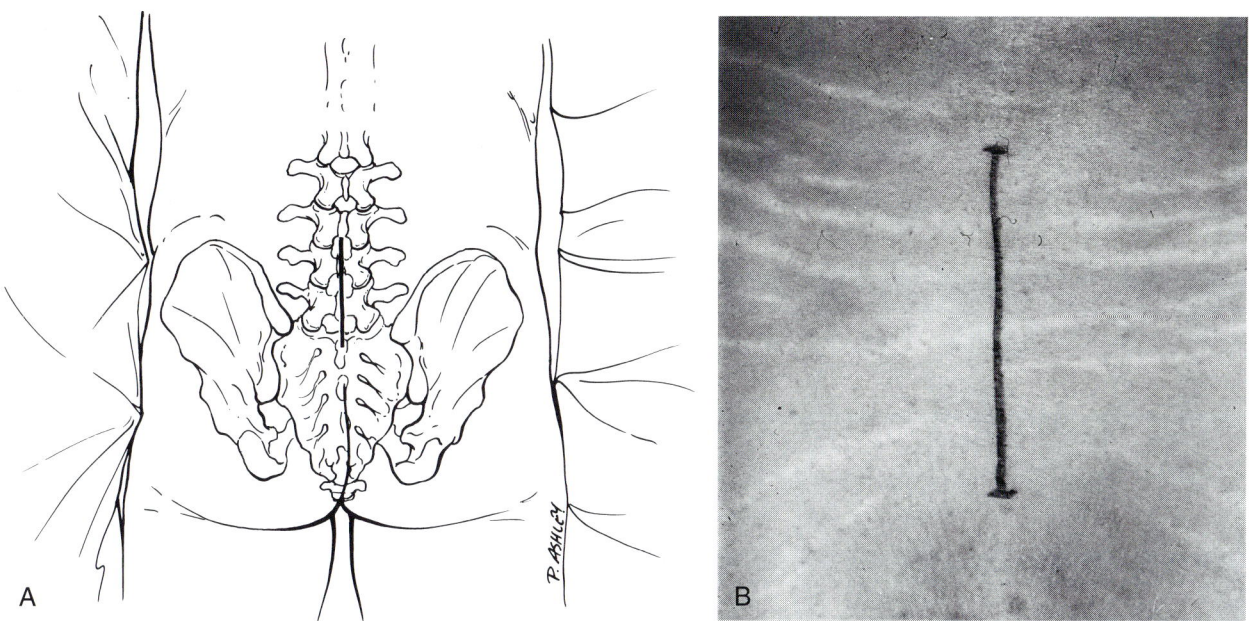

● **Figure 12-2.** *A* and *B,* The utilitarian single midline skin incision, allowing a subsequent paravertebral approach through the fascia and muscles. Harvesting of bone from the iliac crests can also be performed through the same incision.

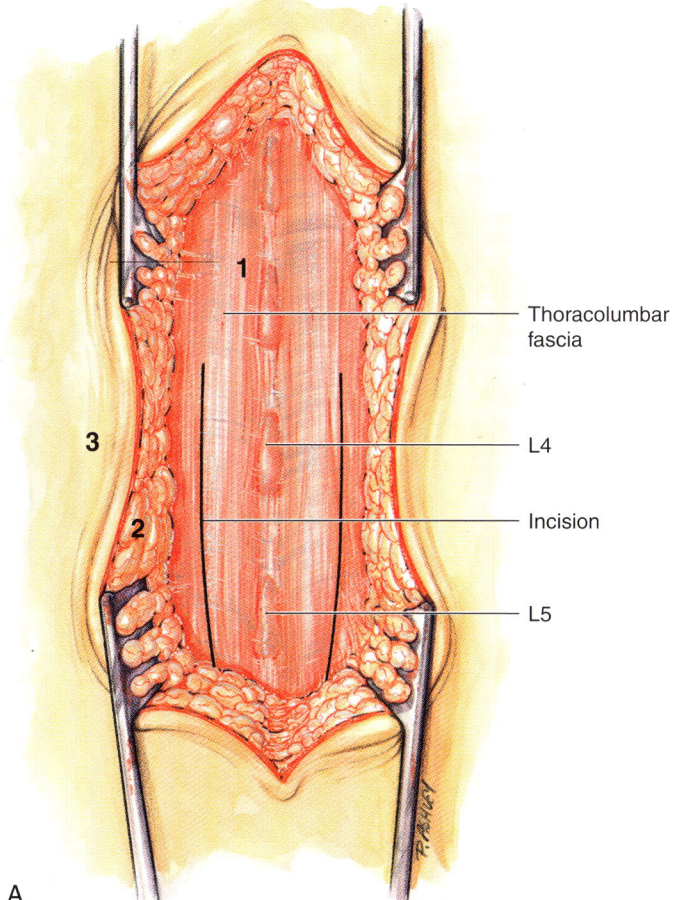

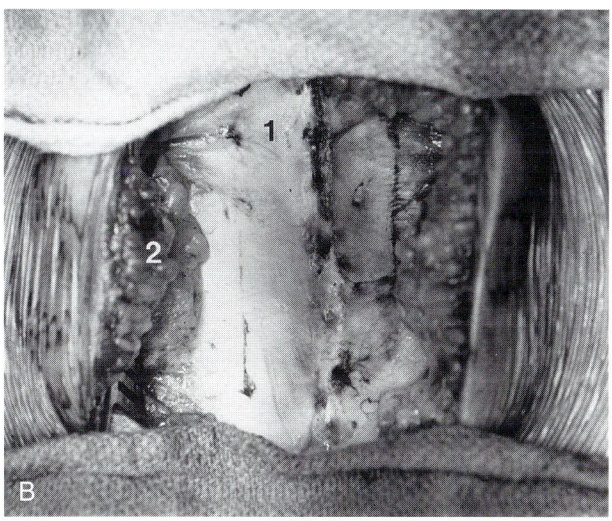

● **Figure 12-3.** *A* and *B,* Exposure of the paravertebral fascia bilaterally through the midline utilitarian skin incision. 1, Paravertebral fascia; 2, subcutaneous fat; 3, skin.

edge of the multifidus muscle, with the ends curving slightly medially, exposing the underlying paravertebral muscles (Figure 12–4). A natural cleavage plane between the most posteromedial muscle (multifidus) and more lateral ones (longissimus) can be identified and entered. With blunt dissection with "peanuts" and two hand-held Hibbs retractors, the paraspinal muscles are split longitudinally, in this relatively avascular plane, to the sacrum. The sacrum can be used as a point of reference, before extending the dissection more cephalad. If the sacrum is not initially identified, or in cases in which the desired approach is not at the L5-S1 level, a transverse process can be palpated deep to the muscle (Figure 12–5). To assess one's position, and thus to minimize the extent of the dissection, a marker is placed on a transverse process, and an anteroposterior or lateral radiograph is obtained. Once the correct level has been verified, dissection over the transverse process is carried medially to the base of the facet joint (see Figure 12–5). Caution must be exercised to ensure that the bony protrusion palpated is a transverse process and not a facet joint. This is a common error, leading to a too medial dissection. Similarly, not feeling the transverse process can lead to a too deep or lateral dissection, possibly causing nerve root injury or an intraperitoneal violation. The lumbar transverse processes should be uncovered of all soft tissue to their tips and around their superior and inferior borders. This facilitates identification of the transverse process as a landmark if subsequent instrumentation is necessary and maximizes the surface area for the bone graft. If the facet joints are to be included in the arthrodesis, a subperiosteal dissection to denude the facets is performed with Bovie cautery, fitted with an extension. For each facet joint included within the fusion, the facet articular

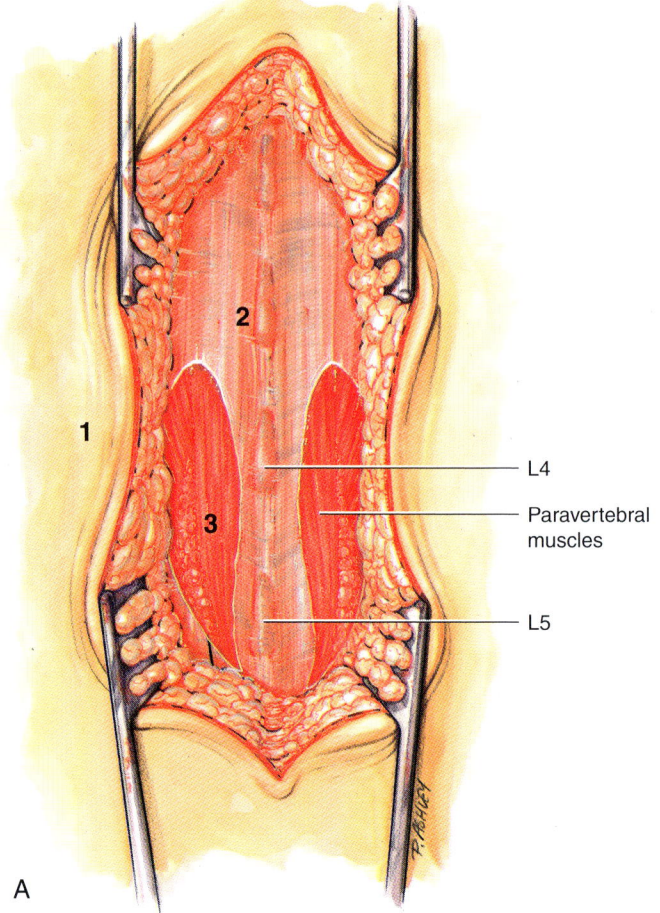
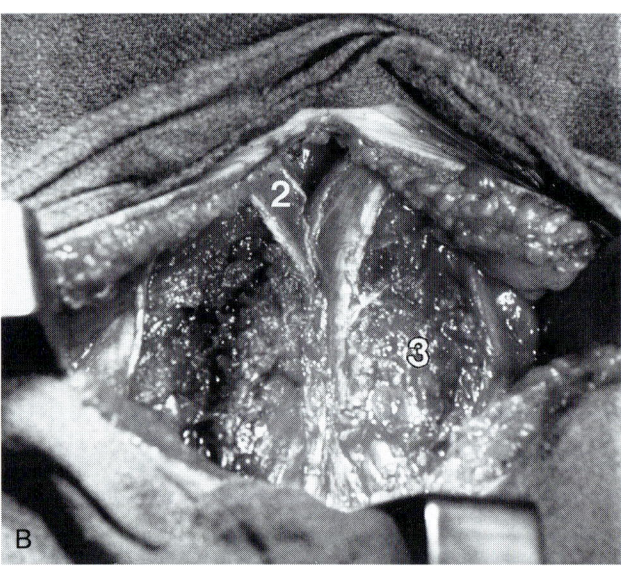

● **Figure 12-4.** *A* and *B* Skin (1) Incision through the paravertebral fascia (2), three fingerbreadths lateral to the midline, exposing the paravertebral muscles (3).

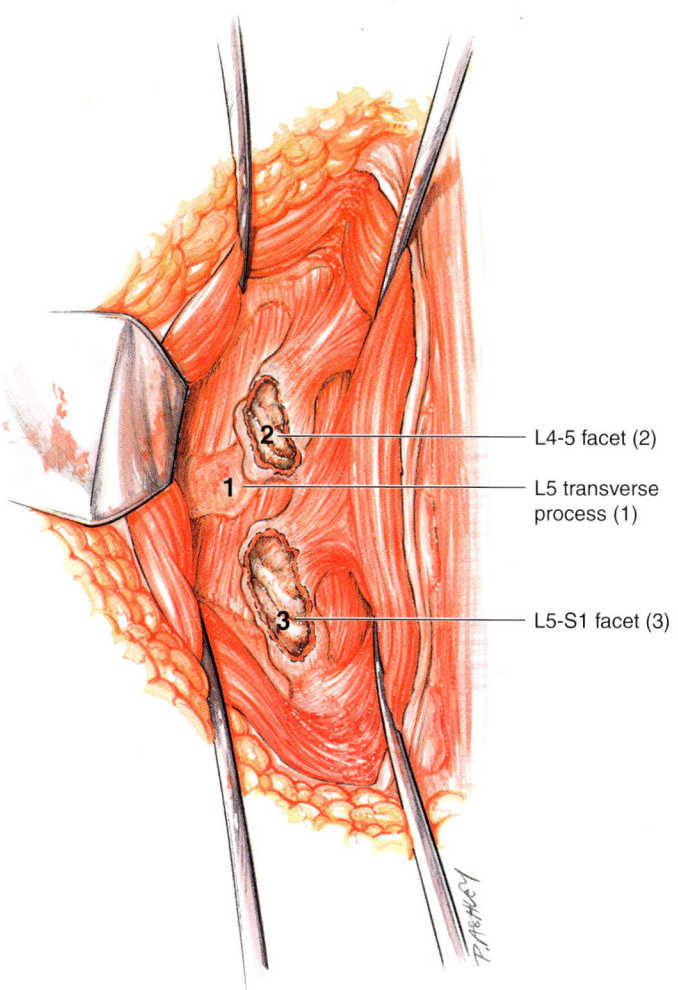

● **Figure 12-5.** Exposure of the posterior elements from L4 to the sacrum. The L5 transverse process (1) is commonly the first structure identified. If the dissection is too medial, the L4-5 (2) or the L5-S1 facet (shown denuded) (3) may be initially palpated.

cartilage should be removed with a narrow rongeur or small curets. Dissection can be carried medially, exposing the lamina and the pars to the base of the spinous processes, if desired. Depending on the surgical indications, the exposure can be extended proximally or distally, with further spreading of the sacrospinalis muscles. In cases of spondylolysis, the pars defect can be identified, encased in a hypertrophic cartilaginous scar, which can be removed with curets and a bur. The underlying "fracture" ends can then be decorticated, in preparation for the subsequent fusion.

The sacral alae should be stripped of soft tissue, with a Cobb dissector, if arthrodesis to this level is planned, exposing the posterior lip of the alae and the anterior edge for fusions to the sacrum. Further exposure in a posterocaudal direction is generally not necessary.

The facet joint located just cephalad to the fusion should be preserved, except for the lateral aspect of the superior articular process of the caudal vertebrae, which should be denuded with its corresponding transverse process. Minimal damage to the facet joint capsule, however, should be incurred. Injury to the nerve roots is unlikely if the exposure remains in the plane of the transverse processes.

If instrumentation is performed, placement of screws in the anteromedially oriented pedicles at L5 and S1 can be difficult in a large patient, owing to the depth of the wound. The sagittal orientation of the paravertebral approach over the lateral masses, however, permits direct visualization of the screw insertion site at the transverse process–facet junction (Figures 12–6 and 12–7). This facilitates not only screw insertion but also instrumentation assembly.

Harvesting of bone from the posterior iliac crest can be undertaken bilaterally, through the same skin incision, without the need for additional incisions. A plane of dissection, between the paravertebral fascia and the subcutaneous tissues, provides access to the iliac crest laterally (see Figure 12–4).

Complications

With adherence to the principles just outlined, complications are unlikely. Violation of the facet joint at the most superior aspect of the dissection occurs if it is erroneously identified as being the transverse process. Deep dissection anterior to the transverse process can lead to violation of the intertransverse membrane. Entry into the retroperiosteum can occur with this maneuver.

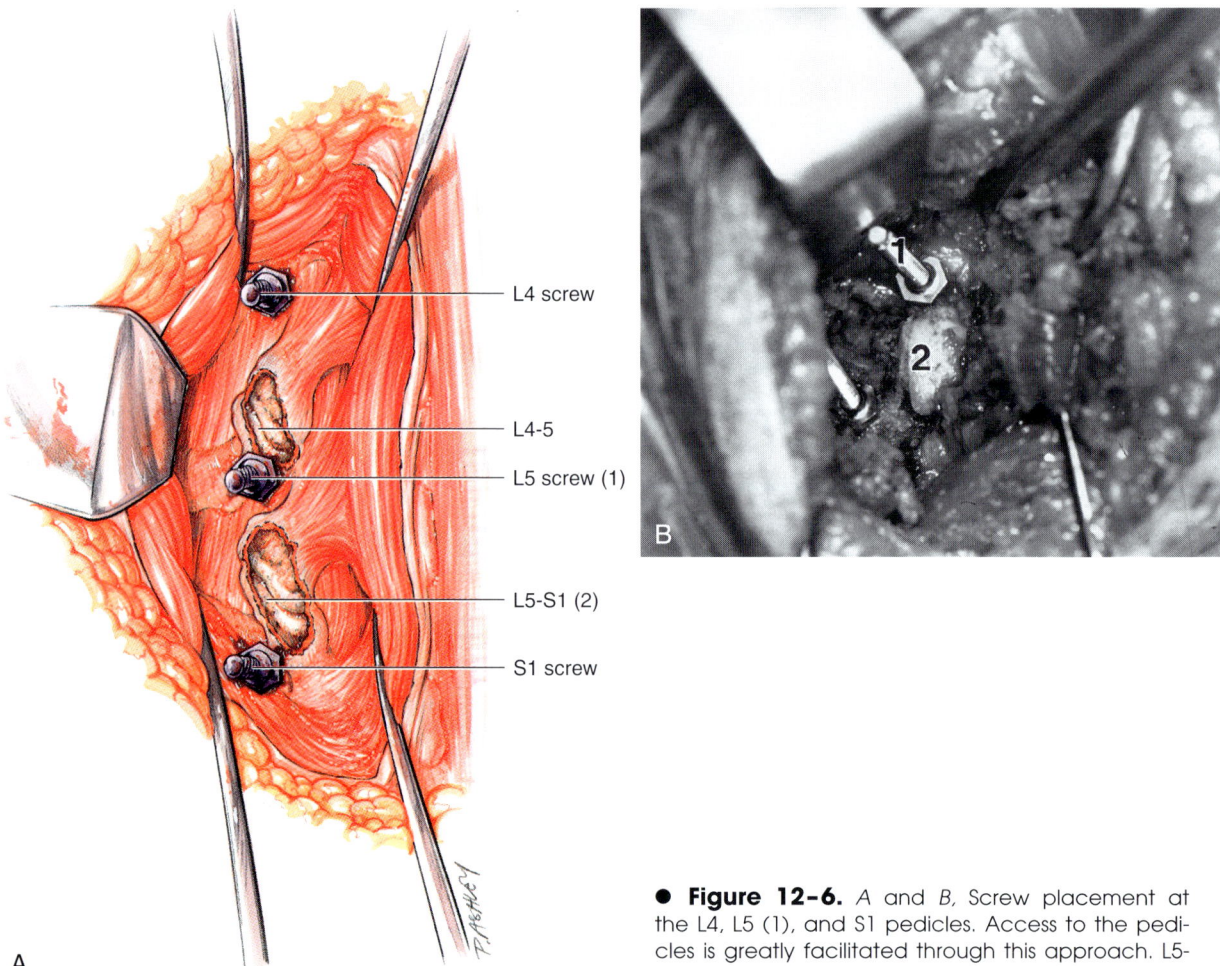

● **Figure 12-6.** *A* and *B*, Screw placement at the L4, L5 (1), and S1 pedicles. Access to the pedicles is greatly facilitated through this approach. L5-S1 facet (2) is shown.

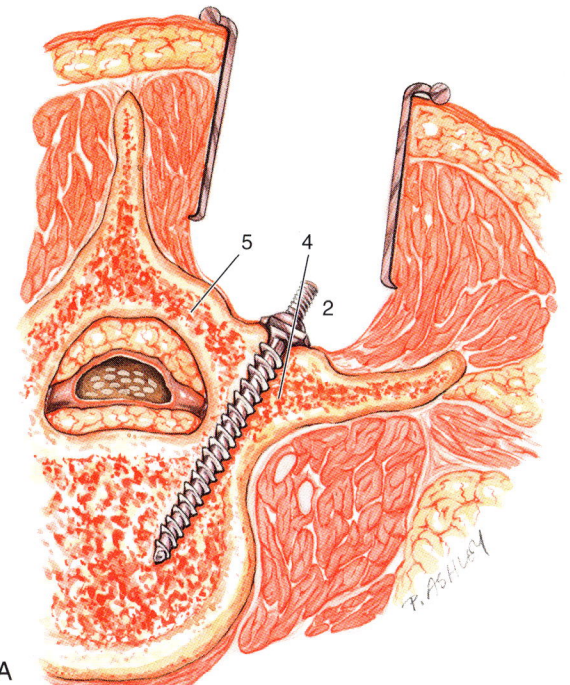
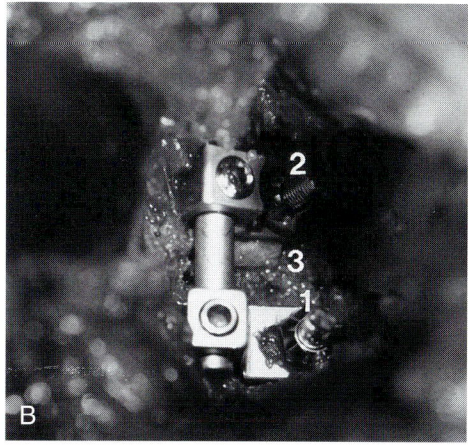

● **Figure 12-7.** *A,* Paravertebral approach at the L5 level, demonstrating an axial cut through the L5 pedicle (4). By using this approach, placement of the L5 pedicle screw (2) is not impeded by the soft tissues. The dissection extends from the tip of the transverse process laterally to the lamina (5) medially. *B,* An L5-S1 fusion with instrumentation through the Wiltse approach. The L5-S1 facet (3) is shown. (1) S1 screw.

Injury to the nerve root can also occur with violation of the intratransverse membrane. Excessive bleeding is likely if meticulous cautery of the pars vessels and facetal artery is not carried out.

Conclusion

The main advantage of the sacrospinalis-splitting approach is that it provides easy access to and visualization of the lateral structures. This diminishes the need for excessive retraction of the soft tissues and thus lessens muscle ischemia. Because the midline and perilaminar soft tissues are left intact, and the lateral muscles are retracted, the vascular supply to the graft may be improved, when compared with a midline approach and exposure over the lamina and facets to the lateral edge of the transverse processes. Bony decortication and fusion, particularly at L4, L5, and S1, are facilitated by this direct approach.

Aside from its traditional usefulness in the treatment of spondylolysis and spondylolisthesis, a limited approach of this kind is also useful for a far-lateral disk herniation.

With the advent of instrumented fusions, in cases in which central decompression and nerve root exploration are not necessary, we have found this approach, by virtue of the orientation of the plane of dissection, to be particularly beneficial (see Figures 12–6 and 12–7). Screw placement in the anteromedially oriented pedicles at L5 and S1 is simplified, and instrumentation assembly is facilitated. Finally, fusion, exploration, and, potentially, instrumentation revision may be easier to perform using this technique.

The main disadvantage of the lateral approach is that visualization of the central canal is limited. Thus, although foraminal stenosis can conceivably be addressed laterally, decompression for central or lateral recess stenosis is difficult, even if complete facetectomies are performed. In cases in which a pathologic process within the spinal canal needs to be addressed, and in which fusion and instrumentation are also desired, a midline approach is preferred.

With the advent of new surgical techniques, this approach is a useful adjunct to the surgical armamentarium.

REFERENCES

1. Wiltse LL, Bateman GJ, Hutchinson RH, Nelson WE: The paraspinal sacrospinalis-splitting approach to the lumbar spine. J Bone Joint Surg Am 50:919, 1968.
2. Wiltse LL: The paraspinal sacrospinalis-splitting approach to the lumbar spine. Clin Orthop 91:48, 1973.

CHAPTER 13

AUTOLOGOUS BONE GRAFT

Cathleen S. Van Buskirk, M.D.
Jerome M. Cotler, M.D.
Todd J. Albert, M.D.

Iliac Bone Graft

Augmentation of the spine with bone is a common operative procedure to effect spinal fusion. Treatment of spinal disorders mandates a thorough knowledge of the human pelvis, which represents the source with the greatest number of disposable bone for grafting. Attributes of the ilium include its cortical rind, which offers innate stability, and the abundant cancellous bone, which offers live bone cells, osteoconductive ability, and osteoinductive ability. The cortical bone of the iliac crest is strong and convex. The greatest source of cancellous bone is found under the posterior-superior iliac spine (PSIS) extending down and around the sciatic notch (Figure 13–1A). Anteriorly on the iliac wing, smaller amounts of cancellous bone are found under the anterior-superior iliac spine (ASIS) and between the cortical tables (Figure 13–1B).

Indications

Indications for a purely cancellous bone graft include use in packing cervical facet joints, transpedicular bone grafting of a vertebral body, and augmentation of any other fusion site. Corticocancellous bone in strips is used for intertransverse process fusions in the thoracic

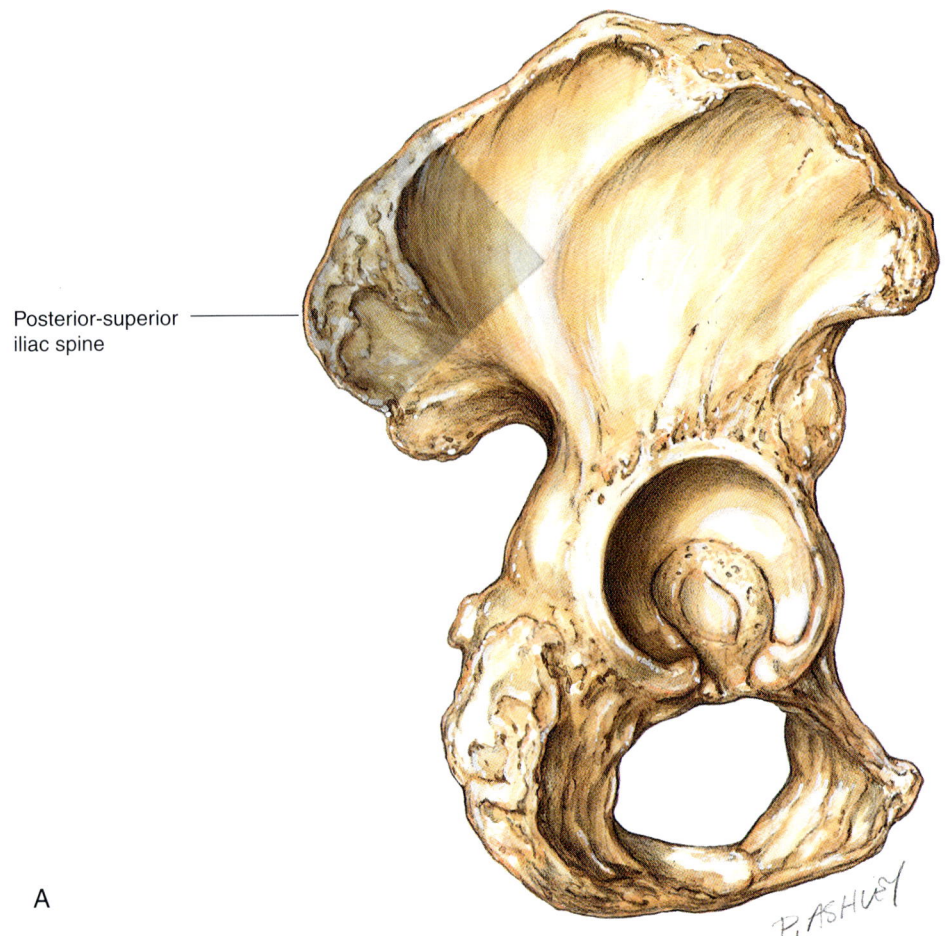

● **Figure 13–1.** *A,* The shaded area represents the most abundant cancellous bone found posteriorly between the inner and outer cortical tables at the level of the posterior-superior iliac spine.

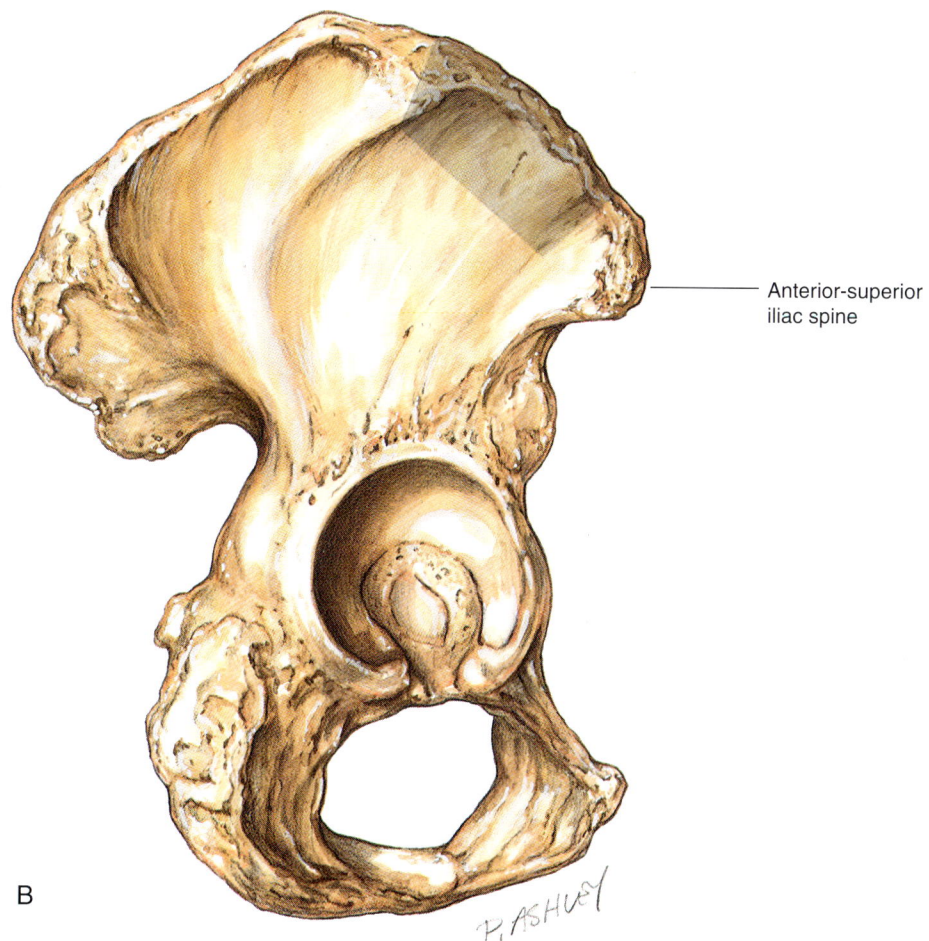

- **Figure 13-1** *Continued B,* The shaded area represents the safe zone anteriorly. Stay at least 2 cm superolateral to the anterior-superior iliac spine to avoid avulsion of its muscular attachments and to avoid injury to the lateral femoral cutaneous nerve.

and lumbar spine, posterior cervical fusions, and occipitocervical fusions. Tricortical grafts are indicated for anterior interbody fusions of the cervical, thoracic, and lumbar spine and in vertebral body reconstructions.

Clinical Anatomy

POSTERIOR APPROACH. The lumbodorsal fascia overlies the latissimus dorsi, external oblique, internal oblique, and transversus abdominus muscles. The lumbodorsal fascia and the fascia overlying the gluteus maximus and medius muscles attach to the iliac crest through a thick band. No muscles cross the iliac crest, thereby resulting in a truly internervous plane.

The nerves at risk through the posterior approach are the superior cluneal nerves, the sciatic nerve, and the superior gluteal nerve. The superior cluneal nerves cross the iliac crest in a cephalad to caudad direction, approximately 8 cm anterolateral to the posterior-superior iliac spine (Figure 13–2). They are purely sensory and innervate the buttock region. The sciatic nerve exits the pelvis through the greater sciatic notch. It is endangered when bone is removed inferior to the posterior-superior iliac spine or when a retractor is placed too

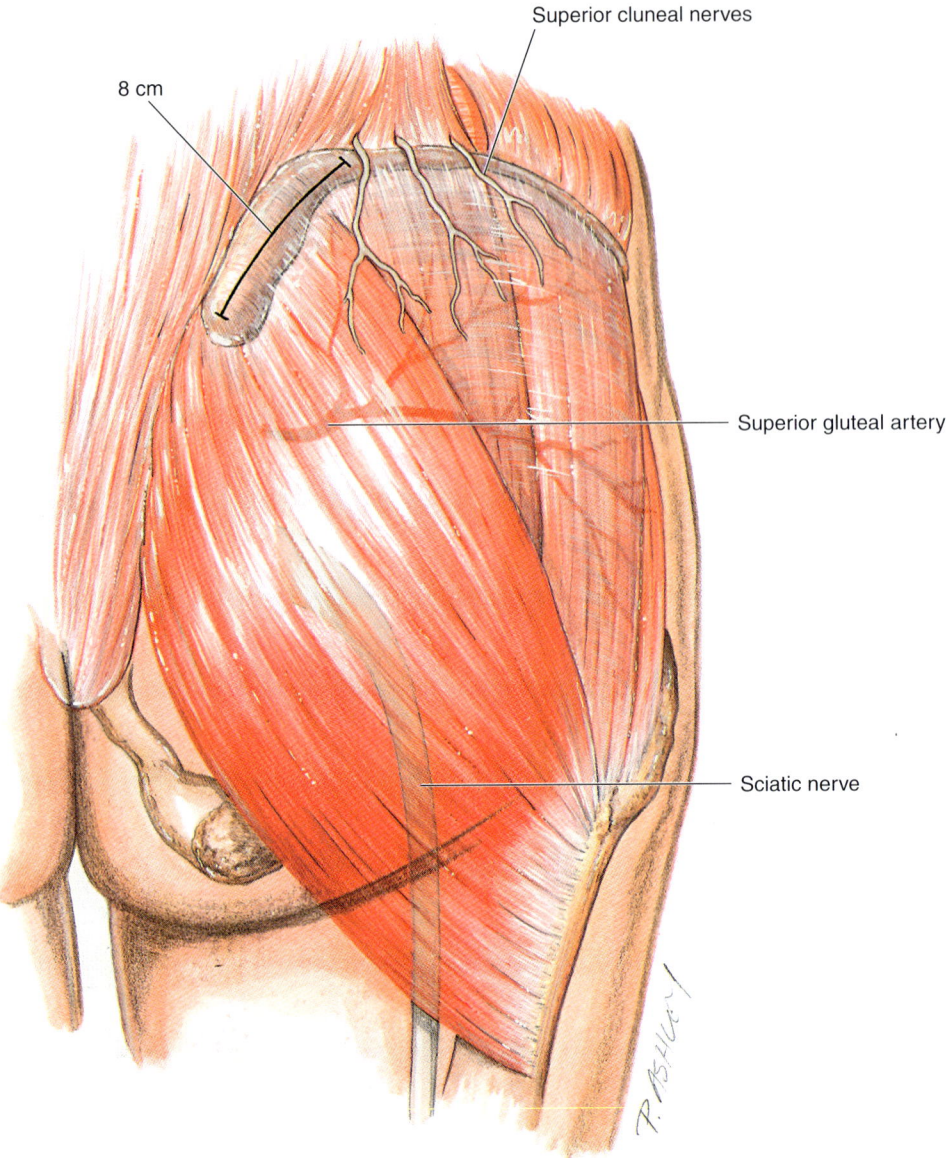

● **Figure 13-2.** Main structures at risk for injury when using a posterior approach to the iliac crest.

deeply. The superior gluteal nerve exits the sciatic notch and traverses laterally between the gluteus medius and gluteus minimus muscles to innervate these two muscles as well as the tensor fasciae latae. The nerve becomes endangered if the sciatic notch is violated and if the dissection of muscle off the posterior iliac crest is not subperiosteal. The superior gluteal artery exits through the most superior aspect of the sciatic notch, follows a course similar to the superior gluteal nerve, and can be injured by the same mechanisms.

Osseous structures at risk during the posterior approach include the sacroiliac joint and the sciatic notch. The sacroiliac joint lies anterior to the posterior-superior iliac spine and can be avoided by paying careful attention to the depth of bone being removed while obtaining an iliac cortical and cancellous graft. The sciatic notch and its neurovascular contents can be avoided by staying cephalad to an imaginary line drawn from the posterior-superior iliac spine, extending directly lateral and then perpendicular to the long axis of the operating table.

ANTERIOR APPROACH. Similar to the posterior iliac crest, no muscles cross the anterior iliac crest. However, one must avoid anterior-superior iliac spine because it gives origin to the sartorius and direct head of the rectus femoris muscles as well as the inguinal ligament. Staying 2 cm proximal to the anterior-superior iliac spine ensures its integrity. Obtaining bone from the inner table requires stripping of the iliacus muscle. This is not problematic unless the dissection strays from a subperiosteal plane or vigorous retraction is applied to the contents of the iliac fossa and abdominal cavity.

The femoral, ilioinguinal, and iliohypogastric nerves lie within the iliac fossa and can be damaged by overzealous retraction. The lateral femoral cutaneous nerve, which is purely sensory, is at greatest risk near the anterior-superior iliac spine. Normally it emerges from the lateral border of the psoas muscle, crosses the anterior surface of the iliacus muscle, and

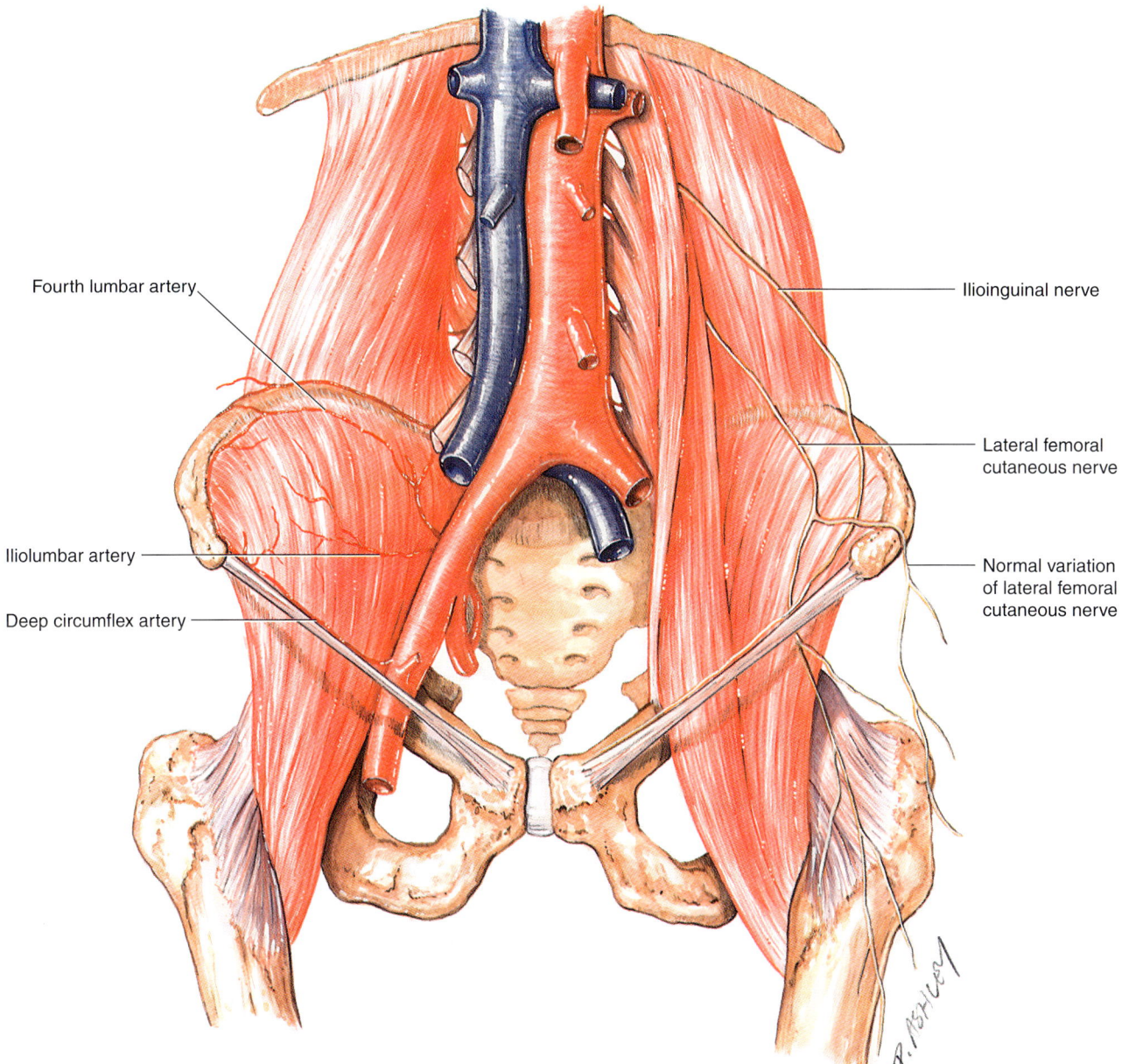

● **Figure 13-3.** Main structures at risk for injury when using an anterior approach to the iliac crest.

courses just medial and inferior to the anterior-superior iliac spine, and deep to the inguinal ligament to enter the thigh (Figure 13–3.) Anomalous pathways of the lateral femoral cutaneous nerve exist. Staying 2 cm lateral to the anterior-superior iliac spine should avoid injury to this nerve.

Three main arteries lies within the iliac fossa and can be injured while the inner table of the ilium is harvested. The iliolumbar artery, the deep circumflex iliac artery, and the fourth lumbar artery can be avoided by adhering to strict subperiosteal dissection.

The ureter and peritoneum have been injured while obtaining iliac grafts. The ureter descends in the retroperiotoneum, makes an acute posteriorly directed turn near the sciatic notch, then courses more ventrally within the pelvis. It is at greatest risk near the sciatic notch and can be injured from both anterior and posterior approaches. The peritoneum is closely adhered to the abdominal wall and iliacus muscle. Care must be taken to avoid inadvertently plunging with osteotomes or gouges.

Surgical Technique

POSTERIOR APPROACH. The posterior approach for obtaining iliac bone graft is used when the patient is undergoing a posterior spinal operation. The patient is prone, and the posterior-superior iliac spine is the key palpable landmark. Some surgeons prefer a vertical skin incision lying approximately 1 cm lateral to the most prominent aspect of the posterior-superior iliac spine, extending from it in a proximal direction and about 10 cm in length (Figure 13–4). Alternatively, the skin incision can be oblique, starting at the poster-

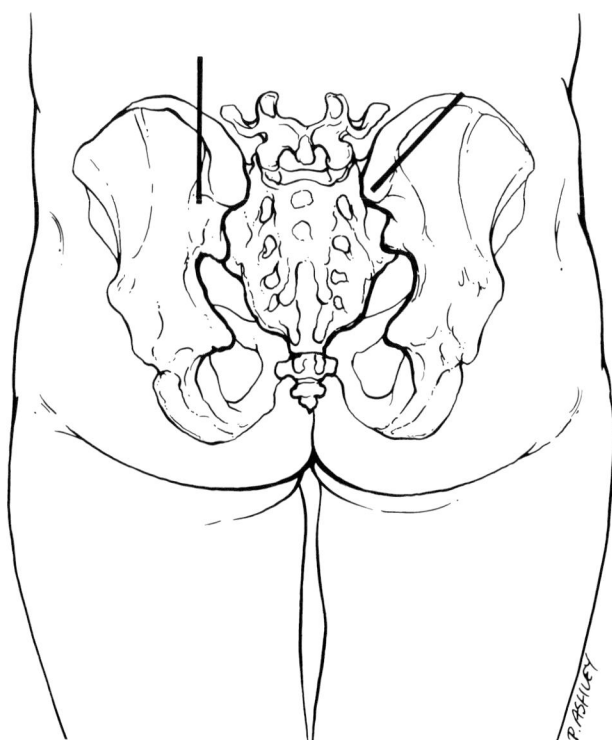

● **Figure 13-4.** Skin incision options for the posterior approach to the iliac crest. The posterior-superior iliac spine is the palpable landmark for both incisions.

ior-superior iliac spine and extending anterolaterally in line with the iliac crest. Dissection is done through the subcutaneous tissues to the lumbodorsal fascia. The surgeon should identify the interval between the latissimus dorsi and abdominal muscles, which are superior and medial to the crest, and the gluteus maximus and medius muscles, which are inferior and lateral to the crest. This interval represents the iliac crest (Figure 13–5). A 6 to 8 cm oblique incision is made directly in line with the iliac crest. Subperiosteal dissection is performed on the outer cortical table, inner table, or both, depending on the desired type of graft required (Figure 13–6). One must keep in mind the location of the sciatic notch. An imaginary line can be drawn from the posterior-superior iliac spine and extended directly lateral; nothing inferior to this line. To avoid injury to the cluneal nerves, the incision should not be more than 8 cm anterolateral to the PSIS (posterior-superior iliac spine). A Taylor retractor is placed to retract the muscles that have been dissected off the crest.

If strips of corticocancellous bone are desired, a large gouge and mallet are used. Bone is removed in a fashion parallel to the iliac crest. To avoid inadvertent penetration of the

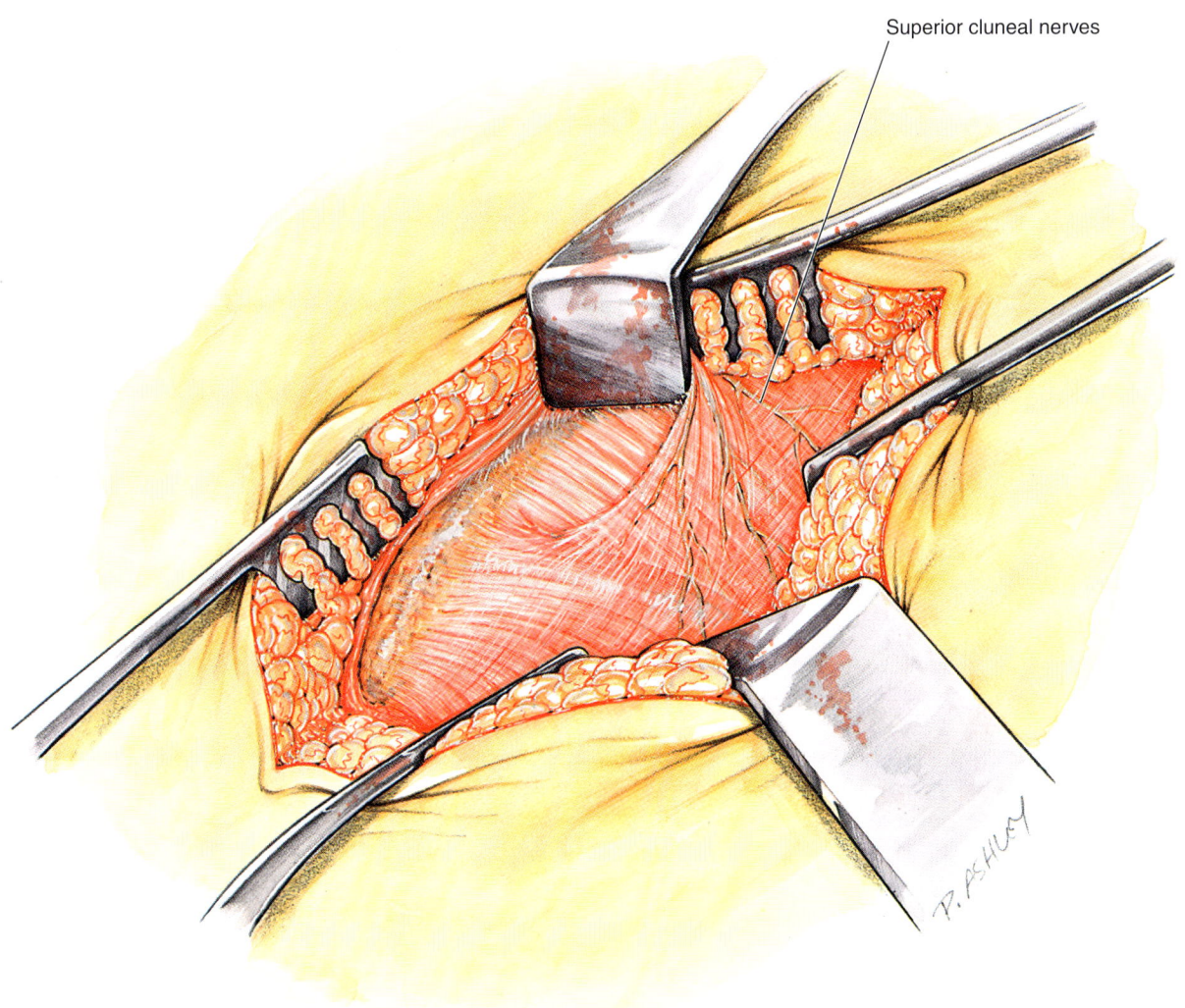

● **Figure 13-5.** The posterior approach uses the interval between the latissimus dorsi and abdominal muscles superiorly and the gluteal muscles inferiorly. These muscles attach to the iliac crest but do not cross it.

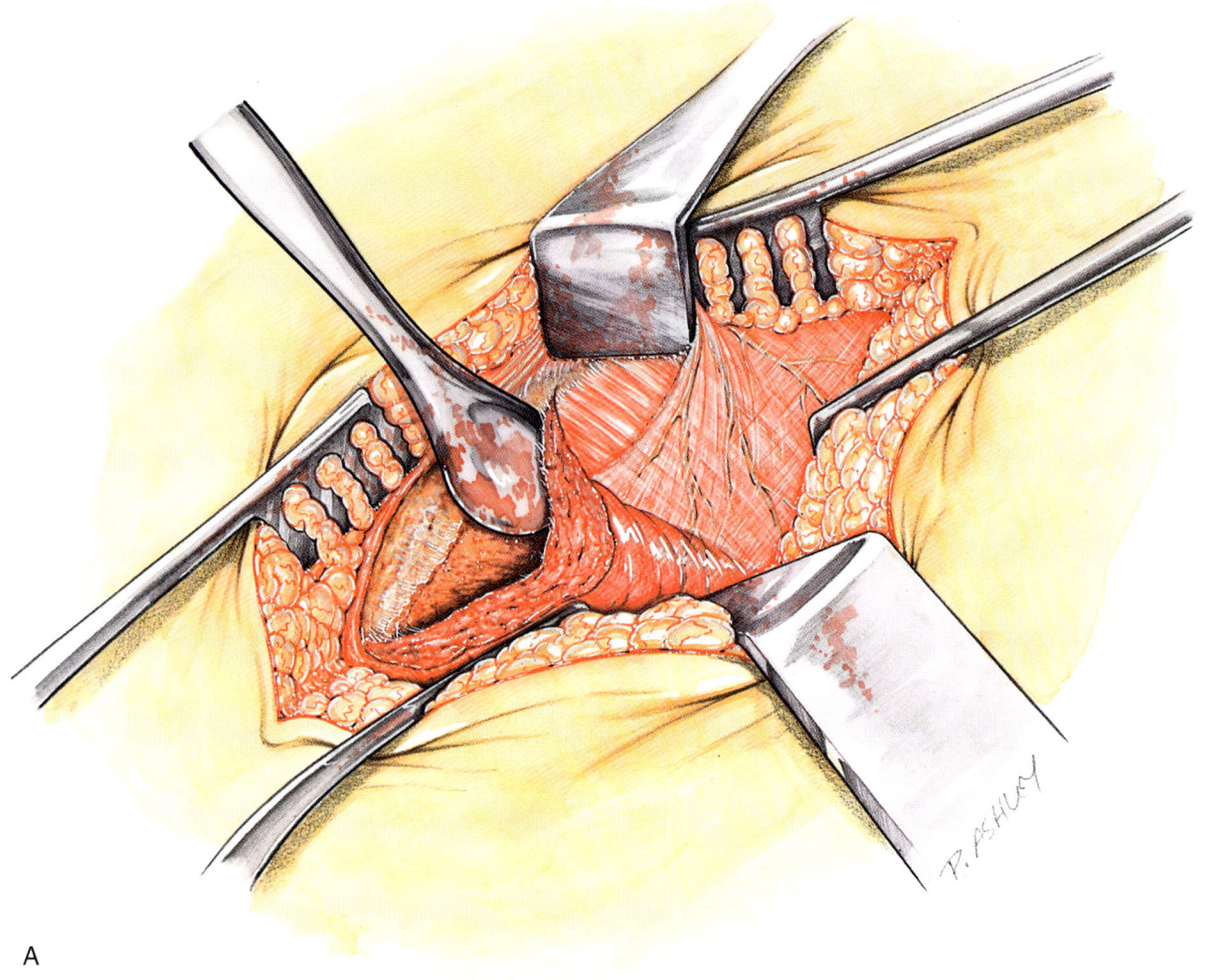

A

● **Figure 13-6.** *A* and *B*, The outer table is exposed by strict subperiosteal dissection. To avoid injury to the superior cluneal nerves, do not dissect more than 8 cm anterolateral to the posterior-superior iliac spine.

sciatic notch, one should always start with the gouge at the posterior-superior iliac spine and proceed in an anterolateral manner. The outer cortex of the ilium along with underlying cancellous bone are taken. If pure cancellous bone is also desired, at this point large gouges and curets are used. Usually there is a large amount of cancellous bone directly under the posterior-superior iliac spine. Cancellous bone is removed until the inner cortical table is visualized. Hemostasis can be obtained by placing thrombin-soaked Gelfoam in the iliac defect or by using bone wax. The wound is closed by suturing the fascial layer to the iliac crest periosteum. Some surgeons prefer to close the wound over a drain.

ANTERIOR APPROACH. The anterior iliac crest is used when a patient is undergoing anterior spinal surgery. The patient is supine, and a small sandbag or rolled towel can be placed under the buttock to raise the side from which the graft will be harvested. The

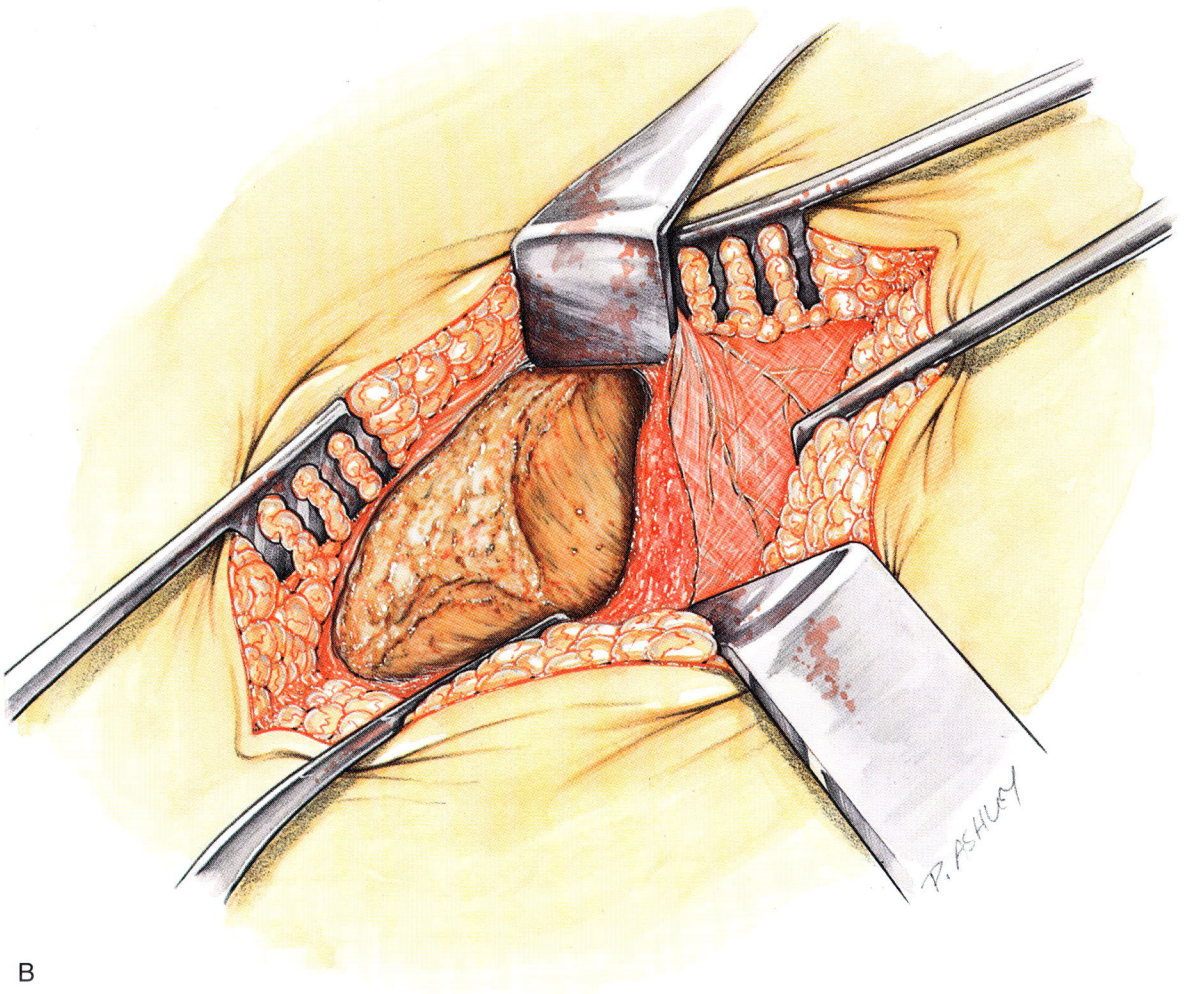

B

● **Figure 13-6** Continued

anterior-superior iliac spine is the key landmark to this approach. The surgeon palpates the anterior-superior iliac spine and begins the skin incision 2 cm superolateral to it. The incision is 5 to 10 cm in length, depending on the amount of graft needed, and follows the natural curve of the iliac crest (Figure 13–7). Self-retaining retractors are placed, and the iliac crest is identified. An incision is made directly onto the crest, taking care not to stray into surrounding muscle. The gluteus medius, gluteus minimus, and tensor fasciae latae are inferior to the crest, and the abdominal muscles are superior to the crest. The muscle attachments are released with electrocautery from either the inner or outer table or both, depending on the type of graft desired. Malleable ribbon retractors are placed in the outer cortical table to retract the gluteus medius, gluteus minimus, and tensor fasciae latae muscles; a malleable ribbon retractor in the inner table retracts the iliacus muscle.

210 • SURGICAL APPROACHES TO THE SPINE

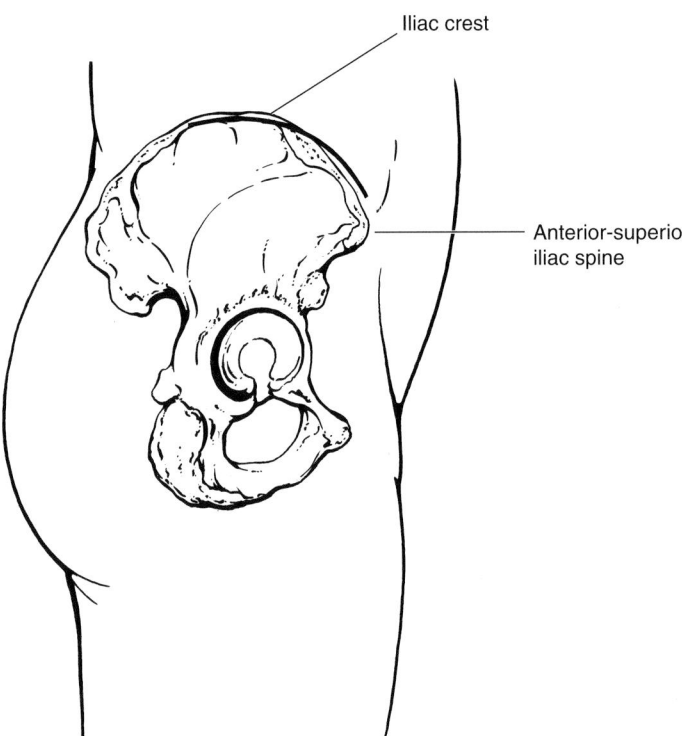

● **Figure 13-7.** Skin incision used for an anterior iliac bone graft. This is an internervous plane, and no muscles cross over the crest.

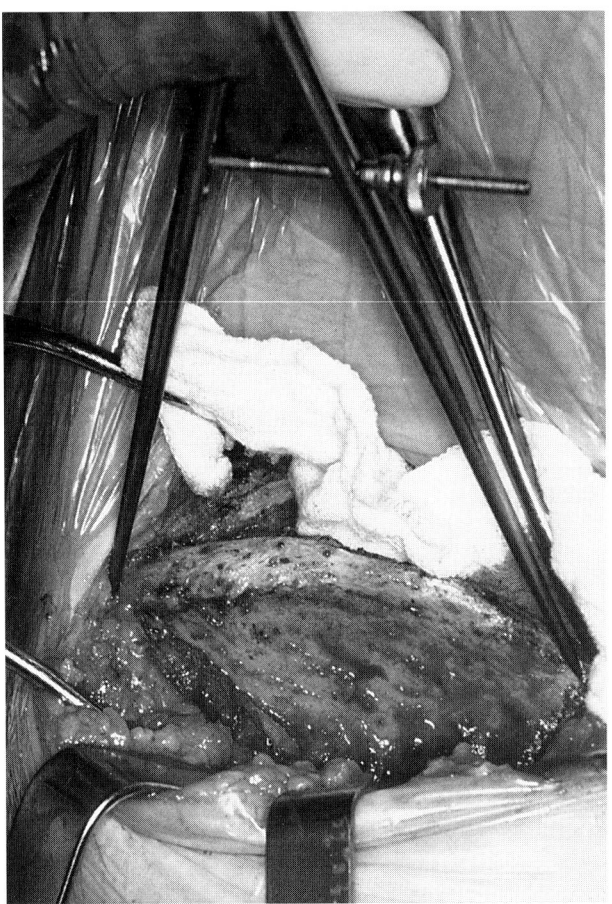

● **Figure 13-8.** Anterior approach for obtaining a tricortical iliac crest bone graft. A caliper is used to mark the intended length of bone and appropriate osteotomy sites.

Corticocancellous and cancellous bone graft are obtained using the same technique described for the posterior approach. If a tricortical iliac graft is necessary for vertebral interbody fusions or for vertebral body reconstructions, one must first determine the size of the required graft. A caliper or template is used to mark the appropriate graft size along the iliac crest (Figure 13–8). One must always remove a slightly larger graft than is necessary. Use of osteotomes and mallets is avoided when possible because these instruments create microfractures and weaken the strength of the graft. Instead, a water-cooled oscillating saw is used to make two parallel vertical cuts through both cortices, keeping in mind the preferred dimensions of the graft (Figure 13–9A). The deep transverse cut is sometimes difficult to make with the oscillating saw; therefore, a curved osteotome may be used to cut through both cortices, taking care to protect the muscles on both sides of the crest. A water-cooled high-speed bur or rongeur is used to sculpt the donor bone to fit the exact needs of the recipient site (see Figure 13–9B). The wound is closed with fascial and muscle reapproximation. The fascia overlying the gluteus medius and tensor fascia latae and the fascia overlying the abdominal muscles are sutured to each other in cases of tricortical iliac crest graft removal, or the fascia is sutured to the periosteum in cases in which corticocancellous strips and cancellous bone were removed.

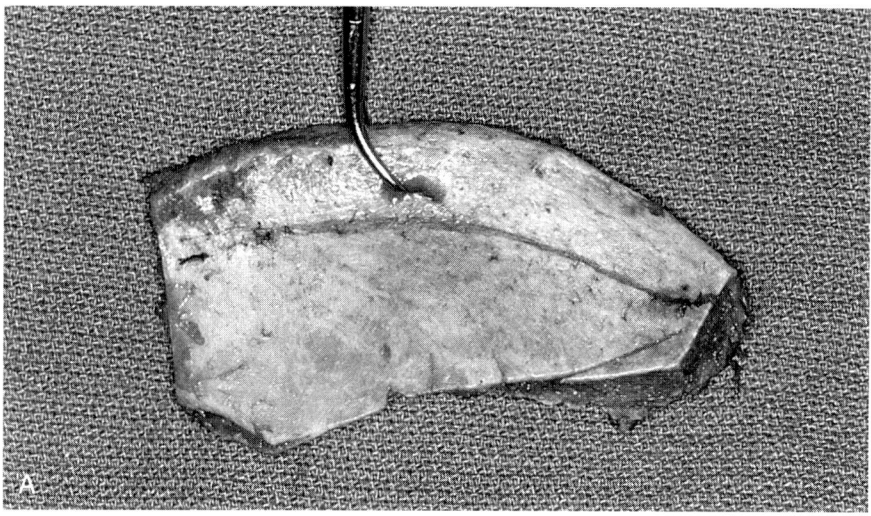

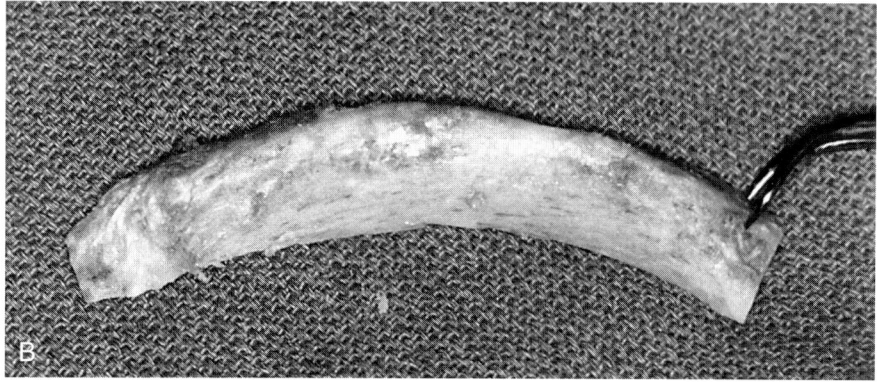

● **Figure 13-9.** *A* and *B*, A tricortical iliac graft is procured by using an oscillating saw for the vertical cuts and an osteotome for the transverse cut. The graft is then contoured using a rongeur and high speed bur to conform to the dimensions of the recipient site.

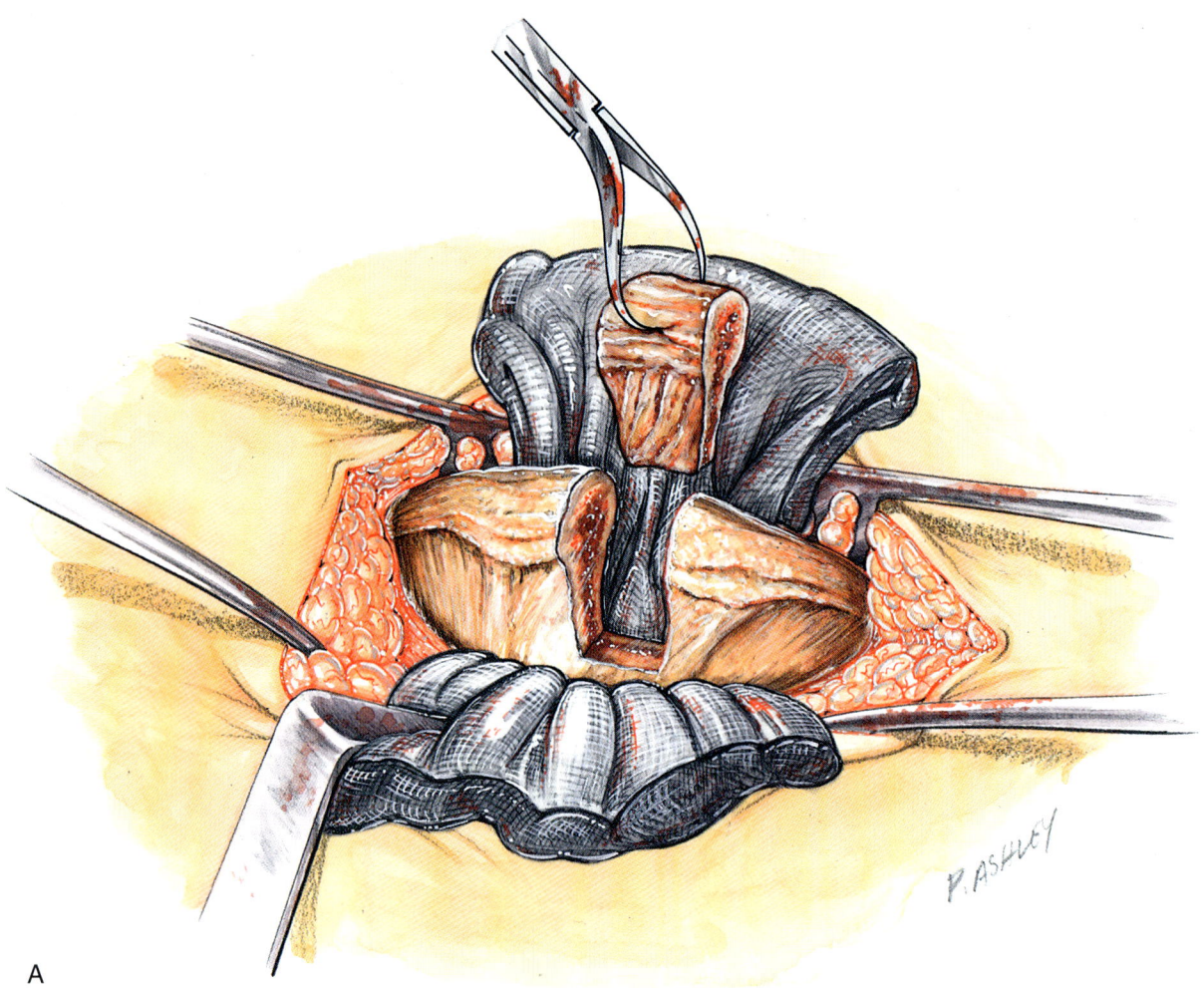

A

- **Figure 13-10.** *A* through *C*, A tricortical iliac graft cut and sculpted to the appropriate size for an anterior cervical fusion after diskectomy. These grafts vary in size, but are commonly 9 mm in length and 13 mm in depth. Note that the cancellous edge is placed posteriorly.

Complications

Complications that occur from obtaining an iliac bone graft range from seemingly minor problems to severe, life-threatening situations. A thorough knowledge of pelvic anatomy, as well as following strict surgical principles, will prevent the majority of these complications.

The superior gluteal artery is vulnerable as it exits the sciatic notch above the piriformis muscle. If injured in this location, the artery can retract into the pelvis and hemostasis becomes difficult to achieve. In this situation, the wound can be packed, the patient repositioned supine, and a retroperitoneal exposure performed to control the bleeding. Alternatively, a portion of bone may be removed to expose the superior edge of the sciatic notch to improve direct visualization of the retracted arterial stump. Other arteries such as the iliolumbar and fourth lumbar arteries can be injured, resulting in hemorrhage, if disssection wanders into muscle rather than staying in a subperiosteal plane.

Nerve injury is one of the more frequently reported complications. The lateral femoral cutaneous nerve usually lies medial and inferior to the anterior-superior iliac spine, however, anomalous pathways have been encountered. Injury to this nerve can result in paresthesias,

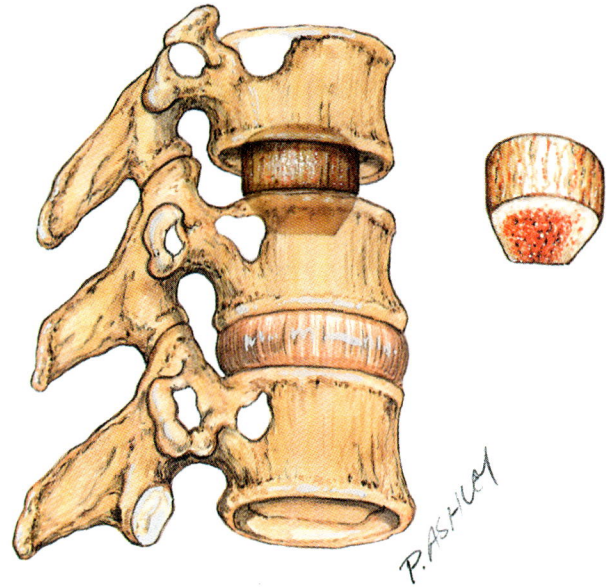

B Anterior cervical interbody fusion (lateral view)

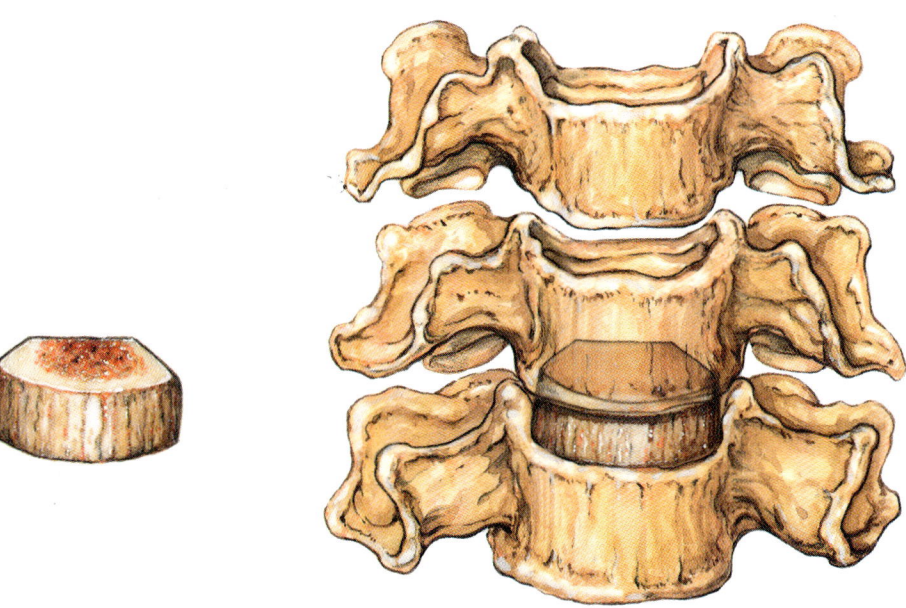

C Anterior cervical interbody fusion (anteroposterior view)

● **Figure 13-10** *Continued*

hyperesthesia, numbness, and pain to the anterolateral thigh. The superior cluneal nerves are most susceptible to injury when a posterior approach is extended more than 8 cm superolateral to the posterior-superior iliac spine. The result of injury can be numbness of the buttock or chronic donor-site pain. Risk to the sciatic nerve can be minimized by staying away from the sciatic notch. The iliohypogastric and ilioinguinal nerves can be injured during an anterior approach by excessive retraction of the iliacus muscle.

Although rare, damage to internal organs, such as the bowel or ureter, have been reported. Furthermore, if the inguinal ligament is detached from the anterior-superior iliac spine, herniation of abdominal contents may occur. Inadequate fascial repair after tricortical graft procurement can also lead to a hernia.

Overaggressive removal of bone beyond specified safe anatomic areas can lead to penetration of the hip joint and sacroiliac joint and to fracture of the anterior-superior iliac spine. Potential also exists for gait abnormality, specifically an abductor lurch, secondary to detachment of the gluteus medius and minimus origins.

Conclusions

Spinal operations often require a concomitant bone graft to promote fusion, and the iliac crest remains the most widely used source of expendable autologous graft. An advantage of autologous bone graft is its ability to provide all three components necessary for bone regeneration: osteogenic cells, osteoinduction, and osteoconduction. Furthermore, autologous grafts imply no added risk of transmitting hepatitis C, the acquired immunodeficiency syndrome, or other unknown infectious processes possible with allografts. The iliac crest, with its unique geometric design, is suitable for a variety of required graft configurations (Figure 13–10). Complications occur with both anterior and posterior graft procurement. Most complications can be avoided by thorough familiarity of the anatomy of the pelvis and by practicing meticulous surgical technique.

Fibular Graft

Indications

A fibular shaft bone graft is used in situations in which a strong structural graft is desired. Specific indications include reconstruction of cervical corpectomies of varying lengths, as

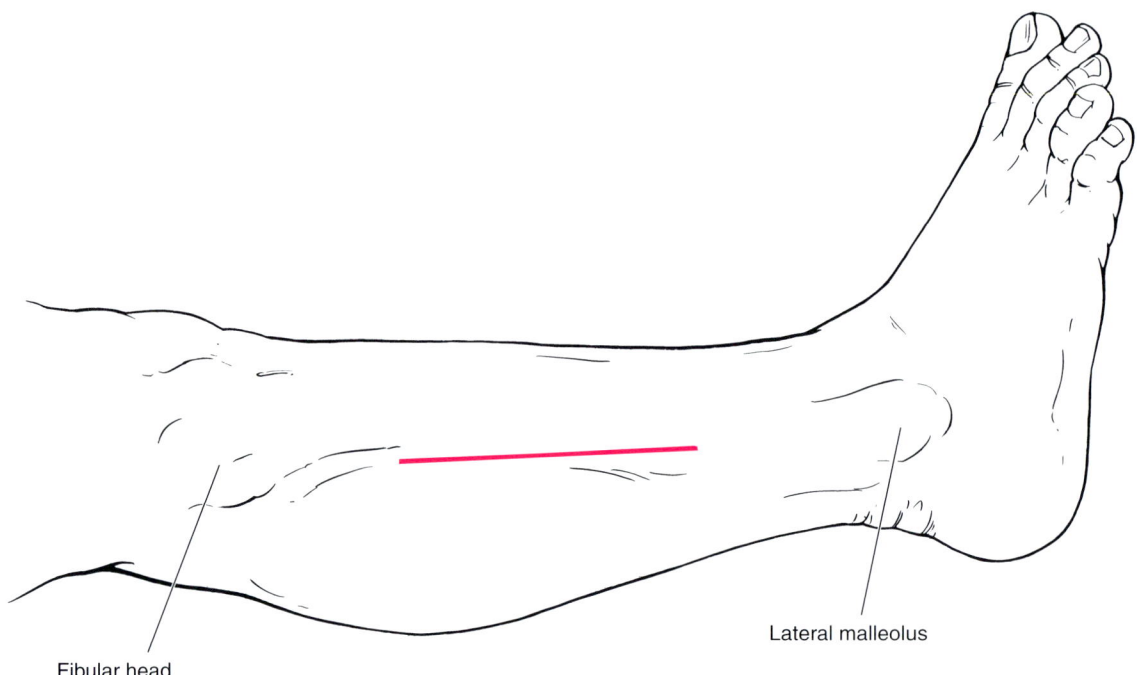

● **Figure 13-11.** The skin incision for obtaining a fibular autograft is directly over the lateral compartment, in the middle third of the leg, and in line with the fibular head and lateral malleolus.

well as thoracolumbar vertebral body resections for tumor, infection, and severe kyphotic deformities. Fibular grafts are nearly entirely cortical and are stronger than iliac crest and rib grafts. Furthermore, the fibula is straight in comparison to the curved nature of the iliac crest and rib. Advantages of the fibular graft include its strength as a strut graft, its availability, and a relatively low morbidity associated with its use. Vascularized fibular grafts have also been used in spinal operations, but with less frequency. Its advantages, compared with a nonvascularized fibular graft, include a more rapid healing response and the capability of the graft to hypertrophy. Disadvantages of a vascularized fibular graft are the technical surgical difficulties and length of operation.

Clinical Anatomy

The palpable bony landmarks of the lateral aspect of the leg are the fibular head proximally and the lateral malleolus distally. The lateral compartment of the leg consists of the peroneus longus and peroneus brevis muscles, the longus being superficial to the brevis. The posterior superficial compartment consists of the gastrocnemius, soleus, and plantaris muscles. The posterior deep compartment is composed of the flexor digitorum longus, posterior tibialis, and flexor hallucis longus muscles. Superficially, the fascial plane lies between the peroneus brevis and soleus muscles. Deeper, the plane is between the peroneus brevis and the flexor hallucis longus muscles. The dorsal cutaneous branch of the superficial peroneal nerve

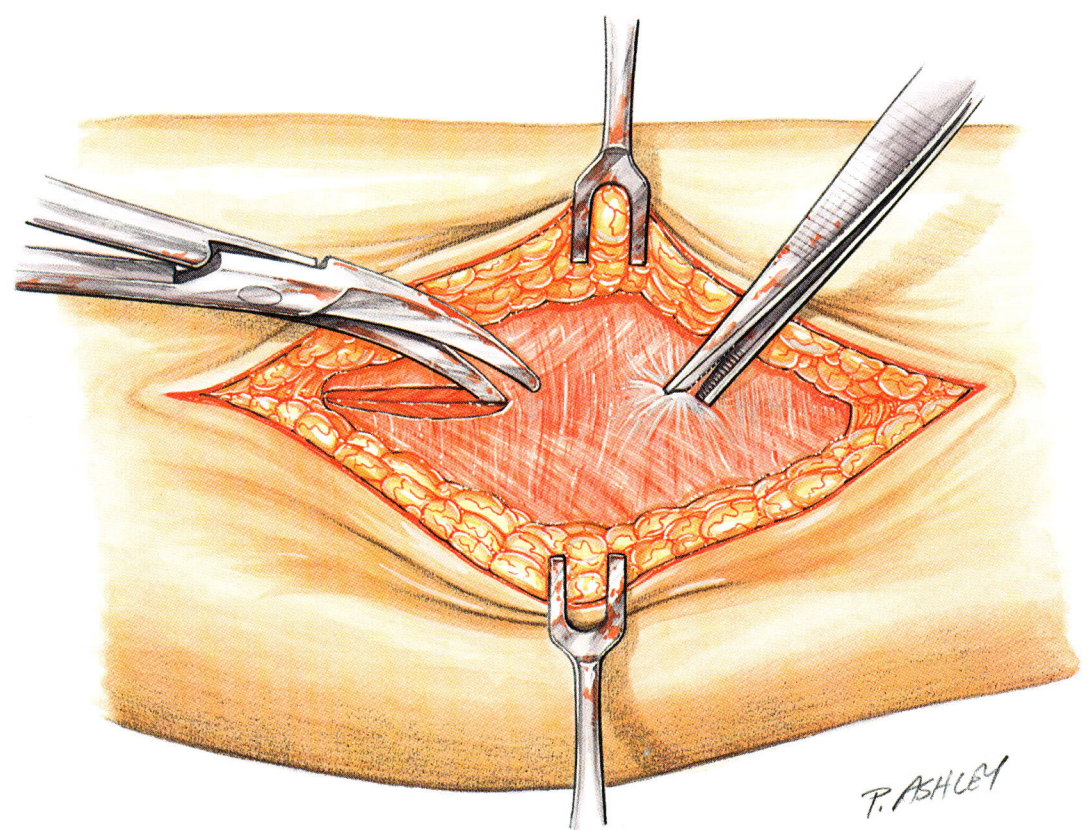

● **Figure 13-12.** The fascia overlying the lateral compartment is incised at the interval between the peroneal muscles and the soleus muscle.

pierces the fascia of the lateral compartment at the junction of the middle and distal thirds of the fibula. The common peroneal nerve wraps around the fibular neck in a posterior to anterior direction. One can avoid injuring this nerve by exposing only the middle third of the fibula and by not retracting in a cephalad direction.

Surgical Technique

The patient may be supine or in the lateral position, depending on the position necessary for the spinal operation. The leg is exsanguinated, and a tourniquet is inflated around the thigh. The fibular head and lateral malleolus are palpated, and a skin incision is made in line with these two landmarks and in the middle third of the leg (Figure 13–11). The incision is brought through subcutaneous tissues down to the fascia overlying the peroneal muscles. The peroneus longus tendon lies superficial to the peroneus brevis muscle. The fascia is then incised at the interval between the peroneal muscles, which are anterior, and the soleus muscle, which lies posteriorly (Figure 13–12). The incision is deepened between the peroneal muscles anteriorly and the flexor hallucis longus muscle posteriorly (Figure 13–13). These muscles are stripped off the fibula in a subperiosteal manner from distal to proximal (Figure 13–14). The required length of the graft is measured and marked. Retractors are placed at the proposed osteotomy sites to protect the surrounding muscular and neurovascular structures. A water-cooled oscillating saw is used to make the proximal and distal osteotomies (Figure 13–15). A periosteal elevator or electrocautery is used to free up any remaining tissue attached to the fibula. Bone wax can be placed on the remaining bone ends to help gain hemostasis. The tourniquet is deflated and further strict hemostasis is obtained.

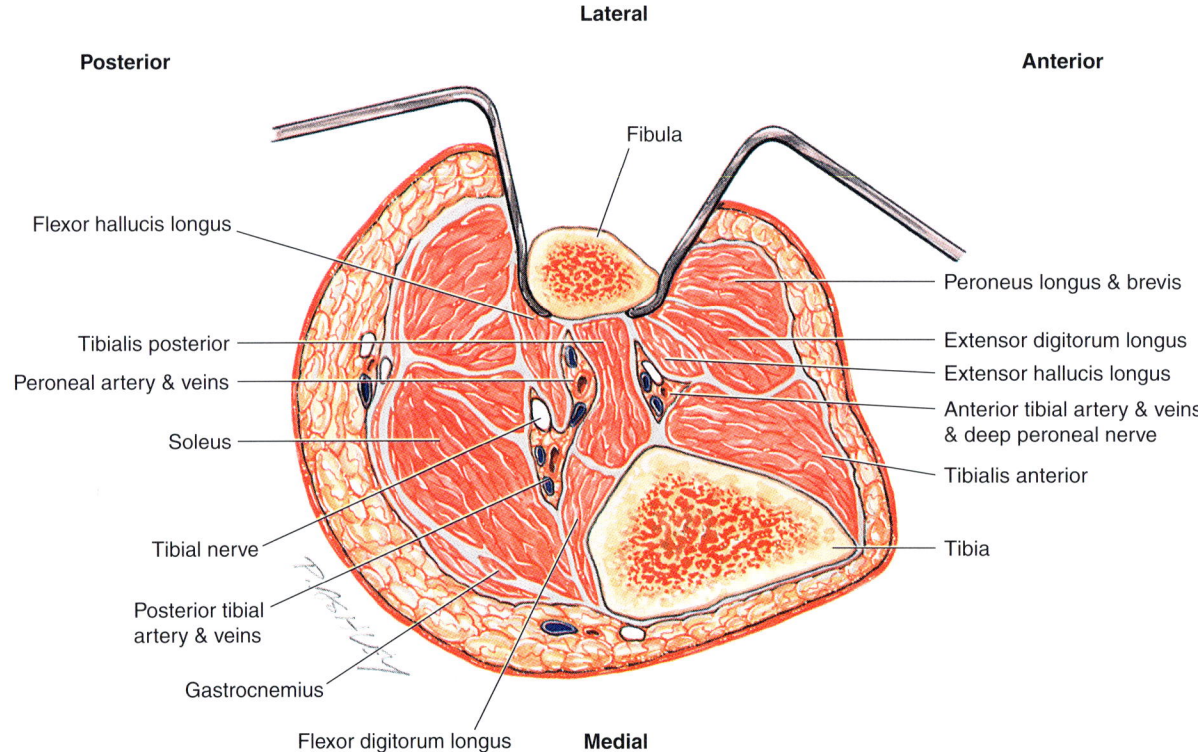

● **Figure 13–13.** Cross section of middle third of leg. The superficial dissection proceeds between the peroneal muscles and the soleus. Deep dissection is between the peroneal muscles anteriorly and the flexor hallucis longus muscle posteriorly.

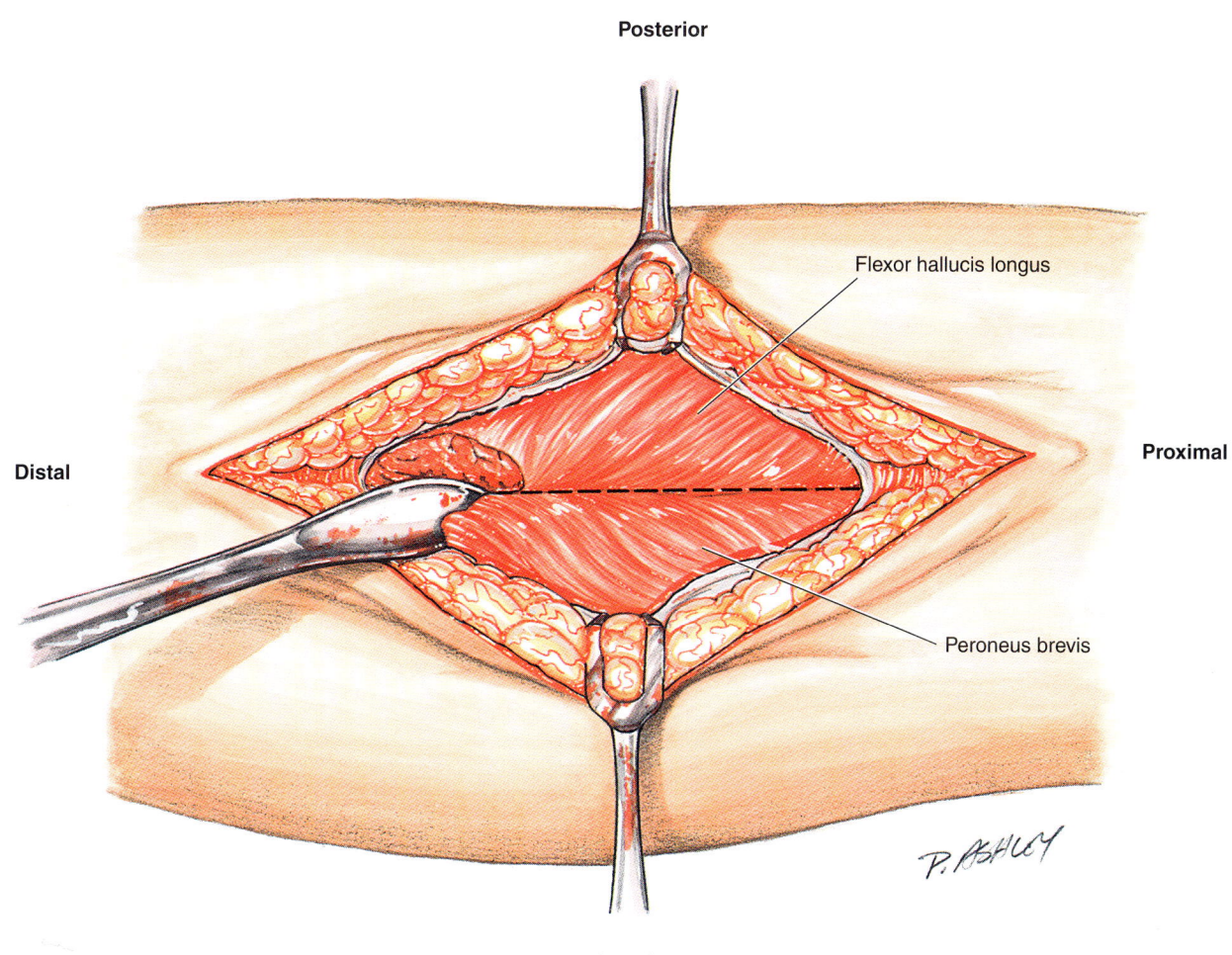

● **Figure 13-14.** Because of the obliquity of the muscular attachments to the fibula, the muscles are stripped in a distal to proximal direction.

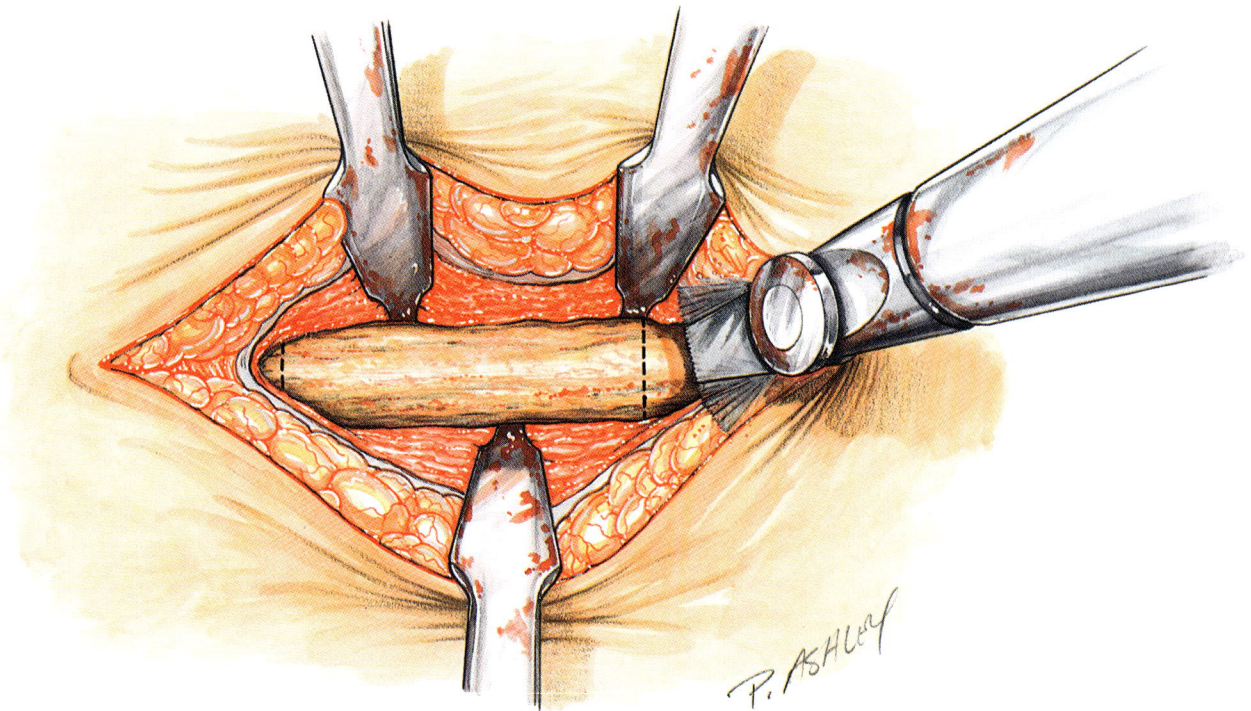

● **Figure 13-15.** The intended length of fibular graft is cut with an oscillating saw, and any remaining soft tissue attachments are released.

Two or three loose sutures are placed in the fascia to reapproximate the edges. The fascia is not closed too tightly to allow for compartment swelling. Subcutaneous tissues and skin are closed in layers.

Complications

Obtaining a fibular bone graft is a fairly straightforward procedure; however, complications can occur. Ankle mortise instability can occur if the fibular graft is taken too distally. A minimum of 6 to 7 cm proximal to the tip of the lateral malleolus should remain uninterrupted to prevent this complication. In children a valgus deformity of the ankle joint can result from proximal migration of the distal fibula after excision of the fibular shaft. Children younger than age 10 therefore require a syndesmotic screw through the fibula and tibia just proximal to the ankle joint to avoid this complication. Compartment syndrome of the leg can develop if the fascia is tightly repaired or if hemostasis is not obtained before closure of the wound. The common, deep, and superficial peroneal nerves may be injured if dissection strays from the middle third of the fibula. The result is a temporary or permanent footdrop, eversion weakness, or cutaneous numbness.

Conclusion

Fibular autograft is an excellent option when structural support from a bone graft is of utmost importance. The largely cortical bone of the fibula is stronger than both iliac crest graft and rib graft. However, the fibula contains very little cancellous bone; therefore,

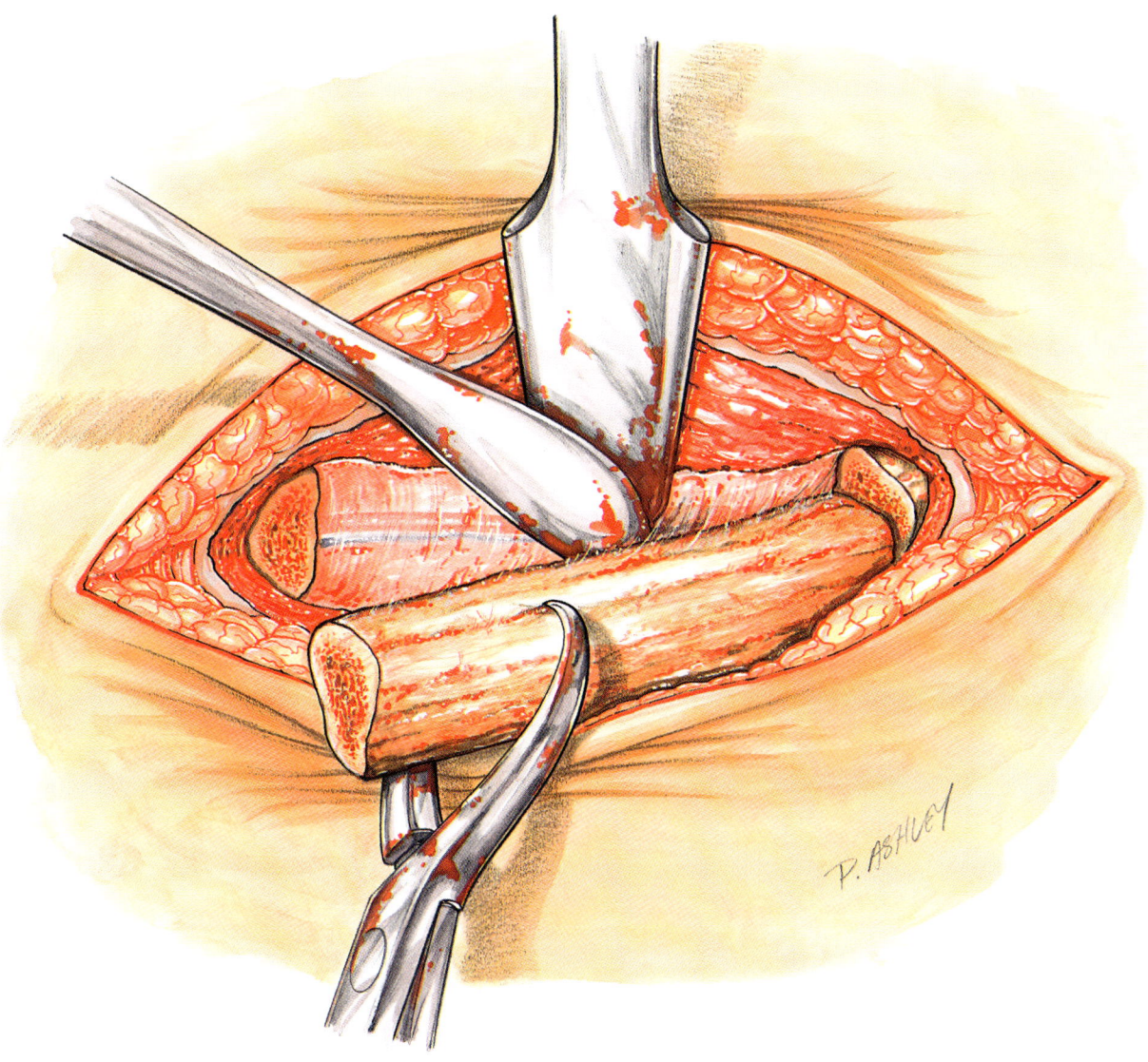

● **Figure 13-15** Continued

healing is by creeping substitution, which can take many months to occur. The middle third of the fibula is expendable, but care must be taken to avoid peroneal nerve injury, disruption of ankle mortise stability, and compartment syndrome.

BIBLIOGRAPHY

1. Arrington ED, Smith WJ, Chambers HG, et al: Complications of iliac crest bone graft harvesting. Clin Orthop Rel Res 329:300, 1996.
2. Balderston RA, An HS: Complications in Spine Surgery. Philadelphia, WB Saunders, 1991.
3. Fowler BL, Dall BE, Rowe DE: Complications associated with harvesting autogenous iliac bone graft. Am J Orthop December, 1995.
4. Freidberg SR, Gumley GJ, Pfeifer BA, Hybels RL: Vascularized fibular graft to replace resected cervical vertebral bodies. J Neurosurg 71:283, 1989.
5. Garfin S: Complications of Spine Surgery. Baltimore, Williams & Wilkins, 1989.
6. Green DP, Hotchkiss RN: Operative Hand Surgery, 3rd ed. New York, Churchill Livingstone, 1993.

Index

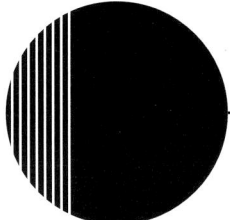

Note: Page numbers in *italics* refer to figures.

A

Abdomen, computed tomography of, *167*
Abscess, spinal, 143
Accessory nerve, spinal, *3, 47,* 56, *58*
Alexander elevator, *122*
Andrews frame, *182,* 194
Anesthesia, for thoracotomy, 118
Annulus fibrosis, anatomy of, *176*
  elevation of psoas in, *153*
  physiology of, 177
Anterior approach(es), to cervicothoracic junction, 61–79
  to lumbar spine, 145–155, 157–171
  to middle and lower cervical spine, 9–24
  to upper cervical spine, 25–52
  to upper thoracic spine, 61–79
Arterial injuries, in iliac bone harvesting, 212
Artery(ies). See specific arteries, e.g., *Carotid artery.*
Articular process, superior, *186*
Articulation, costotransverse, *136*
Atlantoaxial complex, exposure of, *29*
  posterior approach to, 82
  surgical risk in, 82–83
  transarticular fixation of, 92
Auricular nerve, *54*
  dissection of, 55
  in retropharyngeal approach, 48

B

Bone grafts, autologous, *100,* 201–219
  from fibula. See *Fibular grafts.*
  from iliac crest. See *Iliac bone grafts.*
  in foraminotomy, 21, *22*
Bone harvesting, complications of, 212–214
  for fibular grafts, 216
  for tricortical graft, *210,* 211, *211*
  from iliac crest, bilateral, 198
    indications for, 202–203
    with paravertebral approach, *195*
  of corticocancellous bone, *208–209*
Brachiocephalic vessels, 65, 68, *69, 77*
Brooks fusion, for extension injuries, 91, 92
  rotational stability of, 91
  wires in, 92, *97*
Burns' space, 64

C

Cartilage, costal, 160
Carotid artery, *68*
  branches of, *4*
  common, *47, 48*
  exposure of, *3,* 77
  function of, 3
Carotid sheath, at C1 arch, *55*
  at C6 vertebral level, *2, 10*
  in neck cross section, *83*
  retraction of, 65, 68
Carotid tubercle, 12
Cauda equina, *174*
Cervical disk disease, 89
Cervical fusion, tricortical graft in, *212–213*
Cervical region, anatomy of, 1–7, 82–83
  blood vessels in, 2, 3, *3*
  cross section of, *10*
  fascial layers of, 2, *2*
  ganglions in, 5–6
  muscles in, 2–3
  nerves in, 4–5
Cervical spine, anterior approach(es) to, advantages of, 11
  bone grafting in, 21, *22*
  closure techniques in, 21
  complications of, 21, 23
  deep fascial dissection in, 14, 16
  extensile exposure of, 21, *23*
  fascial retraction in, *16*
  for bone grafting, 21, *22*
  in middle and lower regions, 9–24
  in upper region, 25–52
  incision in, 12–13
  landmarks in, *11,* 12
  longus colli elevation in, 16–18
  patient positioning in, 11–12
  platysma section in, 12–13
  preparation for, 11–12
  sternocleidomastoid release in, 13–14
  surgical risk of, 26
  techniques for, 11–21
  traction in, 11
  nonunion of, 112
  posterior approach(es) to, 81–113
    anatomy in, 82–83
    C1 arch location in, *91*
    complications of, 110–112

Cervical spine *(Continued)*
  dural tears in, 111
  embolism in, 112
  in C1-C2 complex, 90–92, 98
  incision in, *84,* 86
  indications for, 82, 90
  interspinous wiring in, 101–103, *102*
  laminae in, 87
  midline plane in, 82, *83, 85, 111*
  neurological complications of, 111, *111*
  occipital nerves in, 91
  occipitocervical fusion in, 98–101
  patient positioning in, 83, 85, 111–112
  rigid internal fixation in, 103, 105–108
  surgical risk in, 82–83
  retropharyngeal approaches to, 47–51
  transoral approaches to, 26–47
  Whiteside's approach to, 53–59
Cervicothoracic junction, anatomy of, 63–64
  anterior approaches to, 61–79
    complications of, 62, 78
    modified, 62, *62,* 64–68
    types of, 62–63
  pedicle entry point in, *109*
  pedicle morphometry in, *110*
  posterior approaches to, 109–110
  sterum-splitting approach to, 76–78
Chassaignac's tubercle, 12
Chest tube(s), in thoracotomy, 124, 129, *129*
Circumflex artery, *205*
Clavicle resection, 68
Cluneal nerve(s), 203, *204,* 207, 213
Cobb retractor, 181, 184
Compartment syndrome, 218
Compression injuries, prevention of, 5
Computed tomography, abdominal, *167*
Costal cartilage, 160
Costotransverse ligaments, 134, *136, 141*
Costotransversectomy, 133–144
  anatomy involving, 134–137
    bones in, 137
    costotransverse ligaments in, 134, *136*
    muscles in, 134, *135*
    neurovascular system in, 134–135
  bone resection in, 138–143, *141–143*
  complications of, 143–144
  incisions in, 137–138, *138*
  muscle dissection in, 138, *139*
  patient positioning in, 137, *138*

221

Costotransversectomy *(Continued)*
  surgical approach to, 137–143
  techniques for, 138–143, *141*
  value of, 134, 144
Cranial nerves, motor, 47–48
Cricothyroid, injuries to, 50
Cushing retractor, 7, 13, *15*
Cutaneous nerve, femoral, 205, *205*, 212–213

D

Diaphragm detachment, 160, 161
Digastric muscle(s), anatomy of, 3
  anterior, *48*
  exposure of, *44, 45*
  posterior belly of, *6, 46, 51*
Dingman mouth gag, 27
Disk, intervertebral, anatomy of, *176,* 177
  herniation of, *192*
Disk space, intervertebral, 21, *22*
Diskectomy, intervertebral, 18, *19,* 21, *21*
  unilateral laminotomy for, 186
Dissection, of paraspinal muscles, 184
  subperiosteal, *29,* 181
Dissector(s), Doyen rib, *123*
  Penfield, 184
Dura mater, 192

E

Embolism, 112
Epiglottis, *41, 49*
Erector spinae muscles, *135, 183*
Esophagus, *68,* 77
  injuries to, 21
Evoked potentials, somatosensory, 83
Extension injury(ies), Brooks fusion for, 91, 92
Eyelid ptosis, 5

F

Facet joints, anatomy of, 184
  misidentification of, 198
  preservation of, 184, 197
Facetectomy, bone removal area in, *90*
  technique for, 89–90
Facial vein(s), *44, 45, 48*
Fat, retroperitoneal, 147, *149, 150*
Femoral cutaneous nerve, 205, *205*, 212–213
Fibular grafts, 214–219
  advantages of, 215, 218
  bone harvesting in, 216
  clinical anatomy in, 215–216
  complications of, 218
  in children, 218
  incision for, *214,* 216
  indications for, 214–215
  landmarks for, 215
  lateral compartment in, 215, *215*
  muscle stripping in, 216, *217*
  patient positioning in, 216
  posterior compartments in, 215
  techniques for, 216–218
  using oscillating saw, 216, *218*
Finochietto rib retractor, *125*
Fixation, of atlantoaxial joint, 92, 98
  rigid internal, 103, 105–108
    benefits of, 103
    hook-plate method of, *108*
    instrumentation for, 103
    screw-plate fixation in, 103, *105*
  transarticular, *98*
Flexion injury(ies), Gallie fusion for, 91–92

Foramen, intervertebral, 175, *175*
Foramen magnum, enlargement of, *100*
  hemorrhage of, 91
Foraminal stenosis, 174
Foraminotomy, anterior technique for, 19–21, *20*
  bone grafting in, 21, *22*
  intervertebral distraction in, 20
  midline approach in, 89
  patient positioning in, *86,* 88–89
  posterior technique for, 88–90, *89*
Fusion, Brooks method, for extension injuries, 91, 92
  rotational stability in, 91
  wires in, *97*
  Gallie method, 91–92
    technique for, *93*
    with cable and locking cinch, *96*
    with flexible wire, *92, 94–95*
  occipitocervical, 98–101

G

Gallie fusion, for flexion injuries, 91–92
  technique for, *93*
  with cable and locking cinch, *96*
  with flexible wire, *92, 94–95*
Ganglia, sympathetic, *169, 170*
  in cervical region, 5–6
  injuries to, 5
Gigli saw, 66–67
Gluteal artery, 204, *204,* 212
Gluteal nerve(s), in iliac bone grafts, 203, 204
Grafts, bone. See *Bone grafts.*

H

Hemorrhage, of foramen magnum, 91
Hemostasis, 181
Hernia, from bone graft harvesting, 213
Horner's syndrome, 5, 21
Hypogastric plexus, *169*
Hypoglossal nerve(s), *51*
  anatomy of, 4, *6*
  exposure of, *3, 47*
  retraction of, *49*
  surgical injuries to, 50

I

Iliac artery, *168–169*
Iliac bone grafts, anterior approach to, anatomy in, 205–206
  arteries in, 206
  incision in, *210*
  landmarks for, 209
  nerves at risk in, 205, 205–206
  patient positioning in, 208–209
  retraction injuries in, 205
  techniques for, 208–211
  cancellous, 202, *202–203*
  complications of, 212–214
  corticocancellous strips in, 202–203
  indications for, 202–203
  posterior approach to, anatomy in, 203–204
    bone harvesting in, 207–208, *208–209*
    incisions in, 206–207
    indications for, 206
    landmarks in, 207, *207*
    nerves at risk in, 203–204
    osseous structures at risk in, 204
    patient positioning in, 206
    techniques for, 206–208
  tricortical, *212–213*

Iliac bone grafts *(Continued)*
  harvesting of, *210,* 211, *211*
  indications for, 203
Iliac crest, bone grafts from, *100,* 202, 214
Iliac veins, 162, 165, *168*
Iliocostalis muscle, 82
Iliohypogastric nerve, 213
Ilioinguinal nerve, *206,* 213
Iliolumbar system, 177–178, *205*
Ilium, as cancellous bone source, 202, *202–203*
Incision(s), for anterior cervical approach, *11,* 11–13
  for costotransversectomy, 137–138, *138*
  for fibular grafts, *214*
  for iliac bone grafts, 206–207, *210*
  for mandibulotomy, *31, 36*
  for posterior lumbar exposure, 179, 181
  for retroperitoneal lumbar exposure, 146, 147, *147,* 161
  for sternum splitting, 76
  for thoracotomy, 70, *70, 117, 120–121,* 123–124, *124*
Injury(ies). See also under anatomy, e.g., *Nerve(s), injuries to.*
  compression, prevention of, 5
  extension, Brooks fusion for, 91, 92
  flexion, Gallie fusion for, 91–92
Intercostal muscle(s), *73–74*
Interspinous ligament(s), *85, 89,* 175, *176*
Intertransverse ligament(s), 175, 184
Intertransverse process, 187
Intervertebral disk, anatomy of, *176,* 177
  herniation of, *192*
Intervertebral disk space, 21, *22*

J

Joint(s), facet, anatomy of, 184
  misidentification of, 198
  preservation of, 184, 197
  sacroiliac, 204
Jugular vein(s), anterior, *14*
  at C6 vertebral level, *2, 10*
  external, *44, 46, 56*
  internal, *3, 47, 48, 57–58, 68, 77*
  ligation of, 7, 13, *15*

K

Kerrison rongeur, 89, 90, 186, 187, 191

L

Laminectomy, bone removal area in, *90*
  decompressive, 184, 186
  interfacet wiring and fusion in, *104*
  technique for, 90
Laminotomy, 186, *191*
Laryngeal muscles, 3
Laryngeal nerve(s), anatomy of, 4, 64
  injuries to, 4
    surgical, 21, 50, *51,* 64
  recurrent, *68,* 77
  superior, *6*
Latissimus dorsi, *135*
Leg, cross section of, *216*
Levator scapulae, *83*
Ligament(s). See also specific ligaments, e.g., *Costotransverse ligaments.*
  longitudinal, *74–75*
  of lumbar spine, 175–176, *176*
  of posterior cervical spine, 82
Ligamentum flavum, *174,* 175, *176,* 188

Ligamentum nuchae, 82, *83*, 86, *89*
Lingual nerve, *49*
Lip split, in mandibulotomy, *39*
  in transoral approach to cervical spine, 26, 31, 43
Longissimus cervicis, 82, *83*
Longitudinal ligaments, 175–176, *176*
Longus colli, *58*
  elevation of, 16–18
  in middle thyroid vein division, 5
  retraction of, 18, *18*, *30*
Lordosis, lumbar, 179
  restoration of, 161, *166*
Lumbar arteries, *205*
Lumbar disease, *166*
Lumbar exposure(s), anterior, 157–171
  for lower spine, 160–162, 165–166
  for tuberculosis treatment, 158
  for upper spine, *159*, 159–160
  general considerations in, 159
  indications for, 158
  patient positioning in, *158*, 159, 160–161
  retroperitoneal approach to, 145–155
  thoracoabdominal approach in, *159*, *160*
  posterior, 173–192
    appropriate level for, 188, 190
    closure of, 187
    complications of, 188, 190–191
    hemostasis in, 179, 181, 190–191
    in fusion with pedicle instrumentation, 186
    in unilateral laminotomy, 186
    incision in, 179, 181
    indications for, 174
    lateral extension in, 182
    obstacles in, 181–182, 184
    pars interarticularis delineation in, 184
    patient positioning in, 179, *182*
    subperiosteal dissection in, 181
    techniques for, 179–188
    transverse process exposure in, 184, *185*
  retroperitoneal vs. transperitoneal approach, 146, 158
  Wiltse approach to, 193–200
Lumbar lordosis, 179
Lumbar spine, anatomy of, 174–179, 192
  articular process of, *174*, 174–175
  blood supply in, 177–178
  iliolumbar system in, 178–179
  intervertebral foramen in, 175, *175*, *176*
  ligaments of, 175–176
  muscles of, 178–179, *180–181*
  nerve roots in, 177, *177*, 190
  stenosis of, 174
Lumbodorsal fascia, 203
Lumbosacral fascia, *183*
Lumbosacral spine, *162*

M

Mandibular nerves, 4–5, *44*, *45*
Mandibulotomy, complications of, 43
  hole pre-drilling in, *35*
  in transoral approach, 26–43
  incisions in, *31*, *36*
  lip split in, *39*
  periosteum elevation in, *33*
  reconstruction plate in, *34*, *42*
  skin division in, *32*
  soft tissue division in, *38*
  tongue split in, *41*
  with sagittal saw, *37*
Manubrium, *76*

Mayfield tongs, *88*
Motor nerves, cranial, 47–48
Mouth floor, division of, *48*
Mouth gag, Dingman, *27*
Multifidus muscle, *83*
Muscles. See also specific muscles, e.g., *Psoas muscle.*
  in retroperitoneal lumbar exposure, 147, 150
  of cervical region, 2, 2–3, 82
  of larynx, 3
  of lumbar spine, *180–181*
  of thoracic spine, 134, *135*
  paraspinal, 184
Myosis, ipsilateral, 5

N

Neck. See also *Cervical* entries.
  cross section of, *83*
Nerve(s). See also specific nerves, e.g., *Auricular nerve.*
  injuries to, 5, 212–213, 218
  of cervical region, *3*, 4–5
  thoracic, 134–135
Nerve palsy, 47
Neurovascular system, in thoracic spine, 134–135, *137*
Nucleus pulposus, *176*, 177

O

Oblique muscle(s), 147, *148*, *164*, *165*
Occipitocervical fusion, approaches to, 98–101
  Ransford loop in, *100*
  Wertheim and Bohlman method in, 98, *99*, 101
Occipitocervical region, 82–83
Odontoid process, *55*
Omohyoid muscle, 3, *65*, *66–67*

P

Palsy, nerve, 47
Paraspinal muscles, 184
Paravertebral fascia, *196*
Paravertebral incisions, 194, *195–196*
Paravertebral muscles, *196*
Parotid gland, *55*, *57*
Pars interarticularis, 184
Pedicle, 186, 192
Periosteum, *33*
Peroneal nerve, 216
Phrenic nerve, *68*
Platysma, *63*, *65*
  at C6 vertebral level, 2, *10*
  dissection of, *12*, *13*
  identification of, *64*
Pleura, 74–75, *126–127*
Posterior approach(es), to cervical spine, 81–113
  to cervicothoracic junction, 109–110
  to lumbar spine, 173–192
Povidone-iodine, *54*
Preperitoneal space, *165*
Pseudarthrosis, 112
Psoas muscle, *151*, *168*
  anatomy of, 147, 150
  elevation of, 151–152, *153*, *154*
  origin of, 150
  posterior view of, *150*
Ptosis, of eyelid, 5

R

Ransford loop, *100*
Reconstruction plate, in mandibulotomy, *34*, *42*
Rectus muscle(s), 162, *164*, *165*
Retractors, Cloward self-retaining, *18*
  Cobb elevator, 181, 184
  Cushing, 7, 13, *15*
  Richardson, 14, *69*
  Taylor, 187, 207
Retroperitoneal approach, to lumbar spine, 145–155
  advantages of, 146
  anatomy of, 147–151
  complications of, 152, 155
  crus of diaphragm in, 150
  incision for, 147, *147*, 161
  muscles in, 147, 150
  patient positioning in, *146*, 146–147, 160–161
  peritoneal tearing in, 155
  safety issues in, 155
  safety of, 166
  sympathetic nervous system in, 151
  vs. transperitoneal approach, 146, 158
  wound closure in, 165–166
Retroperitoneal fat, 147, *149*, *150*
Retroperitoneum, *149*, *150*, *152*, *166*
Retropharyngeal approach, anterior, 47–51
  after dissection, *51*
  complications of, 50–51
  cranial motor nerve injuries in, 47
  nerve palsy in, 47
  techniques for, 47–50
  vertebral exposure in, *50*
  lateral, 53–59
    advantages of, 54, 58
    anatomy of, 54, *55*
    complications of, 58
    history of, 54
    patient positioning for, 54, *54*
    plane of dissection in, *55*
    spinal accessory nerve retraction in, *56*
    techniques for, 54–58
Rhomboid muscle(s), 82, *135*
Rib(s), resection of, 118, *122–123*
  retraction of, 123
Richardson retractor, 14, *69*
Rongeur, Kerrison, 89, 90, 186, 187, 191

S

Sacral alae, 197
Sacral vessels, *169*
Sacroiliac joint, 204
Sacroiliolumbar arteries, *178*
Sacrospinalis muscle, 194
Sagittal saw, *37*
Scalene muscle(s), 57–58
Sciatic nerve(s), 203–204, *204*, 213
Sciatic notch, 203–204, 212
Segmental vessels, 74, *179*
Semispinalis muscle(s), 82
Serratus muscle(s), *73*, 82, *135*
Somatosensory evoked potentials, 83
Spinal abscess, 143
Spinal accessory nerve, *3*, 47, 56, 58
Spinal column, 74
Spinal instability, 144, 191
Spinal stenosis, 174
Spine. See *Cervical spine*; *Lumbar spine*; *Thoracic spine.*
Spinous processes, 82, 83, *85*

Splenius capitis, *83*
Spondylolisthesis, 158, 199
Spondylolysis, 197, 199
Stenosis, spinal, 174
Sternocleidomastoid, *46, 54, 66, 76*
  anatomy of, 2–3, *7, 44,* 63–64
  at C1 arch, *55*
  at C6 vertebra level, *2, 10*
  division of, 65, *65*
  in lateral cervical approach, 56, *57*
  in modified anterior cervicothoracic approach, *62*
  in platysma section, *12, 13, 63*
  release of, 13–14
  retraction of, 64, 69
Sternohyoid muscle, 3
Sternum splitting, 62, 76–78, *77–78*
  skin incision in, *76*
Strap muscles, *65, 66*
Stryker frame, 83, 101
Stylohyoid muscle, *44, 45, 46*
Subclavian vein(s), *66–67, 77*
Submandibular gland, *6, 44, 45, 51*
Submandibular triangle, 3, *3*
Supraspinous ligament, *175, 176*
Swallowing therapy, 47
Sympathetic chain, *74–75*

T

Taylor retractor, 187, 207
Thoracic duct injures, 21
Thoracic inlet, 63, 68
Thoracic instability, iatrogenic, 144
Thoracic nerve(s), 134–135
Thoracic spine, anterior approaches to, 61–79
    proximal thoracotomy in, 63, 69–70
    sternum splitting in, 62, 76–78
    types of, 62–63
  neurovascular anatomy of, 134–135, *137*
  posterior muscles in, 134, *135*
Thoracolumbar junction, *153*
Thoracotomy, 115–131
  anesthesia for, 118
  chest tubes in, *129*
  history of, 116
  incisions for, *117,* 118–119, *120–121,* 123–124, *124*
  indications for, 116
  instruments for, *116*
  left vs. right approach to, 118
  patient positioning in, 118, *119*
  pleural division in, *126–128*
  proximal, 63, 69–70

Thoracotomy *(Continued)*
  incision for, 70, *70*
  latissimus dorsi section in, 70, *71–72*
  patient positioning in, 69, *70*
  rib resection in, 70, *73–74*
  scapula retraction in, 70, *73*
  scapular tip exposure in, *72*
  trapezius sectioning in, 70, *71–72*
  rib resection in, 118, 119, *122–123*
  segmental vessels, *128*
  sutures for, 129–130, *130*
  techniques for, 116–130
Thyroid artery(ies), *6, 51*
Thyroid vein(s), inferior, *77*
  middle, 3, *5*
Trachea, *77*
Tracheoesophageal complex, *68*
Tracheotomy tube, *31*
Traction, 11, 64
Transoral approach(es), cervical incision in, *43*
  complications of, 26, 43, 45, 47
  Dingman mouth gag in, *27*
  pharyngeal mucosa incision in, *28*
  subperiosteal dissection in, *29*
  subplatysmal flap elevation in, *44*
  techniques for, 26, 31, 43–45
  tongue division in, 31, *40, 41*
  with extrapharyngeal exposure, *43,* 43–45
  with lip split and mandibulotomy, 26, 31, 43
Transperitoneal lumbar approach, complications of, 158
  vs. retroperitoneal approach, 146, 158
Transversalis fascia, *65, 147, 149*
Transverse process(es), C1, 56, *57*
  L5, *197*
  models of, *186*
  posterior lumbar exposure of, 184
Transversus abdominis muscle, *147, 149*
Trapezius muscle, *83, 135*
Trauma. See *Injury(ies).*
Trendelenburg position, reversed, 85, *86,* 88
Tubercle, carotid, 12
Tuberculosis, treatment of, 158

U

Ureter, *169*

V

Vagus nerve, *3,* 4, *47, 68*
Veins. See specific veins, e.g., *Jugular vein(s).*

Vertebral artery, *85*
  anatomy of, 7, *92*
  at C1 arch, *55*
  at C6 vertebral level, *2, 10*
  function of, 3
  in neck cross section, *83*
  injuries to, 21, 111
Vertebral body(ies), C1, cross-section of, *55*
  lateral process of, *57, 57–58*
  transverse process of, 56–57
  C1-C2 complex, 90–92, 98
  C4, *49*
  C4-C5, *10, 87, 105*
  C5, *5*
  C5-C7, *109*
  C6, *2, 10*
  exposure of, 78
  L2, *155*
  L2-L3 disk space, 187
  lumbar, 174–175

W

Wertheim and Bohlman method, of occipitocervical fusion, 98, *99,* 101
Wharton's duct, *38, 40*
Whiteside's approach, to upper cervical spine, 53–59
Wilson frame, 194
Wiltse approach, to lumbar spine, 193–200
  advantages of, 199
  cleavage plane in, 196
  complications of, 198–199
  disadvantages of, 200
  facet joint misidentification in, 198
  incisions in, 194, *194,* 195, *195*
  nerve root injuries in, 199
  patient positioning in, 194
  posterior exposure in, *197*
  screw insertion in, 198, *198*
  techniques for, 194–199
Wiring, interfacet, *106–107*
  interspinous, 101–103
    triple-wire technique, *102–103*

X

Xiphoid process, *76*

ISBN 0-7216-4554-2